PRAISE FOR *ESSENTIAL DIABETES LEADERSHIP*

Laurence Chalem has produced a book with a high intellectual level that is also easy to read with impeccable logic. Although he included a couple of off-topic, though interesting digressions, some of the endnotes have such great information that they might have been in the main text as well. His literature searching has a depth and persistence that I envy. Many of the arguments and presentations were the best on sub-topics of diabetes that I have ever seen.

—Joel M. Kauffman, Ph.D.
Emeritus Professor of Chemistry and Biochemistry
University of the Sciences, Philadelphia, PA

This refreshing book, *Essential Diabetes Leadership*, questions the logic of recommending high-carbohydrate diets to diabetics. Among other benefits, the book provides:

- historical perspectives on diabetes and its treatments
- an illuminating allegory to illustrate a potential design flaw of a high-impact diabetes trial
- an assessment of the logic of combating unstable blood sugar levels by dietary bombardments of high-glycemic carbohydrates

The book is all the more poignant and salient because the author is a type I diabetic whose moral compass remains unaffected by the pervasive financial conflicts of interests that so often plague us.

—Philippe P. Hujoel, Ph.D., D.D.S., M.S.D., M.S.
Professor, Dental Public Health Sciences
Adjunct Professor, Epidemiology
University of Washington, School of Public Health

In 2009, Laurence Chalem, like the forward thinking people before him, has thrown down the gauntlet to the American Diabetes Association that their dietary advice is wrong and the proper diet for diabetics is one of carbohydrate restriction, allowing fat and protein to play the major role in food intake. Like a medical doctor, Chalem knows that diabetes, from "just a touch of sugar," to the severe, debilitating insulin demanding form, is a disease in which one cannot properly metabolize carbohydrates. For various reasons insulin production from our pancreas is compromised so the metabolism of sugar cannot occur as intended. I think every medical student in his early years of training asks the question: "Why do we allow excess carbohydrates in the diet of those with diabetes?" The prevailing answer is: "Because the American Diabetes Association says so, and, bowing to this higher god, all your peers do so." Not to allow some 60-70% carbohydrates into our daily diet is heresy.

By the time of graduation you have learned to walk the path of your peers unless you read this book by Laurence Chalem. His 60% fat, 30% protein and 10% carbohydrate diet may be heresy but it is the correct diet for everyone with insulin derangement. A predecessor, Dr. William Harvey started us along this path in 1862 with his successful treatment of morbidly obese Banting. Traditional medicine ridiculed his carbo-restrictive diet and buried it for almost 200 years. Richard Bernstein was diagnosed with insulin dependant diabetes in 1946 when 12 years of age. By the combination of literature research and using himself as a guinea pig, young Bernstein determined that only a severely carbo-restrictive diet would allow control of his excessively brittle blood sugar. He became a doctor because it was the only way he could publish his knowledge in medical journals and is today a specialist in the treatment of diabetes, eating a daily diet much like Banting and Chalem. I regard Laurence Chalem as the re-incarnation of these men with his special knowledge about the proper diet for diabetes. All diabetics and all doctors must read this book. The American Diabetes Association and what you and I have been taught by traditional medicine is wrong. Think for yourself.

—Duane Graveline, M.D., M.P.H.
Former US Air Force Flight Surgeon
NASA flight controller, Mercury and Gemini programs
NASA Scientist Astronaut (1965)
Author: *Lipitor, Thief of Memory*
Statin Damage Side Effects
Statin Damage Crisis
The Dark Side of Statins

ESSENTIAL DIABETES LEADERSHIP

LAURENCE D. CHALEM

ALSO BY LAURENCE D. CHALEM

Thrive With Diabetes: Lead an Optimistic, Fun,
Challenging, Fit, Tenacious, Enlightened, Innovative & Heroic Life

ESSENTIAL DIABETES
LEADERSHIP

LAURENCE D. CHALEM

BookSurge Publishing

Charleston, South Carolina

ESSENTIAL DIABETES LEADERSHIP

Second Edition
Copyright © 2010 by Laurence D. Chalem
All rights reserved.
ISBN: 1-4392-4566-5
ISBN-13: 9781439245668
Library of Congress Control Number: 2009905899

BookSurge Publishing
Charleston, South Carolina
http://www.booksurge.com

Printed in the United States of America
10 9 8 7 6 5 4 3 2 1

About the Author

Laurence D. Chalem (b. 1963), an insulin-dependent — type 1 — diabetic, received his B.A. in Economics (1986), M. Mus. (1994), and M.B.A. (1996) all from the University of Illinois at Urbana-Champaign.

Based in San Jose, California, Mr. Chalem currently serves as global sourcing manager with Cisco Systems, Inc., the worldwide leader in networking that transforms how people connect, communicate, and collaborate. He is the 2009 recipient of the Above-and-Beyond Award, presented by Diversity Best Practices and Working Mother Media, which recognized Network and Affinity Group Leaders whose determination led to the creation, success or turn-around of their group. Laurence served as Co-Chair of the Cisco Disabilities Awareness Network (CDAN) in 2008.

Laurence's HbA_{1c} has been significantly below 7% since 2006. He eats a very low-calorie diet, consisting of approximately 60% fat, largely coconut oil, 30% protein, and less than 10% carbohydrates, typically in the form of vegetables. Besides coconut oil, his favorite oils are macadamia nut, pecan, almond, olive, and avocado, all predominantly mono-unsaturated, and supplements his diet with fish oil. He cooks primarily with coconut oil and real butter.

Financial Disclosure

The author does not receive, and never has received, any form of financial assistance from industry groups that may stand to benefit from the information presented in this book. This includes those from the meat, egg, dairy, nutritional supplement, food, beverage, pharmaceutical, and agricultural industries. The author does not hold, trade, or speculate in the stock of companies whose financial status or share price could potentially be affected by the information presented in this book, with the exception being that he does maintain a 401(k) account managed by a third-party investment company, which, in early 2009, was down over 60%.

Acknowledgements

This, my second book, written over the past year, inspired by further research into four seemingly innocuous footnotes in my previous book, could not have been accomplished without the help, support, advice, and knowledge of other people for whom I am deeply grateful.

The writers and researchers quoted throughout this book to whom that special thank you is due include: Dr. John Barrow, Dr. Richard K. Bernstein, Dr. Jacob Bronowski, Anthony Colpo, Dr. Richard Dawkins, Dr. Mary G. Enig, Sally Fallon, Dr. Barry Groves, Professor Emeritus Robert S. Horn, Dr. Philippe Hujoel, Dr. Joel M. Kauffman, Dr. Malcolm Kendrick, Dr. Henry Lorin, Dr. Kilmer S. McCully, Dr. Joseph Mercola, William Poundstone, Dr. Uffe Ravnskov, Dr. Ron Rosedale, Gary Taubes, and Dr. Eric C. Westman. Without their significant contributions in their respective fields, this book would not have been possible.

Dr. Joel M. Kauffman, Emeritus Professor of Chemistry and Biochemistry at the University of the Sciences, Philadelphia, PA, merits a further, special thank you. Joel took the time to read through and comment upon various versions of the manuscript; this book is far better as a result of acting on his advice. Even a special attribution such as this is hardly adequate to express my appreciation.

Noteworthy also are the many organizations that support the work of the above authors including: the Weston A. Price Foundation; the International Network of Cholesterol Skeptics (THINCS), a group increasingly recognized as the *de facto* authority on the subject of cholesterol; PubMed, a service of the US National Library of Medicine and the National Institutes of Health; Anchor Books; Doubleday; Random House, Inc.; Oxford University Press; Hachette Book Group USA; Little, Brown & Company; and Mercola.com.

Although I deeply appreciate the contributions of the above authors and organizations, please note that acknowledging their quotes, support, help, or genius in this book does not necessarily mean that they are in agreement with my analyses or conclusions. For their analyses and conclusions, you are encouraged to read their books and/or articles as cited in the pages that follow.

Once again, I am deeply indebted to the Wikipedia Foundation and associated Wikipidians that have supplied supporting research. Wikipedia is simply the best resource *and* the best resource online.

A special thank you in this book must go to the reference librarians and staff of the Central Park Library Branch of the Santa Clara City Library, in Santa Clara, California. Consummate professionals all.

Many thanks also to the professionals of Lane Medical Library, Stanford School of Medicine in Palo Alto, California, for allowing access to both their virtual and physical knowledge pathways and destinations. A stroll on campus or up and down University Avenue makes a day's research all the more rewarding.

Once again, I'd like to thank my team at BookSurge Publishing. A thank you also goes to my friends, in reverse alphabetical order this time, Eric Zubiller, Suzanne Ho-Kwan Yuen, Yai Heai Yu, Michael Yao, Haoning Yang, Mami Yamada, Nga Trinh Vu, Tom Tirone, Catherine Liu, Yumi Kuzaki, Robert Holm, Alex Fitzpatrick, Ilan Deen, Lisah Chen, and Scott Brown.

I probably wouldn't have written this book either had it not been for the encouragement of my best friend, Peter Langmar, who modeled that we are not defined by the interests of others, but by our own unique, true and beautiful contributions. I wish he could have been around to see this book published.

And, once again, I'm grateful to my employers, past and present, that provided opportunities to make a difference, and, better yet, make a living. Especially noteworthy is Cisco Systems, Inc. I am deeply indebted to Cisco for providing the best opportunity of my life, which proved invaluable in this book's creation.

For all the people and organizations named above, et al., a warm thank you.

For everyone seeking an optimal solution...

A semi-tractor-trailer driver forgoes the posted signs and proceeds to drive her fourteen-foot tall rig under a thirteen-foot-eight-inch high overpass. Cause and effect, seconds later, the driver realizes that the haul of appliances will be tragically late, and hopes that both her insurance payments and coverage are up to date. Frantic, the driver calls for help.

The emergency operator dispatches all sorts of good Samaritans in response: paramedics, firefighters, tow-truck drivers and police. Traffic backs up for miles, folks get out of their cars in frustration to find out what's keeping them from continuing their lives, and news crews descend on the scene.

All the professionals, adept and knowledgeable specialists in their respective fields—partially blinded by their own self-interest of being the hero—analyze the problem and recommend solutions. The police request further assistance from helicopters, and a tow-truck driver requests a bigger, more powerful tow truck. The mayor of the town pledges millions of dollars in aid as work to pry the truck from the overpass begins.

Even the largest tow truck on the scene isn't powerful enough to pull the 18-wheeler from the overpass. The operator requests assistance from construction crews to dismantle sections of the overpass, with the helicopter standing by to hold a section in mid-air, while the massive tow truck is standing by in front to finally pull the big-rig clear.

Just before the final cut is made on a section of the bridge, one of the occupants of a car a mile behind the action—an eight-year-old boy—finally makes his way to the police officer in charge and says:

> "Why don't you just deflate the tires so that the truck is slightly more than four inches lower and back it out?"

It seems so obvious.

CONTENTS

PREFACE TO THE SECOND EDITION 21

PREFACE 23

AT THE LIBRARY 33

SUPERMASSIVE BLACK HOLES & THE DCCT 63

THE WAY THINGS OUGHT TO BE (PART I) 99

THE WAY THINGS OUGHT TO BE (PART II) 135

DILEMMAS 159

EPILOGUE 177

POSTSCRIPT 193

APPENDIX A: BOOKS ON DIABETES 203

APPENDIX B: REFERENCE BOOKS 227

APPENDIX C: LOW-CARBOHYDRATE ARTICLES 235

APPENDIX D: DCCT BIBLIOGRAPHY 259

NOTES 265

PREFACE TO THE SECOND EDITION

"I find on re-reading it that the picture it presents is close to the one I would paint if I were to start afresh, and write a wholly new book."

JOHN MAYNARD SMITH

Introduction, 1993 Edition of his 1958 book, *The Theory of Evolution*

Unlike legendary Professor John Maynard Smith's above-referenced classic work, thirty-five years have not gone by since my original publication; indeed, I thought about adding content after more like thirty-five days. Nothing new had been discovered in the interim, however, additional commentary and some tidying up were warranted.

Of course, the few grammatical errors found by my conscientious friends have been corrected. Modern spell and grammar checking programs, now a widespread replacement for what is known as manual "light" editing, rarely catch the incorrect usage of function words such as "of" or "if" when the latter rather than the former is intended, and vice-versa. The same goes for "on" and "in." If the "o" and "i" were not so juxtaposed on a keyboard, I would have been free to make other, perhaps more easily recognizable — hence correctable *before* being published — typographical errors.[1] Although I can't with 100% confidence say that between my friends and I we have found and corrected all errors, with slightly more than 107,000 total words between the two covers, foot- and endnotes included, I'm nevertheless confident that if any remain they total < 0.005%.

Just a handful of "heavy" edits were made. One important sentence in the "Epilogue," formerly referring to the role of something higher than the individual versus the individual proper that is acted upon in natural selection, has been corrected with an added note.

Too, several reviewers pointed out how I did not discuss the role of calories in any diet. My response, paralleling answers to other questions in the original Preface, is that I ardently recommend that you read Gary Taubes's masterpiece *Good Calories, Bad Calories* for accurate historical context and current insight into the realm of calories.

Prompting this second edition more so than editing miscellany was the thought-provoking comment that I received, and could not leave well enough alone, that the major hypothesis that I set out to prove was too general; some algorithm maximizes the longevity of a diabetic's happy, healthy life, but what of the individual organs and organ systems? Did I cover them all in good measure? "Postscript" contains my answer.

In the "Note to Oxford Paperback Edition" (1989) of *The Extended Phenotype* (2008), Richard Dawkins imagined that most authors think to themselves: "it doesn't matter if you never read anything else of mine, please at least read *this*." For me, in this book, it is the "Epilogue." And the chapter entitled "Dilemmas." "Supermassive Black Holes & the DCCT" opens our eyes to the major assumption made by nearly all medical textbooks as it relates to advocating a diabetic diet, and I wouldn't have been able to develop that allegory without having first read my way through a hundred or so books "At the Library." I have previously published both parts of "The Way Things Ought To Be," albeit in a different format, in my first book, and rely on them to quote studies when I find myself in a dietary debate.

Apart from the aforementioned adds and changes, I take nothing back. It is my sincere hope that beyond simply reading the words, you too confidently implement the optimal solution, as I do everyday.

PREFACE

"There is nothing to writing," says Red Smith. "All you do is sit down at a typewriter and open a vein."[2] Well, my second book has been as much of a challenge and joy to write as the first—even more so, revealing—and, if you were to measure the glucose in the blood surrounding my keyboard, you would find that it is well within normal range, each and every time you checked. Should the information in this book, as with my first, be helpful, informative and practical enough to empower you to thrive, then on with the bloodletting.

In sitting down to write a second book, as with other authors, the dilemma is fiction or not, and if not, move to another topic, clarify what was already written, somehow compress it, add to it, or provide some combination of the latter three.

Admittedly, when mentioning that I'm an author at social gatherings the inevitable response is "Oh really? What's your book about?" I always hesitate slightly, thinking to myself that the best response would be "It's a romance," or "I'm a mystery novel writer." Saying "It's about diabetes" typically doesn't induce much excitement, let alone make much headway with the fairer sex; I've yet to hear the response "Oh boy! Diabetes, that's so cool!" Romantic sentiment notwithstanding, bringing useful information to folks has a more lasting appeal.

Looking first to fiction, though not straying too far from the central theme of diabetes, perhaps I could write a mystery wherein the hero—a detective—has a form of the disease. Alas, that has been done, albeit without the benefit of a very low-carbohydrate approach, with the lead being one Detective Chief Inspector Endeavour Morse, a fictional character in a series of thirteen detective novels by British author Colin Dexter, developed into a 33 episode television series produced by Central Independent Television from 1987–2000, in which Morse was portrayed by John Thaw.[3] Morse is a senior CID (Criminal Investigation Department) officer with the Thames Valley Police in Oxford, England.

With a thirst for beer, intellectual snobbery and a penchant for the music of Wagner, Morse presents a likeable persona despite his gloomy temperament. Morse dislikes spelling errors and grammatical mistakes, demonstrated by the fact that in every personal or private document written to him he manages to point out at least one spelling mistake. His approach to crime-solving, he asserts frequently, is deductive and one of his key tenets is that "the last person to see the victim alive was the murderer."

Needless to say, Morse dies in a hospital bed from complications of his neglected type 2 diabetes. Not the way things ought to be.

Another idea would be to write a murder-mystery involving the alleged improper use of insulin. That too — and it was non-fiction — has been done.

Claus von Bülow (born Claus Cecil Borberg on August 11, 1926, in Copenhagen, Denmark) was a British socialite of German and Danish ancestry.[4] He was accused of the attempted murder of his wife, Sunny von Bülow (formerly Martha Sharp Crawford), by administering an insulin overdose in 1980. Therein lies the perfect thematic context for a diabetes-related docu-drama; Professor Alan Dershowitz wrote it as *Reversal of Fortune: Inside the von Bülow case* (1985) that was cinematically adapted as *Reversal of Fortune* (1990). Jeremy Irons starred as Claus von Bülow, and Glenn Close as Sunny von Bülow.

The storyline develops thusly: in 1982, von Bülow was tried for the attempted murder of Sunny, which allegedly occurred at her estate, Clarendon Court, in Newport, Rhode Island. At the trial in Newport, von

Preface

Bülow was found guilty and sentenced to thirty years in prison; he appealed, hiring Harvard Law Professor Alan Dershowitz to represent him. Professor Dershowitz and associates rendered doubtful the first trial's most damning evidence and testimony; in 1984 the conviction was reversed; in 1985, after a second trial, von Bülow was found not guilty on all charges.

At the second trial the defense called eight medical experts, all world-class university professors, who testified that Sunny's two comas were not caused by insulin, but by a combination of *ingested*, not injected, drugs, alcohol, and chronic health conditions. The experts were John Caronna, Chairman of Neurology, Cornell; Leo Dal Cortivo, former President, U.S. Toxicology Association; Ralph DeFronzo, Medicine, Yale; Kurt Dubowski, Forensic Pathology, University of Oklahoma; Daniel Foster, Medicine, University of Texas; Daniel Furst, Medicine, University of Iowa; Harold Lebovitz, Director of Clinical Research, State University of New York; Vincent Marks, Clinical Biochemistry, Surrey, Vice-President, Royal College of Pathologists and President, Association of Clinical Biochemistry; and Arthur Rubinstein, Medicine, University of Chicago.

Other experts testified that the hypodermic needle tainted with insulin on the outside, but not inside, would have been dipped in insulin but not injected, as injecting it in flesh would have wiped it clean. Evidence also showed that Sunny's hospital admission three weeks before the final coma showed she had ingested at least 73 aspirin tablets, a quantity that could only have been self-administered, and which indicated her state of mind.

Sunny's family remained convinced of Claus's guilt. For having sided with her father, Cosima von Bülow was disinherited by her maternal grandmother, Annie Laurie (Crawford) Aitken. Von Bülow's two stepchildren from Sunny's previous marriage sued him for $56 million. As a result, von Bülow renounced his claim to Sunny's $75 million personal fortune in exchange for Cosima's reinstatement as joint heiress to the Crawford fortune.

Currently, von Bülow lives in London, writing art and theatre reviews. His ex-wife, Sunny von Bülow, remained comatose at a private nursing home for about 28 years until her death from cardiopulmonary arrest on December 6, 2008, at Mary Manning Walsh Nursing Home in New York City.

These two themes, then, a diabetic detective's casework and an alleged murder and vindication, represent the entire subject of diabetes in the written dramatic literature, fiction or not. Could be that that's all there is — nothing new under the sun — maybe the face of diabetes is far from being able to launch a thousand ships. It's all been done and there is nothing left to say. While we await a cure, we should eat a balanced, low-fat, high complex-carbohydrate diet, take our meds, and enjoy a shortened, complicated lifespan. Our diabetic heroes and anti-heroes alike will succumb to the manifestations of diabetes as if that's the only script. Such is life.

Of course I disagree; but, before I can actually develop a new literary character, there's one more factual book to write on diabetes. Well, actually two. The first, however, a book examining the data that exists on the singular issue of our times — a low-fat, medium protein, high-complex-carbohydrate diet versus a low-carbohydrate, medium protein, high-fat diet — and to demonstrate how we have reached the conclusions we have and whether or not they are justified, exploring in the process the research pertaining to diabetes, obesity, heart disease, blood pressure, et al., has already been written, and quite deftly in fact, by Gary Taubes in *Good Calories, Bad Calories* (2008).

Traversing the continuum from obesity to diabetes, Mr. Taubes writes:

Preface

"Despite the depth and certainty of our faith that saturated fat is the nutritional bane of our lives and that obesity is caused by overeating and sedentary behavior, there has always been copious evidence to suggest that those assumptions are incorrect, and that evidence is continuing to mount."[5]

In *Good Calories, Bad Calories* (First Anchor Books Edition, 2008), Gary Taubes provides the answers to our questions, and puts it all—and I do mean all—into perspective. He places nearly two centuries of assertions, assumptions, observations, research, and experimentation—the biased and the unbiased, reality-based and otherwise—under the microscope. From Banting and Speke, to Rubner, Benedict, and Atwater, to Minkowski, Banting and Bauer, to von Noorden, Rony and Falta, to the German and Austrian community of investigators before World War II such as Schoenheimer, to Newburgh, Wertheimer, Dole, Gordon, Laurell, Krebs, Pennington, Cleave, Burkitt, Stunkard, and Bruch, to Astwood and Mayer, to Atkins, Van Itallie, Bray, Cahill, Hirsch and Reaven, to Greenwood, Ravussin, Bouchard, Levine, Schmidt, Bennet, Friedman, Hill, and many, many more, Mr. Taubes presents a compendious, cohesive, accurate, remarkably flowing historical narrative of the research—and its subsequent influence on the zeitgeist—on obesity, diabetes, heart disease, blood pressure, cancer, dementia, aging, et al., and attributes most of it to metabolic disorder, antagonized and exacerbated by a diet that increases endogenous insulin production.

A calorie is a calorie is a calorie says the dogma, which has been incorrectly compressed into the directional equation $E_i - E_e \rightarrow \Delta E_s$ (defined by Mr. Taubes below) since reason, logic, and common sense went their separate ways decades ago.[*] The research on insulin and fat metabolism

---

[*] Even as I worked on this section, a study appeared in the *New England Journal of Medicine* entitled "Comparison of Weight-Loss Diets with Different Compositions of Fat, Protein, and Carbohydrates" (February 26, 2009), concluding that "Reduced-calorie diets result in clinically meaningful weight loss regardless of which macronutrients they emphasize," even though the range of carbohydrates consumed only went so low as 35% of total calories. George Bray, the lead researcher of that study, wrote a wanting critique of *Good Calories, Bad Calories* in *Obesity Reviews* (published February, 2008, Volume 9, pages 251-263). In good form, Gary Taubes wrote an eloquent response. You can see both the review and response, together with a good analysis of the conflict on *The Blog of Michael R. Eades, MD*, online at

offers a better resolution to the above-referenced diseases, says Taubes, with the efficacy of a low-carbohydrate diet, and it has for several decades.

Thus, the predominant message in *Good Calories, Bad Calories* is that the aforementioned dogma needs to be corrected. As Gary Taubes discusses:

"This faith in the laws of thermodynamics is founded on two misinterpretations of thermodynamic law, and not in the law itself. When these misconceptions are corrected, they alter our perceptions of weight regulation and the forces at work.

The first misconception is the assumption than an association implies cause and effect. Here the context is the first law of thermodynamics, the law of energy conservation. This law says that energy is neither created nor destroyed, and so the calories we consume will be either stored, expended, or excreted. This in turn implies that any change in body weight must equal the difference between the calories we consume and the calories we expend, and thus the positive or negative energy balance. Known as the energy-balance equation, it looks like this:

Change in energy stores = Energy intake - Energy expenditure

The first law of thermodynamics dictates that weight gain — the increase in energy stored as fat and lean-tissue mass — will be *accompanied by* or *associated with* positive energy balance, but it does not say that it is *caused* by a positive energy balance — by "a plethora of calories," as Russell Cecil and Robert Loeb's 1951 *Textbook of Medicine* puts it. There is no arrow of causality in the equation. It is equally possible, without violating this fundamental truth, for a change in energy stores, the left side of the above equation, to be the driving force in cause and effect; some regulatory phenomenon could drive us to gain weight, which would in turn cause a positive energy balance — and thus overeating and/or sedentary behavior. Either way, the calories in will equal the calories out, as they must, but what is cause in one case is effect in the other.

All those who have insisted (and still do) that overeating and/or sedentary behavior *must* be the cause of obesity have done so on the basis of this same fundamental error: they will observe correctly that positive caloric balance must be *associated* with weight gain, but then they will assume without justification that

http://www.proteinpower.com/drmike/statins/gary-taubes-responds-to-george-bray/. Retrieved on 2/28/09.

positive caloric balance is the cause of weight gain. This simple misconception has led to a century of misguided obesity research."[6]

Mr. Taubes continues by discussing the second misinterpretation of the law of energy conservation. In short, that misinterpretation is based upon an assumption of whether those three arguments in the above-equation, namely change in energy stores, energy intake and energy expenditure are related or independent. As Mr. Taubes states: "The question is whether one can actually change energy intake in a living organism without prompting compensatory changes in energy expenditure."[7]

Especially relevant to those that would choose a low-carbohydrate approach to optimize their treatment of diabetes, Mr. Taubes brilliantly takes us through the research on cholesterol, fiber, hunger, satiety, and diets; those that reduce, fatten, and maintain us. Regarding fiber, he states:

"The fiber hypothesis captured the public's nutritional consciousness by virtue of the messianic efforts of a single investigator, a former missionary surgeon named Denis Burkitt, who proposed that this indigestible roughage was a requisite component of a healthy diet. The notion was consistent with Key's hypothesis, which was not the case with Cleave's or Yudkin's hypothesis, and it resonated also with the era's counterculture leanings toward diets heavy in vegetables, legumes, and cereal grains.

Burkitt's fiber hypothesis was based originally and in its entirety on Cleave's saccharine-disease hypothesis, but simply inverted the causal agent. Rather than proclaim, as Cleave did, that chronic disease was caused by the *addition* of sugar and refined carbohydrates to diets that we had evolved naturally to eat, Burkitt laid the blame on the *subtraction* of the fiber from those evolutionarily ideal diets, which in turn led to constipation and then, through a variety of mechanisms, all the chronic diseases of civilization. The fiber deficiency itself was caused either by the removal of fiber during the refining of carbohydrates or by the consumption of refined carbohydrates in lieu of the fibrous, bulky roughage we should be eating. The fiber hypothesis and the refined-carbohydrate hypothesis of chronic disease were photographic negatives of each other, and yet the fiber hypothesis caught on immediately upon appearing in the journals. The refined-carbohydrate hypothesis, which was the only one of the two that was capable of explaining the actual evidence, remained a fringe concept."[8]

The above is indicative of Mr. Taubes' style throughout the book. He presents research in its historical context, replete with sources — his book has a 66 page bibliography — and then goes on to assimilate it into the current milieu. As he continues later in the chapter:

> "Over the last quarter-century, Burkitt's fiber hypothesis has become yet another example of Francis Bacon's dictum of "wishful science" — there has been a steady accumulation of evidence refuting the notion that a fiber-deficient diet causes colon cancer, polyps, or diverticulitis, let alone any other disease of civilization. The pattern is precisely what would be expected of a hypothesis that simply isn't true: the larger and more rigorous the trials set up to test it, the more consistently negative the evidence. Between 1994 and 2000, two observational studies — of forty-seven thousand male health professionals and the eighty-nine thousand women of the Nurses Health Study, both run out of the Harvard School of Public Health — and a half-dozen randomized control trials concluded that fiber consumption is unrelated to the risk of colon cancer, as is, apparently, the consumption of fruits and vegetables. The results of the forty-nine-thousand-women Dietary Modification Trial of the Women's Health Initiative, published in 2006, confirmed that increasing the fiber in the diet (by eating more whole grains, fruits, and vegetables) had no beneficial effect on colon cancer, nor did it prevent heart disease or breast cancer or induce weight loss.

> 'Burkitt's hypothesis got accepted pretty well worldwide, quite quickly, but it has gradually been disproved,' said Richard Doll, who had endorsed the hypothesis enthusiastically in the mid-1970s. 'It still holds up in relation to constipation, but as far as a major factor in the common diseases of the developed world, no, fiber is not the answer. That's pretty clear.'"[9]

Fiber is but one concept elucidated by Mr. Taubes, and the above example takes up only a few pages in a 600+ page book. He also provides quite well-thought-out and developed tutorials throughout his treatise; of particular importance is his enlightening tutorial on triglycerides and cholesterol, with the following setting the stage:

> "The danger of simplifying a medical issue for public consumption is that we may come to believe that our simplification is an appropriate representation of the

biological reality. We may forget that the science is not adequately described, or ambiguous, even if the public-health policy seems to be set in stone. In the case of diet and heart disease, Ancel Keys's hypothesis that cholesterol is the agent of atherosclerosis was considered the simplest possible hypothesis, because cholesterol is found in atherosclerotic plaques and because cholesterol was relatively easy to measure. But as the measurement technology became increasingly more sophisticated, every one of the complications that arose has implicated carbohydrates rather than fat as the dietary agent of heart disease."[10]

From an article in *Science* by John Gofman in 1950, launching the modern era of cholesterol research, Gary Taubes explains how we came to the identification of the three species of lipoproteins, namely, HDL, LDL, and VLDL. This leads to a discussion on which macronutrient raises or lowers which species, which leads to a discussion about Pete Ahrens at Rockefeller University, then to Margaret Albrink, then to validation of their findings by Kuo, Carlson, and Goldstein, then to the expanded hypothesis in 1967 adding chylomicrons to the fold, bringing the number of classes of disorders of lipoprotein metabolism to four. And what does this lead to? It leads to what Mr. Taubes is most famous for bringing to the table:

"The observation that monounsaturated fats both lower LDL cholesterol and raise HDL also came with an ironic twist: the principal fat in red meat, eggs, and bacon is not saturated fat, but the very same monounsaturated fat as in olive oil. The implications are almost impossible to believe after three decades of public-health recommendations suggesting that any red meat consumed should at least be lean, with any excess fat removed."[11]

It is challenging to describe a description, but I will say that he provides a tutorial of triglycerides and cholesterol that has previously been unseen in the literature. It's his use of context, sources, and style that one is able to read it and walk away with a true understanding of the complexities and relationships involved.

In short, my knowledge of triglycerides and cholesterol—and your knowledge too—is much more in tune with reality as a result of reading his tutorial; that it is carbohydrates pushing metabolism toward the production of *atherogenic* lipoproteins and not the consumption of saturated fat that drives atherosclerosis. Other books, as we will see, take it from there to describe the actual means of atherosclerosis development. It is *not* developed from plaque made up of particles of fat and cholesterol that stick to the artery walls like sewage inside a pipe; rather, it is arterial muscle tissue, white blood cells, collagen, calcium, blood platelets, and more, that gets trapped as boils within the first and second layers of the arterial wall that serves as the genesis of atherosclerosis. Subsequent clot formation after the contents of the plaque — better described as a boil — bursts through the arterial wall is the most likely cause of an ischemic coronary event.

Those other great books describing the pathogenesis of coronary heart disease that I will point out later, notwithstanding, *Good Calories, Bad Calories* should be at the top of your must-read list.

But the book you're reading now isn't focused on heart disease or with obesity *per se* as it is with diabetes, the flip side of the same coin. In the immediate pages that follow, we will spend some time reviewing information channels, and the information therein, putting ourselves in the position of a person recently diagnosed with diabetes, and figuring out where to go to get accurate, intelligent, correct, optimal information. We will then find out that there are obstacles in our way, some quite large and influential; but, we needn't let ourselves be bothered by them. Armed with the proper information, we can influence back, and an optimal solution can be implemented, enabling us to thrive.

AT THE LIBRARY

Finding credible information, let alone an optimal treatment, for diabetes shouldn't be a terribly difficult task. The options of said optimal treatment, however, permutations of direct or indirect influencers of blood sugar are finite but vast. So how does one find then categorize the differing options, narrowing the field to such optimal solution, in spite of credible, though oftentimes divergent information? Well, there really are only a few places that house and disseminate such information: a doctor, the internet, a friend, other health-providers such as a nurse or dietician, a bookstore, a national library[12] such as the US Library of Congress, a private library, or a regional, state, city, university, or local library.

There certainly must be good information about diabetes somewhere on the internet,[13] and it does provide the added benefit of being accessible by anyone on the globe with a connection and an interface. Trouble is, navigating to all the relevant sites, documenting, cataloging, then analyzing and drawing conclusions about a best practice from the internet, unless you have a specific site in mind already, is a near-impossible task, as we shall see.

Searching the term "diabetes" on five well-known search engines in early 2009, I found the following number of relevant pages: 82,000,000 on

GOOGLE, 395,000,000 on YAHOO, 49,000,000 on MSN, 12,769,380 on LYCOS, and 11,380,000 on ASK. Working alone, and assuming that I'm able to successfully navigate to each site, spending no more than ten minutes total reading through each site, documenting my findings, and navigating to the next site, for eight hours each day, including weekends, it would take 4,703 *years* to work through the GOOGLE search results, 22,546 years to catalogue YAHOO's, 2,842 years for MSN, 729 years to get through the results from LYCOS, and 650 for ASK. I'll leave this problem to a more ambitious researcher with substantially more resources at hand to solve.

Before I move on, however, it is important to remember that we have put ourselves in the shoes of a recently diagnosed person with diabetes, and thus are tying to find the optimal solution to our disease. But the search results, if that task is ever completed, from the internet will not be presented to us categorized as "good" or "bad," "effective" or "ineffective," "true" or "not true." It is up to the searcher to make that determination. This concept is best summarized by Hal Abelson, Ken Ledeen, and Harry Lewis, in their book *Blown to Bits: Your Life, Liberty, and Happiness After the Digital Explosion* (2008):

> "The web is no longer a library. It is a chaotic marketplace of the billions of ideas and facts cast up by the bits explosion. Information consumers and information producers constantly seek out each other and morph into each other's roles. In this shadowy bits bazaar, with all its whispers and its couriers running to and fro, search engines are brokers. Their job is not to supply the undisputed truth, nor even to judge the accuracy of material that others provide. Search engines connect willing producers of information to willing consumers. They succeed or fail not on the quality of the information they provide, because they do not produce content at all. They only make connections. Search engines succeed or fail depending on whether we are happy with the connections they make, and nothing more. In the bazaar, it is not always the knowledgeable broker who makes the most deals. To stay in business, a broker just has to give most people what they want, consistently over time."[14]

Skipping doctors, friends, family, relatives, other health-care providers, periodicals, and bookstores as sources of objective information for the moment, let's take a look at a national library. My apologies in advance for being US-centric; take heart, however, as there is most likely a national library in your country, though, perhaps with a different classification system.[15]

As with most other topics of discussion, a few words—okay, maybe more—are needed to get into the subject. So let's now briefly take a look at the history and pertinent facts of the Library of Congress; the best summary can be found at Wikipedia, which is where I found what follows.[16]

The Library of Congress is the *de facto* national library of the United States and the research arm of the United States Congress. Located in three buildings in Washington, D.C., it is the largest library in the world by shelf space and holds the largest number of books.[17]

The Library of Congress was established by Congress in 1800 and was housed in the United States Capitol for most of the 19th century. After much of the original collection had been destroyed during the War of 1812, Thomas Jefferson sold the library 6,487 books, his entire personal library, in 1815.[18] After a period of decline during the mid-19th century the Library of Congress began to grow rapidly in both size and importance after the American Civil War, culminating in the construction of a separate library building and the transference of all copyright deposit holdings to the Library. During the rapid expansion of the 20th century the Library of Congress assumed a preeminent public role, becoming a "library of last resort" and expanding its mission for the benefit of scholars and the American people.

The Library's primary mission is investigating inquiries made by members of Congress through the Congressional Research Service; although it is open to the public, only legislators, Supreme Court justices and other high-ranking government officials may check out books. Through the United States Copyright Office, the Library of Congress also receives copies of every book, pamphlet, map, print, and piece of music registered in the United States. As the *de facto* national library, the Library of Congress promotes literacy and American literature through projects such as the American Folklife Center, American Memory, Center for the Book and Poet Laureate.

The Library of Congress was established on April 24, 1800, when President John Adams signed an Act of Congress providing for the transfer of the seat of government from Philadelphia to the new capital city of Washington. Part of the legislation appropriated $5,000 "for the purchase of such books as may be necessary for the use of Congress..., and for fitting up a suitable apartment for containing them..." Books were ordered from London and the collection, consisting of 740 books and 30 maps, was housed in the new Capitol.[19] Although the collection covered a variety of topics, the bulk of the materials were legal in nature, reflecting Congress' role as a maker of laws.

Thomas Jefferson played an important role in the Library's early formation, signing into law on January 26, 1802 the first law establishing the structure of the Library of Congress. The law established the presidentially appointed post of Librarian of Congress and a Joint Committee on the Library to regulate and oversee the Library, as well as giving the president and vice president the ability to borrow books.[20] The Library of Congress was destroyed in August 1814, when invading British troops set fire to the Capitol building and the small library of 3,000 volumes within.[21]

Within a month, former President Jefferson offered his personal library[22] as a replacement. Jefferson had spent 50 years accumulating a wide variety of books, including ones in foreign languages and volumes of philosophy, science, literature, and other topics not normally viewed as part of a legislative library, such as cookbooks, writing that, "I do not know that it contains any branch of science which Congress would wish to exclude from their collection; there is, in fact, no subject to which a Member of Congress may not have occasion to refer. In January 1815, Congress accepted Jefferson's offer, appropriating $23,950 for his 6,487 books.[23]

The collections of the Library of Congress include more than 32 million cataloged books and other print materials in 470 languages; more than 61 million manuscripts; the largest rare book collection in North America, including the rough draft of the Declaration of Independence, a Gutenberg Bible (one of only four perfect vellum copies known to exist);[24] over 1 million US government publications; 1 million issues of world newspapers spanning the past three centuries; 33,000 bound newspaper volumes; 500,000 microfilm reels; over 6,000 comic book[25] titles; the world's largest collection of legal materials; films; 4.8 million maps; sheet music; 2.7 million sound recordings; more than 13.7 million prints and photographic images including fine and popular art pieces and architectural drawings; the Betts Stradivarius; and the Cassavetti Stradivarius.

The Library developed a system of book classification called Library of Congress Classification (LCC), which is used by most US research and university libraries, although most public libraries continue to use the Dewey decimal system.

The Library serves as a legal repository for copyright protection and copyright registration, and as the base for the United States Copyright Office. Regardless of whether they register their copyright, all publishers are required to submit two complete copies of their published works to the Library—this requirement is known as *mandatory deposit*.[26] Parties wishing not to publish, need only submit one copy of their work. Nearly 22,000 new items published in the U.S. arrive every business day at the

Library. Contrary to popular belief, however, the Library does not retain all of these works in its permanent collection, although it does add an average of 10,000 items per day. Rejected items are used in trades with other libraries around the world, distributed to federal agencies, or donated to schools, communities, and other organizations within the United States.[27] As is true of many similar libraries, the Library of Congress retains copies of every publication in the English language that is deemed significant.

Guinness World Records currently lists the Library of Congress as the "World's Largest Library." This apparently is based on the shelf space the collection occupies; the Library of Congress states that its collection fills about 530 miles (850 km), while the British Library, reports about 388 miles (625 km) of shelves.[28] The Library of Congress holds about 130 million items with 29 million books against approximately 150 million items with 25 million books for the British Library.[29]

The Library of Congress is usually quoted as occupying, if digitized and stored as plain text, 20 terabytes of information (10 in other quotations), based on the amount of cataloged books in the Library of Congress classification system (20 million in 2007[30]) and estimating one megabyte of text per book.[31] This leads many people to conclude that 20 terabytes is equivalent to the entire holdings of the Library, but this is misleading because the Library contains many items in addition to books, such as manuscripts, photographs, maps, and sound recordings,[32] that, if digitized, would amount to much more information. The Library currently has no plans for systematic digitization of any significant portion of its books.

The Library makes millions of digital objects, comprising tens of terabytes, available at its American Memory site. American Memory is a source for public domain image resources, as well as audio, video, and archived Web content. Nearly all of the lists of holdings, the *catalogs* of the library, can be consulted directly on its web site. Librarians all over the world consult these catalogs, through the Web or through other media better suited to their needs, when they need to catalog for their collection a book published in the United States. They use the Library of Congress Control Number to make sure of the exact identity of the book.

The Library of Congress provides an online archive of the proceedings of the U.S. Congress at THOMAS, including bill text, Congressional Record text, bill summary and status, the Congressional Record Index, and the United States Constitution. The Library also administers the National Library Service for the Blind and Physically Handicapped, a talking and Braille library program provided to more than 766,000 Americans.

The Library of Congress is physically housed in three buildings in Washington, D.C.,[33] and is open to the general public for academic research and tourists. Only those who are issued a Reader Identification Card may enter the reading rooms and access the collection. The Reader Identification Card is available in the Madison building to persons who are at least 16 years of age upon presentation of a government issued picture identification (e.g., a driver's license, state ID card or passport). However, only members of Congress, Supreme Court Justices, their staff, Library of Congress staff and certain other government officials can actually remove items from the library buildings. Members of the general public with Reader Identification Cards must use items from the library collection inside the reading rooms only; they cannot remove library items from the reading rooms or the library buildings.

Since 1902, libraries in the United States have been able to request books and other items through interlibrary loan from the Library of Congress if these items are not readily available elsewhere. Through this, the Library of Congress has served as a "library of last resort," according to former Librarian of Congress Herbert Putnam.[34]

The Library of Congress Classification (LCC) is a system of library classification developed by the Library of Congress.[35] It is used by most research and academic libraries in the U.S. and several other countries. It is not to be confused with the Library of Congress Subject Headings or Library of Congress Control Number. Most public libraries and small academic libraries continue to use the Dewey Decimal Classification (DDC). The classification was originally developed by Herbert Putnam in 1897, just before he assumed the librarianship of Congress. With advice from Charles Ammi Cutter, it was influenced by Cutter Expansive Classification, and the DDC, and was specially designed for the special purposes of the Library of Congress. The new system replaced a fixed location system developed by Thomas Jefferson. By the time of Putnam's departure from his post in 1939, all the classes except K (Law) and parts of B (Philosophy and Religion) were well developed. It has been criticized as lacking a sound theoretical basis; many of the classification decisions were driven by the particular practical needs of that library, rather than epistemological considerations.

Although it divides subjects into broad categories, it is essentially enumerative in nature. It provides a guide to the books actually in the library, not a classification of the world.

The National Library of Medicine classification system (NLM) uses the classification scheme's unused letters *W* and *QS–QZ*. Some libraries use NLM in conjunction with LCC, eschewing LCC's R (Medicine). Others prefer to use the LCC scheme's *QP-QR* schedules and include Medicine *R*.

Here is the classification system with the letters and corresponding subject areas of the Library of Congress:

A   General Works
B   Philosophy, Psychology, and Religion
C   Auxiliary Sciences of History
D   General and Old World History

E	History of America
F	History of the US and British, Dutch, French, and Latin America
G	Geography, Anthropology, and Recreation
H	Social Sciences
J	Political Science
K	Law
L	Education
M	Music
N	Fine Arts
P	Language and Literature
Q	Science
R	Medicine
S	Agriculture
T	Technology
U	Military Science
V	Naval Science
Z	Bibliography, Library Science, and General Information Resources

We're almost ready to search diabetes at the Library of Congress, and need one more piece of information, the subclasses. Of course, all the above classes have a group of subclasses, but here are the ones for Medicine, Class R:

- Subclass R Medicine (General)
- Subclass RA Public aspects of medicine
- Subclass RB Pathology
- Subclass RC Internal medicine
- Subclass RD Surgery
- Subclass RE Ophthalmology
- Subclass RF Otorhinolaryngology
- Subclass RG Gynecology and obstetrics
- Subclass RJ Pediatrics
- Subclass RK Dentistry
- Subclass RL Dermatology
- Subclass RM Therapeutics. Pharmacology
- Subclass RS Pharmacy and materia medica

- Subclass RT Nursing
- Subclass RV Botanic, Thomsonian, and eclectic medicine
- Subclass RX Homeopathy
- Subclass RZ Other systems of medicine

So now let's search the Library of Congress database, available online, and see what we find.

First visiting http://www.loc.gov/index.html, the Library of Congress home page, then navigating to the catalogue page at http://catalog.loc.gov/, one can search by keyword, title, author, or subject. The most general search would be by subject, at which one finds 3,359 matches for the keyword "diabetes."

On closer inspection of the search results, eight of our 3,359 books are from the 18th century, 1762-1798, to be exact, under the subclass RC, internal medicine, and five of those rare books, all dissertations entitled *Dissertatio Medica Inauguralis, De Diabete,* are written in Latin. The authors and their books' published dates, are, respectively, William Stevenson (1762), George Jessop (1771), William Boyd, M.D. (1773), Joseph Hart Myers (1779), and James Vernon, M.D. (1796). *Tentamen Medicum Inaugurale, De Diabete,* by Alexander Marcet (1797), is the sixth book, leaving two books by John Rollo to complete the century. One of his books is simply entitled *Cases of the Diabetes Mellitus* (1797), and the other, also published in 1797, has the enormous title:

> *An account of two cases of the diabetes mellitus, with remarks, as they arose during the progress of the cure: to which are added, a general view of the nature of the disease and its appropriate treatment, including observations on some diseases depending on stomach affection, and a detail of the communications received on the subject since the dispersion of the notes on the first case / by John Rollo; with the results of the trials of various acids and other substances in the treatment of the lues venerea, and some observations on the nature of sugar, &c.,* [etc.] *by William Cruickshank.*

This book is particularly important, as Dr. John Rollo (d. 1809), a Scots physician and Surgeon General of the Royal Artillery, pioneered the systematic treatment of the disease by a restricted diet. Using a urine glucose test devised by Dobson,[36] he came up with the first effective treatment for diabetes: a diet high in what he called "animal food" (fat and meat) and low in "vegetable matter" (grains and breads). This diet prolonged life for many diabetics, those with what we now call type 2, and with modifications, was the only treatment for diabetes until the 1920s.[37]

Moving on to the 19th century, there were 27 books listed in the Library of Congress search database, with publishing dates in the 1802 to 1897 timeframe. But before I continue with a synopsis of books from this era, I think it is here that we shall diverge with a brief tale of the GOOGLE Book Search.[38] It's an important tale to tell, because, as we will find, GOOGLE makes many of these books available, at least those in the public domain, to read free of charge on the internet.

In December of 2004, GOOGLE announced a partnership with several major libraries to make digital copies of their collections and permit the text of the literature to be searched online by the GOOGLE search engine.[39] GOOGLE is providing its partnering libraries with a digital copy of the donor institution's collection.

The Print Library Project is only one of several initiatives by the company to enhance the breadth of its online search capabilities. It was originally a component of "GOOGLE Book Search," which included the Library Project and its "Partner Program," an online book marketing program designed to help publishers and authors promote their books by displaying a limited number of sample pages in connection with a user's word search. The Library Project was described on its website:

> "When you click on a search result for a book from the Library Project, you'll see the Snippet View which, like a card catalog, shows you information about the book plus a few snippets — a few sentences of your search term in context. You may also

see the Sample Pages View if the publisher or author has given us permission or
the Full Book View if the book is out of copyright. In all cases, you'll see 'Buy this
Book' links that lead directly to online bookstores where you can buy the book."[40]

After some academic and commercial publishers objected to the Library
Project, GOOGLE took a brief hiatus from scanning to allow publishers
time to identify works that they, i.e., the copyright holders, do not want to
be included in the digital database. This has been referred to an "opt out"
plan. The general rule of copyright law requires a prospective user to seek
permission for use; GOOGLE has reversed the process by announcing its
intention to digitize entire collections of the contributing libraries *unless* a
content owner opts out by acting to *withhold* permission. This contributes
to the content holders' claim that GOOGLE is engaged in massive
copyright infringement.

The complaint filed by plaintiff publishing companies (the Publishers)
accuses defendant GOOGLE of massive copyright infringement.[41] By
digitizing copyrighted works without permission, GOOGLE is alleged to
violate the copyright holders' exclusive rights to copy and/or display
protected work.[42] Plaintiffs contend that GOOGLE's project is strictly
commercial because it "pays" for the libraries' collections by delivering
digital copies back to them; and, GOOGLE will realize significant
advertising revenues as a consequence of its enhanced search capabilities.

Defendant GOOGLE essentially contends that its opt out program negates
any infringement liability. But, if infringement were found, GOOGLE
argues that its activity is protected by copyright's fair use doctrine.
GOOGLE cites the U.S. Court of Appeals for the Ninth Circuit's decision
in *Kelly v. Arriba Soft Corp.* as support for the proposition that Internet
search engines' indexing activities constitute a fair use.[43]

Although the Library of Congress is not a participant in GOOGLE's book
search project, they are, nonetheless, a part of this tale. Like many other
great research libraries, the Library of Congress has been moving into the

digital world. One way they're doing it is through a scanning project that, as of January, 2009, has put 25,000 books online for anyone to read or download.

The Alfred P. Sloan Foundation is funding the $2 million project, and the scanning is being done by the Internet Archive. The San Francisco-based nonprofit group aims to preserve cultural artifacts such as musical recordings and Web pages, as well as books, and make them available online.

The books being digitized in this project are all at least 75 years old and thus out of copyright. The scanned books from the Library of Congress are available online at the Internet Archive, http://www.archive.org/details/texts.[44]

The important take-away here is that regardless of whether a book was scanned by GOOGLE or the Internet Archive, or any other entity for that matter, the odds increase each day that a given book—in whole or passages selected by the publisher—is available to read on the internet, in text within a browser, or portable document format (.pdf).[45]

So let's now return to the books from the Library of Congress dating to the 19th century. There were 27 books listed in the LOC search database, with publishing dates in the 1802-1897 timeframe. They are listed here. And, yes, some of these can be found and read online.

Title: *An essay on the disease commonly called diabetes*
Author: Washington, William   Year: 1802

Title: *Medical reports of cases and experiments, with observations, chiefly derived from hospital practice: to which are added, an enquiry into the origin of canine madness; and thoughts on a plan for its extirpation from the British isles*
Author: Bardsley, Samuel Argent   Year: 1807

Title: *Cases of diabetes, consumption, &c., with observations on the history and treatment of disease in general*

Author: Watt, Robert   Year: 1808

Title: *English olive-tree, or, A treatise on the use of oil and the air bath: with miscellaneous remarks on the prevention and cure of various diseases, gout, rheumatism, diabetes, &c.*

Author: Trinder, William Martin   Year: 1812

Title: *De diabete mellito*

Author: Bennewitz, Heinrich Gottlob   Year: 1824

Title: *An inquiry into the nature and treatment of diabetes, calculus, and other affections of the urinary organs: with remarks on the importance of attending to the state of the urine in organic diseases of the kidney and bladder: and some practical rules for determining the nature of the disease from the sensible and chemical properties of that secretion*

Author: Prout, William   Year: 1825

Title: *An inquiry into the nature and treatment of diabetes, calculus, and other affections of the urinary organs; with remarks on the importance of attending to the state of the urine in organic diseases of the kidney and bladder: and some practical rules for determining the nature of the disease from the sensible and chemical properties of that secretion. From the 2d London ed., rev. and much enl.: with notes and additions by S. Colhoun.*

Author: Prout, William   Year: 1826

Title: *Hospital facts and observations: illustrative of the efficacy of the new remedies, strychnia, brucia, acetate of morphia, veratria, iodine, &c. in several morbid conditions of the system: with a comparative view of the treatment of chorea, and some cases of diabetes: a report on the efficacy of sulphureous fumigations in diseases of the skin, chronic rheumatism, &c.*

Author: Bardsley, James Lomax   Year: 1830

Title: *Du diabète sucré*

Author: Chaloin, Louis Ernest   Year: 1853

Title: *Diabetes mellitus*

Author: Clapp, Sylvanus   Year: 1854

Title: *Case of diabetes mellitus*

Author: Jones, Joseph   Year: 1858

Title: *On diabetes, and its successful treatment*

Author: Camplin, John Mussendine   Year: 1858

At the Library

Title: *On diabetes, and its successful treatment. From the 2d London ed.*
Author: Camplin, John Mussendine   Year: 1861

Title: *Zur lehre vom diabetes mellitus*
Author: Engmann, Wilhelm   Year: 1869

Title: *On the origin of diabetes, with some new experiments regarding the glycogenic function of the liver*
Author: Lusk, William Thompson   Year: 1870

Title: *Ueber diabetes mellitus*
Author: Wünnenberg, Ludwig   Year: 1870

Title: *De la glycosurie, ou, Diabète sucré: son traitement hygiénique: avec notes et documents sur la nature et le traitement de la goutte, la gravelle urique, sur l'oligurie, le diabète insipide avec excès d'urée, l'hippurie, la pimélorrhée, etc.*
Author: Bouchardat, Apollinaire   Year: 1875

Title: *Considérations sur la pathogénie et sur le traitement du diabète*
Author: Dumoulin, Auguste   Year: 1877

Title: *A treatise on Bright's disease and diabetes*
Author: Tyson, James   Year: 1881

Title: *De la gymnastique de l'hydrothérapie*
Author: Hoffmann, Louis   Year: 1882

Title: *Does the present state of knowledge justify a clinical and pathological correlation of rheumatism, gout, diabetes, and chronic Bright's disease?*
Author: Tyson, James   Year: 1886

Title: *Diabetes. Mellitus and insipidus*
Author: Smith, Andrew Heermance   Year: 1889

Title: *Diabetes: its causes, symptoms, and treatment*
Author: Purdy, Charles Wesley   Year: 1890

Title: *Cookery for the diabetic*
Author: Poole, W.H.   Year: 1891

Title: *Ueber coma diabeticumm im anschluss an die narcose*
Author: Müller, Wilhelm   Year: 1894

Title: *Die Zuckerkrankheit und ihre Behandlung*
Author: von Noorden, Carl   Year: 1895

Title: *Kliniske undersøgelser over kvælstofudskilningens forhold til den diætetiske behandling ved diabetes mellitus*
Author: Lauritzen, Marius   Year: 1897

One such book, *Diabetes: Its Causes, Symptoms, and Treatment*, by Charles Wesley Purdy, is available on the internet. And it should come as no surprise, that more than a century ago, in 1890, Charles Purdy wrote:

"Prophylactic [preventive] measures are advisable for people of diabetic parentage, or for those whose families present marked tendencies to the disease. In such cases it is wise to adopt a system of diet which limits the use of starchy and saccharine foods to the most moderate proportions. Occupations should be selected which entail the least possible mental pressure and excitement; and, if practicable, a residence should be chosen as near the sea-level as possible, with a mean temperature range of about 70 F. The observance of the above conditions will insure the individual the best chances of avoiding the disease.

Until future investigation shall have revealed some agency through which we are able to check the excessive formation of sugar in the liver, our chief resource against the disease must consist in withholding from the system that which it is capable of converting into sugar, and in supplying that which it is capable of assimilating as nourishment. The accomplishment of this object is the essential aim of the dietetic treatment of diabetes.

Physiological chemistry as well as experience have shown us that the chief source of sugar-production in the system is the carbohydrate foods, more especially starches and sugar. In nearly all mild cases of diabetes, and in most cases of recent origin, the avoidance of these foods arrests the excretion of sugar, as well as the more prominent symptoms of the disease. The sugar-forming powers of the organism in diabetes are feeblest in their operation upon nitrogenous materials, and therefore animal foods are the least susceptible of conversion into sugar. Next in order rank the green parts of certain vegetables, which quite strongly resist sugar transformation. Finally, the starchy and saccharine members of the carbohydrate group are the most easily transformed into sugar of all, and are therefore the most dangerous for use. Practically, then, the more completely we are able to eliminate the starchy and saccharine foods from the diet, the more completely we are able to hold the disease under control. At first sight this might seem to be a very simple matter; but when we come to furnish a diet-list that strictly conforms to the above principle, it will be found a most difficult problem to solve, owing to the very wide diffusion of starch and sugar throughout the organic world.

Of the other foods derivable from the vegetable kingdom, the cereals and seme of the tubers are the most dangerous. Potatoes, beets, parsnips, carrots, among the latter; and, of the former, rice, sago, oatmeal, cornmeal, buckwheat, rye, barley, peas, and beans, should be prohibited without compromise in most, if not in all, cases. In the strict form of dieting we are obliged to avoid the whole list. In cases of moderate severity we may, however, draw upon one class of vegetables greens. Green vegetables consist mostly of cellulose, and contain little, sometimes almost no, starch. They are rendered still less objectionable if boiled before being eaten, as the hot water dissolves out much of the remaining starch and sugar. The starch and sugar contents of vegetables vary considerably, according to the degree of cultivation and the nature of the soil and climate in which they are grown. As a rule, a high degree of domestic cultivation favors an increase of the starch and sugar, while high temperature and sunny skies have an opposite tendency. Among the least objectionable vegetables may be mentioned lettuce, cucumbers, olives, mushrooms, Brussels-sprouts, cabbage, spinach, and water-cresses.

Most nuts except chestnuts may be permitted, the list including almonds, walnuts, Brazil nuts, filberts, butternuts, and cocoanuts.

Great differences prevail in practice with regard to the use of fruits in diabetic conditions, some authorities allowing them freely, while others curtail them. Some fruits, such as apples and strawberries, really contain very little sugar, and in the case of apples the sugar is in such form that it is often well assimilated by diabetics.

The truth is that it is more difficult to make a rule which will apply universally with regard to the use of fruits than with any other class of foods in these cases; and therefore it must to some extent be a matter of experiment in each individual case. It may be stated, however, in a general way, that mild cases will bear a moderate use of such fruits as apples, tomatoes, and strawberries; but in severe cases it is best to prohibit their use without exception."[46]

Purdy's treatment is particularly salient even today, but I will hold off on my comments for the moment, as surveying books is the primary task at hand.

The interesting observation to bring up here is that although the Library of Congress holds the most books in the world, it does not contain every book. While searching for an electronic version of <u>William</u> Washington's book *An Essay of the Disease Commonly Called Diabetes* online, which I did not find, I fortuitously found the book entitled *Diabetes Mellitus and Its Treatment,* by Richard Thomas <u>Williamson</u>, M.D., M.R.C.P., published in 1898. Interestingly, this book is not in the collection of the Library of Congress, however, it is an important book.

In the chapter "General Principles of Treatment," Dr. Williamson writes:

> "Potatoes should be excluded from the diet first, then bread, and gradually all carbohydrates should be cut off. In the place of bread, the aleuronat and cocoa-nut cakes mentioned on p. 357 may be given."[47]

He states that the chief object to be aimed at in the treatment is to diminish the amount of sugar in the urine and blood, and to diminish the amount of urine, and to relieve thirst. And that object may be attained by removal of the carbohydrates from the diet. Reflecting on the work of John Rollo, Dr. Williamson writes:

> "Ever since Rollo published his book on diabetes in 1797, and pointed out the value of restriction of the carbohydrates in the food, it has been acknowledged that of all forms and methods of treatment this dietetic one is the most important."[48]

He also writes:

> "All authors agree as to the great value of fat in the severe forms of diabetes; and, in addition to fatty food, cod-liver oil, lipanin [an artificial cod-liver oil substitute], and other fats may be given."[49]

> "Most articles of food from the animal kingdom may be taken freely by diabetic patients. Butchers' meat and flesh meat of various kinds, poultry, game, and fish, may be taken in any form. But in the cooking thereof flour or bread crumbs should not be used, if a very strict diet is indicated; aleuronat may be used in place of flour, however, and butter and fats may be freely employed.

The following articles may also be allowed freely: tongue, ham, bacon, potted beef, and chicken, preserved meats of various kinds, sardines, tinned and preserved fish, beef extracts, beef-tea, meat juices, broth, soups, and jellies (when prepared without the addition of any saccharine or starchy materials).

Eggs in various forms are most useful articles of diet. An egg weighing about 600 grs. contains about 90 grs. of albumin and 75 grs. of fatty material. When hard boiled they can be taken with comparatively large quantities of butter. The "buttered" egg or omelet is a useful form...Honey, of course, ought never to be taken. Butter, cheese, and cream may be allowed in large quantities." [50]

"Fats, both animal and vegetable, are the most valuable articles of diet for diabetic patients, especially for those who suffer from the severe forms of the disease, and may be allowed in large quantities.

The more important articles of diet, containing a large quantity of fat, are butter, cream, bacon, cheese, eggs, suet." [51]

"Cocoa-nuts contain a small quantity of sugar, but this may be removed easily, and cocoa-nut flour may be used for the preparation of biscuits." [52]

Dr. Williamson concludes his discussion on "cocoa-nuts" with recipes consisting of water, "cocoa-nut," eggs, and cream for "excellent" cakes, biscuits and buns made without sugar or carbohydrates that a diabetic can tolerate quite well, prepare inexpensively at home, and prefer more, i.e., they taste better, than most diabetic cakes offered at the time.

In the Appendix, Richard Thomas Williamson presents the following list of articles of diet and beverages, arranged in a tabular form, which ought to be sanctioned or forbidden, when for diagnostic or therapeutical purposes a very strict diet is desirable: [53]

Sanctioned	Forbidden
Butchers' meat of all kinds (except liver); potted and preserved meats. Ham, tongue, bacon. Poultry, game. Fish (fresh, dried, and preserved); sardines, shrimps. Broths, animal soups, and jellies (prepared without the addition of saccharine or starchy materials). Eggs, cheese, cream. Butter, suet, oils, and fats. Custard (without sugar). Reliable bread substitutes (gluten bread, almond and aleuronat cakes). Green vegetables--mustard and cress, watercress, endive, lettuce, spinach, turnip-tops, cabbage, broccoli, Brussels sprouts, spring onions. Nuts (walnuts, almonds, filberts, hazel nuts, Brazil nuts), but not chestnuts. Water, soda-water, and mineral waters. Tea, coffee. Dry sherry, claret, Burgundy, hock, Moselle, Ahr wines, most Rhine wines, Austrian and Hungarian table wines (all in moderate quantities, however). Brandy in small quantities.	Sugar; saccharine and farinaceous articles of food. Pastry and farinaceous puddings. Rice, sago, arrowroot, tapioca, macaroni, vermicelli, semolina. Potatoes. Wheaten bread and biscuits. Carrots, turnips, parsnips, beetroot, beans, peas, large onions. Liver. Oysters, cockles, mussels, the "puddings" of crabs and lobsters. Honey. All sweet fruit and dried fruits. Port, Tokay, champagne, and sweet wines. Must, fruit juices and syrups. Sweet lemonade. Liqueurs. Beer, ale, porter, and stout. Rum and sweetened gin. Cocoa and chocolate. Milk in large quantities.

Articles of Food in Diabetes
From Williamson, M.D., M.R.C.P., R.T. *Diabetes Mellitus and Its Treatment*. Edinburgh & London: Young J. Pentland; New York: The Macmillan Company, 1898, pages 406-407.

Again, no need to comment on this list of foods sanctioned or forbidden in the diabetic's diet, other than to say that we will revisit it again in a later chapter. For now, let's conclude our discussion of the LOC book search.

From the 18th century's eight books on diabetes, at least from the perspective of the Library of Congress, the 19th century's growth rate of 237.5% — there are now an additional 27 books on the shelf — pales in comparison with the next century. Between the beginning and end of the 20th century, there are now an additional 1,930 books published and stocked on the shelves. That represents a century-to-century growth rate of slightly more than 7,048%. Instead of keeping you in suspense, let me mention here that, although we're far from the end of the 21st century, the

Library of Congress already holds an additional 1,367 from this century. Add to that the 27 books in the LOC diabetes search results that are undated, and we have the grand total of 3,359 books that we originally found in the database. Books from the 20th century make up a majority 57%, and those of the 21st century, not a decade old — 10% young at the time of this writing — make up 41% of the collection.

Let me surprise you, and, perhaps, quell your fears, by noting that I won't be listing or going through any of the afore-mentioned 1,930 20th, or 1,367 21st century books here. True, I am not the same caliber investigator as a Gary Taubes, Barry Groves, or host of other past- and present-day saints. But we know what truly separates these books from those of the prior centuries. Those writers in the 20th century, to borrow and alter Charles Purdy's words, were the future investigators that revealed the agency through which we are able to check the excessive formation of sugar in the liver. Moreover, the identification of beta cells — those little heaps of cells — within the islets of Langerhans in the pancreas as the center of insulin production, tied inexorably to the diabetes condition, and leading to the purification and dissemination of analog insulin for patient self-management, is the primary driver of the burgeoning — scientific, dietetic, therapeutic, historical, and otherwise informational — diabetes book growth in the 20th century.

3,359 sources are considerably less than the millions found online, but still pose some practical problems. First, unless you're an elected official, you cannot "check-out" any books from the Library of Congress; that's a perk reserved for any voracious reader winning office. Yes, you can read any of them — while you're there — but, you cannot bring any books out of the library for any period of time. And, of course, you have to be in Washington, DC. I've toyed with the idea of taking a sabbatical there, finding a relatively inexpensive hotel, and reading through the list of 3,359 books. Assuming three hours per book, which would include documenting my findings, at eight hours a day, seven days a week, my sabbatical would have to be almost three-and-a-half years. Sounds more like retirement. Even if I skim each book for an hour, I would still need more than a year to complete the task. And that wouldn't include sight-seeing. A two to three year's sabbatical, however, is an intriguing thought.

So, like me, the average diabetic looking for information is relegated to visiting something more local to learn the totality of the world of diabetes. And so it is here that we really begin our journey.

What type of information is available about diabetes at the local library? I hypothesized that most books contain good information about the disease, i.e., etiology, physiology, impact on society, history, A_{1c} tutorials, nutritional options, etc., and that there would also be some books advocating a specific diet. So to test that hypothesis, I decided to visit my local library.

Before the results are provided, let's take a brief detour to find out a little more about libraries, what are now recognized as entitlements of a free society.

The first library in America was founded in 1638, at Harvard University. A few churches also established small parish libraries in the colonial period, but these had little effect on the average man.[54]

"Libraries developed first in the American colonies as private collections and then within higher education institutions. These early libraries were small for three reasons: relatively few materials were published in the New World, funds were limited, and acquiring materials was difficult. Even as late as 1850, only 600 periodicals were being published in the United States, up from 26 in 1810. Monographic publishing was equally sparse, with most works being religious in nature."[55]

"Academic libraries preceded public libraries in the United States. Established in 1833, the Peterborough Town Library in New Hampshire usually is identified as the first free, publicly owned and maintained library in the united States. A library established in Franklin, Massachusetts, though funds from Benjamin

Franklin to purchase 116 volumes, was opened to all inhabitants of the town in 1790. Though public, it was not supported by public funding. Social libraries, limited to a specific clientele and supported by subscriptions, had existed in the colonies for more than 100 years. One of the more well known is the Philadelphia Library Company, founded by Benjamin Franklin in 1731 and supported by fifty subscribers to share the cost of importing books and journals from England. Other social libraries were established and supported by philanthropists and larger manufacturers to teach morality, provide a more wholesome environment, and offer self-education opportunities to the poor and uneducated drawn to cities. Circulating libraries were commercial ventures that loaned more popular materials, frequently novels, for a fee. When considered together, these early libraries were furnishing the collections that libraries provide today—materials that are used for information, education, and recreation."[56]

As of 2008, there were 30,022[57] total United States Libraries, categorized as armed forces, college and university, electronic, government, community college, law, medical, public and state, religious, and special, including industry and company libraries as well as libraries serving associations, clubs, foundations, institutes, and societies. Add to those 30,022 the 80 total libraries administered by the United Stated in its territories, and the 3,685 total Canadian libraries, and we have a grand total of 33,787 libraries listed in the *American Library Directory*.[58]

During the last week of 2008, and into the first few weeks of 2009, I visited the Santa Clara City Library, 2635 Homestead Road, in Santa Clara, California. Not an average library as it turns out, but a very good library with 354,579 book titles and 724 periodical subscriptions[59] in its collection, giving it a 2008 HAPLR score of 897, putting it in the 99th percentile of all libraries.[60]

Where would these books on diabetes be located? Let's quickly review the Dewey Decimal Classification System to find out.

"The Dewey Decimal Classification (DDC) is the most widely used library classification system in the world. It is used in more than 135 countries, and has been translated into over 30 languages. In the United States, 95% of all public and school libraries, 25% of all college and university libraries, and 20% of special libraries use the DDC.

The DDC was conceived by Melvil Dewey in 1873 and first published in 1876. The first edition was 44 pages long: 14 pages of front and back matter, 12 pages of summaries and schedules, and 18 pages of index. The first edition of the Abridged DDC appeared in 1894." [61]

"In the DDC, basic classes are defined by traditional academic disciplines or fields of study. No principle is more basic to the DDC than this: the parts of the Classification are arranged by discipline, not by subject." [62]

"At the broadest level, the DDC is divided into ten *main classes*, which together cover the entire works of knowledge. These classes are divided into ten *divisions* and each division into ten *sections*, although not all the numbers for the divisions and sections have been used." [63]

"The ten main classes are:

000   Generalities
100   Philosophy, parapsychology and occultism, psychology
200   Religion
300   Social Sciences
400   Language
500   Natural sciences and mathematics
600   Technology (Applied sciences)
700   The arts   Fine and decorative arts
800   Literature (Belles-lettres) and rhetoric
900   Geography, history, and auxiliary disciplines

The first digit in the numbers listed above indicates the *main class*. Although each number contains three digits, only the first digit is significant in this list. The remaining zeroes fill out the notation to the required digits.

Each main class consists of ten *divisions*, also numbered 0 through 9. The number of significant digits here is two, the second digit indicating the division. 6$\underline{0}$0 is used for general works on the applied sciences, 6$\underline{1}$0 for the medical sciences, 6$\underline{2}$0 for engineering, 6$\underline{3}$0 for agriculture.

Each division has ten *sections*, again numbered 0 through 9. The third digit in each three-digit number indicates the section. Thus 63$\underline{0}$ is used for general works on agriculture, 63<u>1</u> for specific techniques, 63<u>2</u> for plant injuries, 63<u>3</u> for field and plantation crops." [64]

Thus, books on diabetes are found in the main class <u>6</u>00, Technology (Applied sciences), division 6<u>1</u>0, Medical sciences, section 61<u>6</u>, Diseases, and, finally, into the subsection 616.<u>4</u>, Diseases of the endocrine system.

One other topic must be discussed before tending to the business at hand, and that is that books on library shelves are by no means a static affair. Libraries have distinct operational guidelines that vary from library to library, inclusively known as "collection development and management."

"Selection of materials for libraries has been around as long as libraries have, though records of how decisions were made in the ancient libraries of Nineveh, Alexandria, and Pergamum are nonexistent. One can assume that the scarcity of written materials and their value as unique records made comprehensive, completeness, and preservation guiding principles. Libraries served primarily as storehouses rather than as instruments for the dissemination of knowledge. Comprehensiveness, completeness, and preservation have continued as library goals through the growth of commerce, the Renaissance, invention of movable type, expanding lay literacy, the Enlightenment, the public library movement, and the proliferation of electronic resources. Size continues to be a common, though only one, measure of a library's greatness." [65]

The Santa Clara City Library utilizes its own guide for weeding out older, obsolete, and/or warn-out books contained and discussed in *Circulating Collection Management Manual* (1999). This manual starts off with four collection policies: Freedom To Read, Library Bill of Rights, Materials Selection Policy, and Circulating Collection policy. Most notable is the General Weeding Guidelines regarding Medical Sciences, classified as 610-619:

"Recognizing that much medical information is already dated by the time it is published in book form, the library buys nearly everything available within the collection guidelines, attempting to provide the most current material possible in a rapidly changing field…Material is selected primarily for the general reader, patient, parent, or other non-professional." [66]

And so here we are where we started this discussion, at the Santa Clara City Library, looking for books on diabetes. Peering at the shelf of books contained within the 616.4 classification, I found 75 books published from 1997 to 2008.[67] An additional 19 reference books—not surprisingly in the reference section—published from 1998 to 2008, that included significant articles on diabetes, were also found. General diet or other health books neither on the shelf in section 616.4, nor in the reference section, were disregarded. Reading through the books off the shelf, I was surprised to find that, with but one exception, each and every book advocated a specific diet. Of the 75 books off the shelf, only 10 advocated a low-carbohydrate diet to treat the disease. One book, *The First Year: Type 2 Diabetes. An Essential Guide for the Newly Diagnosed* (2001), contained only objective information, and all the rest—64—an astounding 85% of the books off the shelf, advocated a low-fat, high-carbohydrate diet to treat a disease manifested by impaired carbohydrate metabolism. I've included the entire list of both "books off the shelf," which I've simply labeled as "Books on Diabetes," and "Reference Books" in, respectively, Appendices A & B, complete with the evidence; that is, the specific references in those books that determine whether it advocates a low-fat or a low-carbohydrate diet.

By the way, general agreement about what it means to have a low-fat, low-carbohydrate, or even a low-protein diet has never really been attained, so let's try to bring some clarity. From a purely mathematical standpoint, if you have three parameters—in our case the three parameters are carbohydrate, protein, and fat—and, additionally, three levels—low, medium, and high—the first question to ask is how many combinations are there? The answer is 3x3x3, of course, which is 27 total combinations. But we then have to define what it means to have a low, medium, or high level. Again, there isn't any general agreement in the literature of those distinctions. To help with our discussion, let's define "low" as a range of 0%-30%, medium as a range of 30%-40%, and high as a range of 40%-100%

of total calories. With only three variables, 50% of any one variable would be a plurality, and slightly over 50% would be a majority; therefore by definition any percentage greater than 50% has to be high. We could consider anything in the 40%-50% range to be either in the "high-medium" area or the "low-high," but I've chosen that range to simply be within the "high" amount.

We can now see from Table 1 those 27 total combinations of low, medium, and high for the three different parameters of carbohydrate, protein and fat. But notice that there are only 22 total real possibilities given the above definitions. Note that the ranges given above (low = 0%-30%, medium = 30%-40%, high = 40%-100%) do not work for any specific percentage in number 1 (low carbohydrate, low protein, low fat); that is, since the low range is 0%-30%, even at the far end of that range — 30% — if the three parameters of carbohydrate, protein and fat were each 30%, the total is only 90%, not 100%, so we are forced to drop that as a valid option. The same holds true for numbers 18 (medium carbohydrate, high protein, high fat), 24 (high carbohydrate, medium protein, high fat), 26 (high carbohydrate, high protein, medium fat), and 27 (high carbohydrate, high protein, high fat). These numbers, then, the five discounted options, have all been highlighted. Thus the total amount of real possibilities of combinations of low, medium, and high portions of carbohydrate, protein, and fat are 22.

	Carbohydrate	Protein	Fat
1	Low	Low	Low
2	Low	Low	Medium
3	Low	Low	High
4	Low	Medium	Low
5	Low	Medium	Medium
6	Low	Medium	High
7	Low	High	Low
8	Low	High	Medium
9	Low	High	High
10	Medium	Low	Low
11	Medium	Low	Medium
12	Medium	Low	High
13	Medium	Medium	Low
14	Medium	Medium	Medium
15	Medium	Medium	High
16	Medium	High	Low
17	Medium	High	Medium
18	Medium	High	High
19	High	Low	Low
20	High	Low	Medium
21	High	Low	High
22	High	Medium	Low
23	High	Medium	Medium
24	High	Medium	High
25	High	High	Low
26	High	High	Medium
27	High	High	High

Table 1
The 27 total combinations of low, medium, and high for the three
different parameters of carbohydrate, protein and fat. The five
discounted options, numbers 1, 18, 24, 26, & 27 have been
highlighted gray.

Back to our discussion. We found that 64 books—85% of the books off the shelf, advocated a low-fat, high-carbohydrate diet to treat a disease manifested by impaired carbohydrate metabolism. None described high protein intake, so we are safe to conclude that these books all refer to either medium or low protein, which is not particularly relevant to our discussion.

And the reference books, those written and commented on exclusively by doctors, faired much, much worse. With but one tenuous exception—the diabetes section in *Childhood Diseases and Disorders Sourcebook* (2003) didn't advocate a diet *per se*, it stated that "…A child or teen needs to follow a meal plan developed by a physician, diabetes educator, or a registered dietician," but, of course, in 2003, a physician, diabetes educator, or a registered dietician would most likely have advocated a low-fat diet—18 out of the 19 reference books *advocated*, not simply informed about, but *advocated* a low-fat, and by definition, a high-carbohydrate diet to best treat a disease characterized by, at best, impaired, and, at worst, non-existent carbohydrate metabolism.

Kind of makes me wonder that if there were a section written devoted to cigarette, alcohol, or drug abuse, would these same reference books tout cigarettes, alcohol, and drugs as the basis for treatment?

Granted, our results are just from one library, and not from a random sample of, say, 30 from the population of 30,000+ libraries. Nonetheless, the odds that I found the one library with a large majority of shelved books, or all reference books, written advocating a high-carbohydrate diet, out of all the libraries out there is rather small. Yes, it would be interesting to survey a random sample of this nation's libraries, perhaps even others around the globe, to find the true mean and variance of the numbers of diabetes books on the shelves that advocate low- or high-carbohydrate diets, and then the mean and variance of the reference books, but I have neither the time nor resources necessary to devote to that task.

The more relevant question anyway is why do nearly all the reference books, those credible, driving forces behind replication by also-rans, why is it that they advocate a high-carbohydrate, low-fat diet?

And so we move to the next chapter to answer that question. Contrary to its title, however, you needn't own a telescope to read it.

SUPERMASSIVE BLACK HOLES & THE DCCT

When a star runs out of nuclear fuel, it will collapse. If the core, or central region, of the star has a mass that is greater than three suns, no known nuclear forces can prevent the core from forming a deep gravitational warp in space called a black hole. A black hole is a dense, compact object whose gravitational pull is so strong that—within a certain distance of it—nothing can escape, not even light. Black holes are thought to result from the collapse of certain very massive stars at the ends of their evolution.[68]

A black hole does not have a surface in the usual sense of the word. There is simply a region, or boundary, in space around a black hole beyond which we cannot see. This boundary is called the event horizon.[69]

Anything that passes beyond the event horizon is doomed to be crushed as it descends ever deeper into the gravitational well of the black hole. No visible light, nor X-rays, nor any other form of electromagnetic radiation, nor any particle, no matter how energetic, can escape. The radius of the event horizon, proportional to the mass, is very small, only 30 kilometers for a non-spinning black hole with the mass of 10 Suns.[70]

Can astronomers see a black hole? Not directly. The only way to find one is to use circumstantial evidence. Observations must imply that a sufficiently large amount of matter is compressed into a sufficiently small region of space so that no other explanation is possible. For stellar black holes, this means observing the orbital acceleration of a star as it orbits its unseen companion in a double or binary star system.[71]

Searching for black holes is tricky business. One way to locate them has been to study X-ray binary systems. These systems consist of a visible star in close orbit around an invisible companion star which may be a neutron star or black hole. The companion star pulls gas away from the visible star.[72]

As this gas forms a flattened disk, it swirls toward the companion. Friction caused by collisions between the particles in the gas heats them to extreme temperatures and they produce X-rays that flicker or vary in intensity within a second.[73]

Many bright X-ray binary sources have been discovered in our galaxy and nearby galaxies. In about ten of these systems, the rapid orbital velocity of the visible star indicates that the unseen companion is a black hole. The X-rays in these objects are produced by particles very close to the event horizon. In less than a second after they give off their X-rays, they disappear beyond the event horizon.[74]

However, not all the matter in the disk around a black hole is doomed to fall into the black hole. In many black hole systems, some of the gas escapes as a hot wind that is blown away from the disk at high speeds. Even more dramatic are the high-energy jets that radio and X-ray observations show exploding away from some stellar black holes. These jets can move at nearly the speed of light in tight beams and travel several light years before slowing down and fading away.[75]

Do black holes grow when matter falls into them? Yes, the mass of the black hole increases by an amount equal to the amount of mass it captures.

The radius of the event horizon also increases by about 3 kilometers for every solar mass that it swallows. A black hole in the center of a galaxy, where stars are densely packed, may grow to the mass of a billion Suns and become what is known as a supermassive black hole.[76]

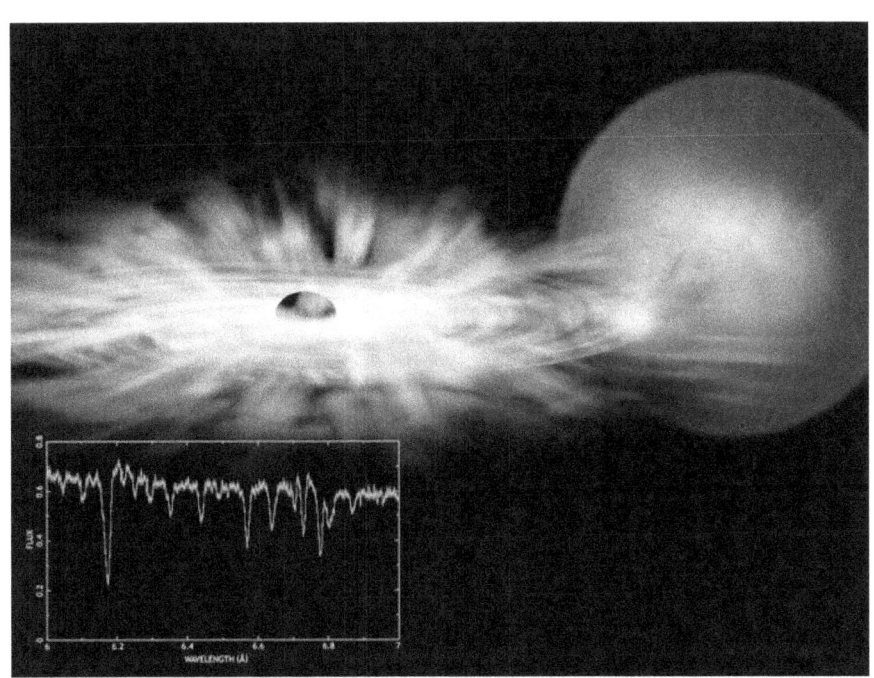

The X-ray spectrum (see inset) of a binary star system consisting of a black hole and a normal star indicates that turbulent winds of multimillion degree gas are swirling around the black hole. As the illustration shows, much of the hot gas is spiraling inward toward the black hole, but about 30 percent is blowing away.

The temperature and intensity of the winds imply that powerful magnetic fields must be present. These magnetic fields, likely carried by the gas flowing from the companion star, create magnetic turbulence that generates friction in the gaseous disk and drive winds from the disk that carry momentum outward as the gas falls inward. Magnetic friction also heats the gas in the inner part of the disk to X-ray emitting temperatures. Image credit: Illustration: NASA/CXC/M.Weiss; X-ray Spectrum: NASA/CXC/U.Michigan/J.Miller et al.

Recently Chandra* has found evidence that black holes with masses of about a thousand Suns can be formed in dense star clusters by processes that are not yet understood.[77]

Kitty Ferguson, in her accessible book on black holes entitled *Prisons of light: Black Holes*, explains that a black hole is not the destiny of all suns:

> "In the late 1920s, Subrahmanyan Chandrasekhar, a young Indian physicist then at the University of Cambridge, calculated that is a star's mass is less than 1.4 times the mass of our sun, gravity will not be able to overpower this exclusion principle repulsion among the electrons. The star shrinks and becomes a white dwarf, but, because of the exclusion principle, it shrinks no further. That star will not become a black hole. We now call this mass of 1.4 solar masses the "Chandrasekhar limit." Only in a star whose mass is *more* than the Chandrasekhar limit will gravity overcome the exclusion principle among the electrons and be the victor in this second competition."[78]

Supermassive black holes with the mass of many millions of stars are thought to lie at the center of most large galaxies. The evidence comes from optical and radio observations which show a sharp rise in the velocities of stars or gas clouds orbiting the centers of galaxies. High orbital velocities mean that something massive is creating a powerful gravitational field which is accelerating the stars. X-ray observations indicate that a large amount of energy is produced in the centers of many galaxies, presumably by the in-fall of matter into a black hole.[79]

---

* Since its launch on July 23, 1999, the Chandra X-ray Observatory has been NASA's flagship mission for X-ray astronomy, taking its place in the fleet of "Great Observatories." NASA's premier X-ray observatory was named the Chandra X-ray Observatory in honor of the late Indian-American Nobel laureate, Subrahmanyan Chandrasekhar. Known to the world as Chandra, which means "moon" or "luminous" in Sanskrit, born October 19, 1910 in Lahore, died August 21, 1995, in Chicago, was widely regarded as one of the foremost astrophysicists of the twentieth century. Chandra was an Indian born American astrophysicist, a Nobel laureate in physics along with William Alfred Fowler for their work in the theoretical structure and evolution of stars, and nephew of Indian Nobel Laureate Sir C. V. Raman. Chandrasekhar served on the University of Chicago faculty from 1937 until his death. He became a naturalized citizen of the United States in 1953. Abridged biography courtesy of Wikipedia, available online at: http://en.wikipedia.org/wiki/Subrahmanyan_Chandrasekhar. Retrieved on 2/22/09.

How could a supermassive black hole form in the center of a galaxy? One idea is that an individual star-like black hole forms and swallows up enormous amounts of matter over the course of millions of years to produce a supermassive black hole. Another possibility is that a cluster of starlike black holes forms and eventually merges into a single, supermassive black hole. Or, a single large gas cloud could collapse to form a supermassive black hole.[80]

Recent research, including results from Chandra suggests that galaxies and their black holes do not grow steadily, but in fits and starts. In the beginning of a growth cycle, the galaxy and its central black hole are accumulating matter. The energy generated by the jets that accompany the growth of the supermassive black hole eventually brings the infall of matter and the growth of the galaxy to a halt. The activity around the central black hole then ceases because of the lack of a steady supply of matter, and the jets disappear. Millions of years later the hot gas around the galaxy cools and resumes falling into the galaxy, initiating a new season of growth.[81]

Admittedly, this is a cursory introduction to the subject. If you are interested as much as I am in learning where, why, and how we are, let alone what else is out there, you would be best served by reviewing much more information.

A quick search on the Library of Congress returned 390 books written on black holes, and, surprisingly, only 9 on supermassive black holes. In addition to Kitty Ferguson's book cited above, see *Gravity's Fatal Attraction: Black Holes in the Universe*, by Mitchell Begelman and Martin Rees (New York: Scientific American Library, 1996). For a particularly good history underlying Chandrasekhar's anticipation of the existence of black holes, and the clash of personalities at the time of his discoveries, see *Empire of the Stars: Obsession, Friendship, and Betrayal in the Quest for Black Holes*, by Arthur I. Miller (New York: Houghton Mifflin Company, 2005).

See also *The Black Hole at the Center of our Galaxy,* by Fulvio Melia (New Jersey: Princeton University Press, 2003). In addition, you could read any book by Stephen Hawking[82] to gather a better understanding of our existence and that of black holes. These works include: *A Brief History of Time* (Tenth Anniversary Edition, New York: Bantam Books, 1996), *Black Holes and Baby Universes and Other Essays* (New York: Bantam Books, 1994) and *The Theory of Everything: The Origin and Fate of the Universe* (Beverly Hills, CA: New Millennium Press, 2002).

Two books worth mentioning that are not focused on black holes, but, nevertheless, are worth your reading time because they answer so many questions, and even propose others, are *The Origins of the Future: Ten Questions for the Next Ten Years,* by John Gribbin (New Haven, CT: Yale University Press, 2006), and *Just Six Numbers: The Deep Forces that Shape the Universe,* by Martin Rees (New York: Basic books, 2000). Both are written accessibly for the lay reader like me, and both do a good job of putting things — the universe — into perspective. That we exist at all is the result of some very fine tuning, and that the search for answers inevitably leads to more questions, *ad infinitum.*

And, of course, I cannot leave the subject of black holes and supermassive black holes without mentioning the 19,100,000 and 1,360,000 individual results, respectively, when performing a search on GOOGLE.

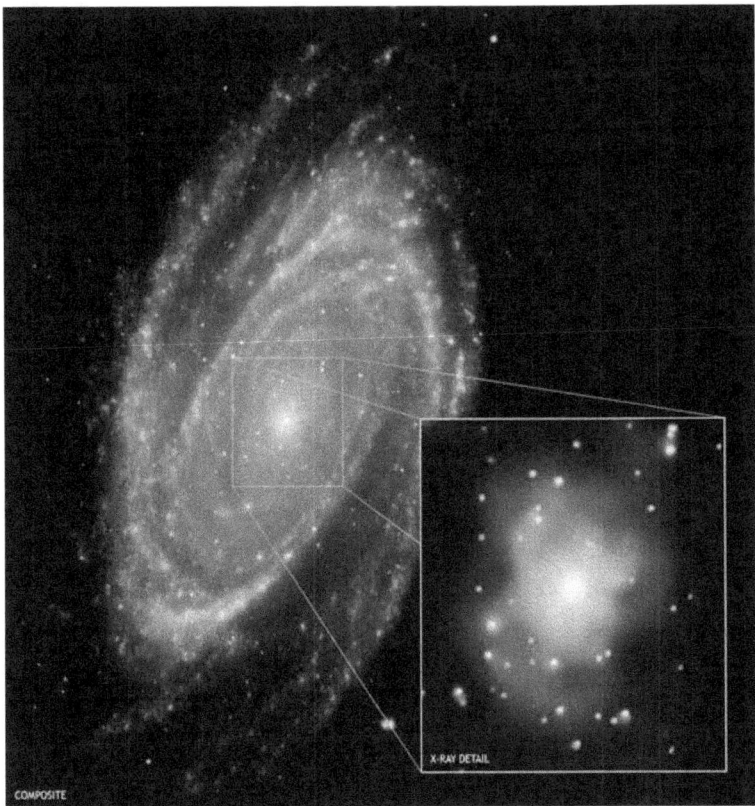

This composite NASA image of the spiral galaxy M81, located about 12 million light years away, includes X-ray data from the Chandra X-ray Observatory, optical data from the Hubble Space Telescope, infrared data from the Spitzer Space Telescope and ultraviolet data from GALEX. The inset shows a close-up of the Chandra image. At the center of M81 is a supermassive black hole that is about 70 million times more massive than the Sun. A new study using data from Chandra and ground-based telescopes, combined with detailed theoretical models, shows that the supermassive black hole in M81 feeds just like stellar mass black holes, with masses of only about ten times that of the Sun. This discovery supports the implication of Einstein's relativity theory that black holes of all sizes have similar properties, and will be useful for predicting the properties of a conjectured new class of black holes.

The supermassive black hole in M81 generates energy and radiation as it pulls gas in the central region of the galaxy inwards at high speed. Therefore, the model that Markoff and her colleagues used to study the black holes includes a faint disk of material spinning around the black hole. This structure would mainly produce X-rays and optical light. A region of hot gas around the black hole would be seen largely in ultraviolet and X-ray light. A large contribution to both the radio and X-ray light comes from jets generated by the black hole. Multiwavelength data is needed to disentangle overlapping sources of light.

Image Credit: X-ray: NASA/CXC/Wisconsin/D.Pooley and CfA/A.Zezas; Optical: NASA/ESA/CfA/A.Zezas; UV: NASA/JPL-Caltech/CfA/J.Huchra et al.; IR: NASA/JPL-Caltech/CfA

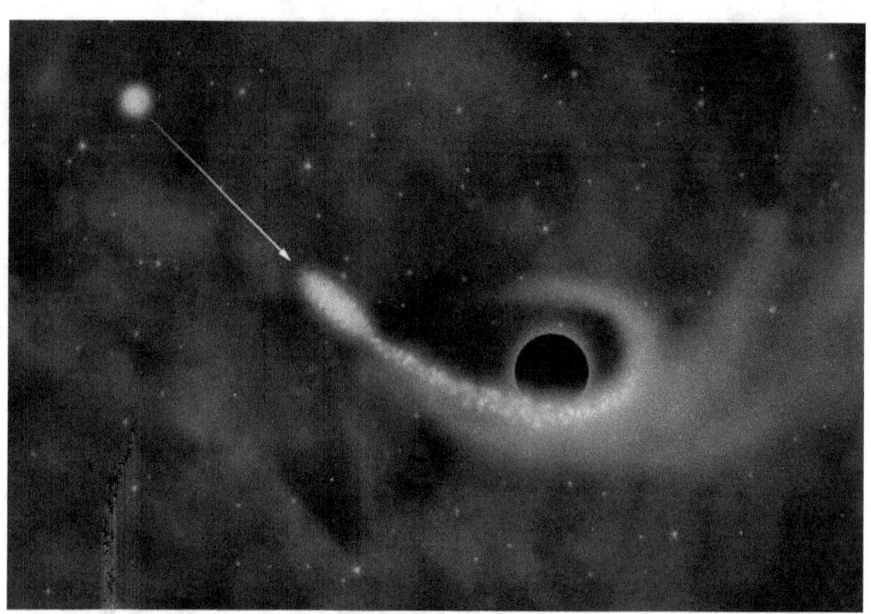

The illustration above depicts a supermassive black hole ripping apart a star and consuming a portion of it, a long-predicted astronomical event confirmed by NASA's Chandra and the European Space Agency's XMM-Newton X-ray Observatories.

Astronomers believe a doomed star came too close to a giant black hole after being thrown off course by a close encounter with another star. As it neared the enormous gravity of the black hole, the star was stretched by tidal forces until it was torn apart. This discovery provides crucial information about how these black holes grow and affect surrounding stars and gas.

Illustration: NASA/CXC/M.Weiss

Having read my brief overview, and perhaps endeavored to read a few of the aforementioned cited books, you are now as much of an expert on black holes as I, and we are ready to develop a couple of metaphors, then apply our learning to find an optimal solution to our diabetes conundrum.

There are stellar black holes and supermassive black holes.

Stellar black holes in the realm of diabetes include the use of fiber and carbohydrates in the diet. Carbohydrates have typically been restricted in diabetes diets throughout the century, and only recently has it been such a controversial topic. For example, in "General Treatment of Diabetes," (1970), written by D. A. Pyke, M.D., F.R.C.P., the author states:

> "The only important recent advance in the dietary treatment of diabetes is that it has now been widely agreed that diets should be reckoned in 10 g. carbohydrate portions and that, except in the obese, fat and protein need not be restricted. Control of diabetes, even in the obese, is often achieved by carbohydrate restriction alone, before there is any weight reduction. Though it may be a useful encouragement to a fat patient to lose weight that this will control his diabetes, this is in fact seldom essential; the important measure is carbohydrate restriction."[83]

The above article is in sharp contrast to numerous biased articles written in the decades previous, and after, such as "Low-Fat Diet and Therapeutic Doses of Insulin in Diabetes Mellitus," (1955), where the author, Inder Singh states assuredly that:

> "There is no indication that healthy people taking a diet rich in carbohydrates are especially liable to diabetes; in fact numerous observations show improvement of carbohydrate tolerance following its greater intake."[84]

That conclusion was based on a study of 80 "insulin-sensitive" diabetics, but if you were to see the actual BG levels of those studied, you would be aghast at how high they were. Of the 80 people studied, 25 started with relatively normal BG levels, but the majority of them had starting BG levels over 125, with some in the 200, 300, and 400 mg/dL range, and one even starting at 600. By the end of the glucose tolerance test, that individual was at 1,000.[85]

Clearly, the standards back in 1955 weren't quite so high. Let us turn to 1976, however, when the high-carbohydrate diet was gaining some momentum. In "Beneficial Effects of a High Carbohydrate, High Fiber Diet on Hyperglycemic Diabetic Men," (1976), the authors, Tae G. Kiehm, M.D., James W. Anderson, M.D., and Kyleen Ward, R.D., state the following:

> "A "diabetic" diet is an essential feature in the treatment of diabetes and traditionally this diet has been restricted in carbohydrate.[86] Although recently it has been recommended that the carbohydrate content of the diabetic diet be increased,[87] no data are available that provide compelling evidence for increasing the carbohydrate content of the diabetic diet. However, several studies[88] suggest that a high-carbohydrate may be beneficial in treating some patients. Because diets containing 75 to 85% of calories as carbohydrate have been associated with improved glucose metabolism of normal individuals and patients with mild diabetes, we have studied the therapeutic utility of a 75% carbohydrate diet in treating diabetic patients requiring either insulin or oral hypoglycemic agents."[89]

Here is a summary of that study:

> "High carbohydrate diets rich in dietary fiber were fed to 13 hyperglycemic diabetic men; five men required 15 to 28 units of insulin per day, five men required sulfonylureas, and three men required 50 to 55 units of insulin. All 13 men were fed weight maintaining American Diabetic Association diets containing 43% of calories as carbohydrates for 1 week and then were fed 75% carbohydrate diets with 15 g. of crude dietary fiber for approximately 2 weeks. After 2 weeks on the 75% carbohydrate diet, sulfonylureas were discontinued in all five men, insulin was discontinued in four men and decreased from 28 to 15 units in 1 man from the group requiring less than 30 units per day. Fasting plasma glucose values were significantly lower (P<0.001)[*] in all 10 men. However, insulin requirements and

---

[*] In statistical hypothesis testing, the p-value is the probability of obtaining a result at least as extreme as the one that was actually observed, assuming chance alone. In this case, P<0.001 means that the odds of the results happening by chance alone are 0.1%.

fasting plasma glucose values were not changed in the three men requiring 40 to 55 units of insulin. Fasting serum cholesterol values were significantly (P<0.001) lower and mean fasting serum triglyceride values were 15% lower on the high carbohydrate diet than on the American Diabetic Association diet in these 13 men. Thus a high carbohydrate diet with generous amounts of fiber may be the treatment of choice of diabetic patients requiring sulfonylureas or less than 30 units of insulin per day." [90]

In "High-Carbohydrate Diets and Insulin-Dependent Diabetics," (1979), by R W Simpson, J I Mann, J Eaton, R D Carter, and T D Hockaday, the authors concluded: "Thus several measures of carbohydrate and lipid metabolism appear to be more satisfactory when patients receive a HC [High-Carbohydrate] diet, which is an acceptable alternative to that still recommended to most insulin-requiring patients." [91]

In "A high Carbohydrate Leguminous Fibre Diet Improves All Aspects of Diabetic Control," (1981), by Simpson HC, Simpson RW, Lousley S, Carter RD, Geekie M, Hockaday TD, and Mann JI, the authors concluded that "a diet high in complex carbohydrate and leguminous fibre improves all aspects of diabetic control, and continued use of a low carbohydrate diet no longer appears justified." [92]

In "Digestible Carbohydrate—an Independent Effect on Diabetic Control in Type 2 (Non-Insulin-Dependent) Diabetic Patients?" (1982), by H. C. R. Simpson, R. D. Carter, S. Lousley, and J. I. Mann, the authors stated that "Many studies have shown high carbohydrate, high fibre diets to benefit diabetic control, the improvement being attributed mainly to an effect of fibre," without footnote identifying any of those studies. And they concluded "These results indicate that a diet rich in carbohydrate, but restricted in fibre, does not cause overall deterioration of diabetic control or lipid metabolism in stable Type 2 diabetic patients, and suggest that digestible carbohydrate has an effect on basal blood glucose independent of fibre." [93]

In "What Carbohydrate Foods Should Diabetics Eat?" (1984), by JI Mann, the author stated:

> "...Epidemiological evidence suggested that the standard diabetic diet, low in carbohydrate and relatively high in fat, might actually increase the risk of cardiovascular disease, the most frequent cause of death among diabetics. Furthermore, several studies suggested that diets relatively high in fibre rich carbohydrate reduced hyperglycemia in diabetic patients. Though there remains some disagreement about the precise quantity of carbohydrate which should be included in the diabetic diet, the diabetic associations of many Western countries, including the United States, Britain, Canada, Australia, and Finland, have affirmed the importance in the management of diabetes and recommend an increase in unrefined carbohydrate (especially fibre rich carbohydrate) with a reduction in the fat intake." [94]

Further in the article, he asks two fundamental questions:

> "Does this mean that wholemeal bread and potato should be eliminated from or at least discouraged in the diabetic diet, or that suitability of foods for the diabetic may in future be determined in the laboratory?
>
> The answer to both questions must be no, at least in the light of present knowledge. Wholemeal bread and potatoes have formed a substantial part of several experimental diets which have over weeks or months shown an appreciable improvement in diabetic control." [95]

He concludes this article with the following statement, subtly insinuating that it's not a diabetic's diet that should drive the insulin use, but, rather, it's the prescribed exogenous insulin use that should drive the diet:

> "Finally, every commentary on dietary advice for diabetics should restate the most important principles: energy intake should be adjusted to maintain the ideal body weight and in the insulin dependent diabetic a regular meal pattern should be established to match the injected insulin. [96]

But are these studies credible? Hardly. Dr. Uffe Ravnskov points out Jim Mann's conflicts of interest in his latest book. He writes:

"All [these] studies were co-authored by Jim Mann, a professor in Human Nutrition and Medicine at the University of Otago, a WHO expert in nutrition and the main advisor for the Sugar Research Advisory Service (SRAS), an information service established in 2002 and funded by the New Zealand Sugar Company with the aim 'to encourage appropriate use and enjoyment of sugar as part of a healthy and balanced diet.' Jim Mann is also the main author of the European guidelines for the treatment and prevention of diabetic patients. But you will look in vain for any information about the author's possible competing interests in that paper or in his other publications." [97]

We find more answers, especially those centered on what it means to be insulin resistant, in Gary Taubes's discussion of geneticist James Neel, the thrifty-gene hypothesis creator that would later reject his own idea. Focused on what constitutes insulin resistance, Gary Taubes wrote that "Neel suggested three scenarios of these insulin-secretory responses that could constitute a pre-disposition to obesity and/or type 2 diabetes—each of which, he wrote, would be a physiological 'response to the excessive glucose pulses that result from the refined carbohydrates/over-alimentation of many civilized diets.'" [98] Of those three scenarios, one stands out as coming closest to reality:

"Here an appropriate amount of insulin is secreted in response to the "excessive glucose pulses" of a modern meal, and the response of the muscle cells to the insulin is also appropriate. The defect is in the relative sensitivity of muscle and fat cells to the insulin. The muscle cells become insulin-resistant in response to the "repeated high levels of insulinemia that result from excessive ingestion of highly refined carbohydrates and/or over-alimentation," but the fat cells fail to compensate. They remain stubbornly sensitive to insulin. So, as Neel explained, the fat tissue accumulates more and more fat, but "mobilization of stored fat would be inhibited." Now the accumulation of fat in the adipose tissue drives the vicious cycle.

This scenario is the most difficult to sort out clinically, because when these investigators measure insulin resistance in humans they invariably do so on a whole body level, which is all the existing technology allows. Any disparities between the responsiveness of fat and muscle tissue to insulin cannot be measured. This is critical, because for the past thirty-five years the American Diabetes Association has recommended that diabetics eat a diet relatively rich in carbohydrates based on the notion that this makes them more sensitive to insulin, at least temporarily, so the diet appears to ameliorate the diabetes. This effect was initially reported in 1971, by the University of Washington endocrinologists Edwin Bierman and John Brunzell, who then waged a lengthy and successful campaign to persuade the American Diabetes Association to recommend that diabetics eat more carbohydrates rather than less. If Neel's third scenario is correct, however, a likely explanation for why carbohydrate-rich diets appear to facilitate blood-sugar control after meals is that they increase the insulin sensitivity of the fat cells specifically, while the muscle tissue remains insulin-resistant." [99]

Here might be the opportune time to tell the tale of James Van Gundia Neel (March 22, 1915 – February 1, 2000) and his refinement. [100]

James Neel, a professor of Human Genetics at the University of Michigan Medical School, proposed the "thrifty genotype" hypothesis in 1962 in his paper "Diabetes Mellitus: A 'Thrifty' Genotype Rendered Detrimental by 'Progress'?" Neel intended the paper to provoke further contemplation and research on the possible evolutionary and genetic causes of diabetes among populations that had only recently come into regular contact with Westerners. [101]

The genetic paradox Neel sought to address was this: diabetes conferred a significant reproductive, and thus evolutionary, disadvantage to anyone who had it; yet the populations Neel studied had diabetes in such high frequencies that a genetic predisposition to develop diabetes seemed plausible. Neel sought to unravel the mystery of why genes that promote diabetes had not been naturally-selected out of the population's gene pool. [102]

Neel proposed that a genetic predisposition to develop diabetes was adaptive to the feast and famine cycles of Paleolithic human existence, allowing humans to fatten rapidly and profoundly during times of feast in order that they might better survive during times of famine. [103]

While Neel considered the "thrifty genotype" notion worth further investigation, he also proposed in 1962, yet did not develop until years later, a counter-hypothesis. namely that "this frequency of obesity and diabetes is a relatively recent phenomenon" in which case the question would become "what changes in the environment are responsible for the increase?"[104]

In the decades following the publications of his first paper on the "thrifty genotype" hypothesis, Neel investigated the frequency of diabetes and, increasingly, obesity in a number of other populations, and, as a proper scientist, sought out observations that might disprove or discount his "thrifty gene" hypothesis.

Neel's further investigations cast doubt on the "thrifty genotype" hypothesis. If a propensity to develop diabetes were an evolutionary adaptation, then diabetes would have been a disease of long standing in those populations currently experiencing a high frequency of diabetes. However, Neel found no evidence of diabetes among these populations earlier in the century.[105] And when he tested younger members of these populations for glucose intolerance—which might have indicated a predisposition for diabetes—he found none.[106]

In 1989, Neel published a review of his further research based on the "thrifty genotype" hypothesis and in the Introduction noted the following: "The data on which that rather soft hypothesis was based has now largely collapsed."[107] However, this sentence clearly could only be applied to his original hypothesis, because later in the same paper where he continued to refine his concepts, Neel noted "...the concept of a "thrifty genotype" remains as viable as when first advanced..." He went on to advance that the thrifty genotype concept be thought of in the context of a "compromised" genotype that effects several other metabolically-related diseases.

This refinement is actually just a return by Neel to the alternative hypothesis to which he had alluded twenty years earlier—that modern, very-high levels of obesity and diabetes among formerly native populations were a relatively recent phenomenon most likely caused by changes in diet. Given that some "thrifty gene" populations, like the Inuit, experienced a rise in obesity and diabetes in conjunction with a *reduction* of the proportion of fat and protein in their diets, Neel surmised that the dietary causes of obesity and diabetes lay in carbohydrate consumption, "specifically the use of highly refined carbohydrate."[108]

The central premise of the thrifty gene hypothesis—that famines were common and severe enough to select for thrifty genes has been recently challenged.[109] Many of the populations that later developed high rates of obesity and diabetes appeared to have no discernible history of famine or starvation (for example, Pacific Islanders whose "tropical-equatorial islands had luxuriant vegetation all year round and were surrounded by lukewarm waters full of fish.").[110] Moreover, one of the most significant problems for the "thrifty gene" idea is that it predicts that modern hunter gatherers should get fat in the periods between famines. Yet data on the body mass index of hunter-gatherer and subsistence agriculturalists clearly show that between famines they do not deposit large fat stores.[111]

We return now to see that Gary Taubes provides the last word on carbohydrates when he states:

> "It is not the case, despite public-health recommendations to the contrary, that carbohydrates are required in a healthy human diet. Most nutritionists still insist that a diet requires 120 to 130 grams of carbohydrates, because this is the amount of glucose that the brain and central nervous system will metabolize when the diet is carbohydrate rich. But what the brain uses and what it requires are two different things. Without carbohydrates in the diet, the brain and central nervous system will run on ketone bodies, converted from dietary fat and from the fatty acids released by the adipose tissue; on glycerol, also released from the fat tissue with the breakdown of triglycerides into free fatty acids; and on glucose, converted from the protein in the diet. Since a carbohydrate-restricted diet, unrestricted in calories, will, by definition, include considerable fat and protein, there will be no shortage of fuel for the brain. Indeed, this is likely to be the fuel mixture that our brains evolved to use, and our brains seem to run more efficiently on this fuel mixture

than they do on glucose alone. (A good discussion of the rationale for a minimal amount of carbohydrates in the diet can be found in the 2002 Institute of Medicine [IOM] report, *Dietary Reference Intakes*. The IOM sets an "estimated average requirement" of a hundred grams of carbohydrates a day for adults, so that the brain can run exclusively on glucose, "without having to rely on a partial replacement of glucose by [ketone bodies]." It then sets the "recommended dietary allowance" at 130 grams to allow margin for error. But the IOM report also acknowledges that the brain will be fine without these carbohydrates, because it runs perfectly well on ketone bodies, glycerol, and the protein-derived glucose.)"[112]

Let's take a look at the IOM report:

"The lower limit of dietary carbohydrate compatible with life apparently is zero, provided that adequate amounts of protein and fat are consumed. However, the amount of dietary carbohydrate that provides for optimal health in humans is unknown. There are traditional populations that ingested a high fat, high protein diet containing only a minimal amount of carbohydrate for extended periods of time (Masai), and in some cases for a lifetime after infancy (Alaska and Greenland Natives, Inuits, and Pampas indigenous people) (Du Bois, 1928; Heinbecker, 1928). There was no apparent effect on health or longevity. Caucasians eating an essentially carbohydrate-free diet, resembling that of Greenland natives, for a year tolerated the diet quite well (Du Bois, 1928). However, a detailed modern comparison with populations ingesting the majority of food energy as carbohydrate has never been done.

It has been shown that rats and chickens grow and mature successfully on a carbohydrate-free diet (Brito et al., 1992; Renner and Elcombe, 1964), but only if adequate protein and glycerol from triacylglycerols are provided in the diet as substrates for gluconeogenesis. It has also been shown that rats grow and thrive on a 70 percent protein, carbohydrate-free diet (Gannon et al., 1985). Azar and Bloom (1963) also reported that nitrogen balance in adults ingesting a carbohydrate-free diet required the ingestion of 100 to 150 g of protein daily. This, plus the glycerol obtained from triacylglycerol in the diet, presumably supplied adequate substrate for gluconeogenesis and thus provided at least a minimal amount of completely oxidizable glucose.

The ability of humans to starve for weeks after endogenous glycogen supplies are essentially exhausted is also indicative of the ability of humans to survive without an exogenous supply of glucose or monosaccharides convertible to glucose in the liver (fructose and galactose). However, adaptation to a fat and protein fuel requires considerable metabolic adjustments.

The only cells that have an absolute requirement for glucose as an oxidizable fuel are those in the central nervous system (i.e., brain) and those cells that depend upon anaerobic glycolysis (i.e., the partial oxidation of glucose to produce lactate and alanine as a source of energy), such as red blood cells, white blood cells, and medulla of the kidney. The central nervous system can adapt to a dietary fat-derived fuel, at least in part (Cahill, 1970; Sokoloff, 1973). Also, the glycolyzing cells can obtain their complete energy needs from the indirect oxidation of fatty acids through the lactate and alanine-glucose cycles.

In the absence of dietary carbohydrate, de novo synthesis of glucose requires amino acids derived from the hydrolysis of endogenous or dietary protein or glycerol derived from fat. Therefore, the marginal amount of carbohydrate required in the diet in an energy-balanced state is conditional and dependent upon the remaining composition of the diet. Nevertheless, there may be subtle and unrecognized, untoward effects of a very low carbohydrate diet that may only be apparent when populations not genetically or traditionally adapted to this diet adopt it. This remains to be determined but is a reasonable expectation.

Of particular concern in a Western, urbanized society is the long-term consequences of a diet sufficiently low in carbohydrate such that it creates a chronically increased production of β-hydroxybutyric and acetoacetic acids (i.e., keto acids). The concern is that such a diet, deficient in water-soluble vitamins and some minerals, may result in bone mineral loss, may cause hypercholesterolemia, may increase the risk of urolithiasis (Vining, 1999), and may affect the development and function of the central nervous system. It also may adversely affect an individual's general sense of well being (Bloom and Azar, 1963), although in men starved for an extended period of time, encephalographic tracings remained unchanged and psychometric testing showed no deficits (Owen et al., 1967). It also may not provide for adequate stores of glycogen. The latter is required for hypoglycemic emergencies and for maximal short-term power production by muscles (Hultman et al., 1999).

EVIDENCE CONSIDERED FOR ESTIMATING THE AVERAGE REQUIREMENT
FOR CARBOHYDRATE

The endogenous glucose production rate, and thus the utilization rate, depends on the duration of starvation. Glucose production has been determined in a number of laboratories using isotopically labeled glucose (Amiel et al., 1991; Arslanian and Kalhan, 1992; Bier et al., 1977; Denne and Kalhan, 1986; Kalhan et al., 1986; King et al., 1982; Patel and Kalhan, 1992). In overnight fasted adults (i.e., postabsorptive state), glucose production is approximately 2 to 2.5 mg/kg/min, or approximately 2.8 to 3.6 g/kg/d. In a 70-kg man, this represents approximately 210 to 270 g/d. In the postabsorptive state, approximately 50 percent of glucose production comes from glycogenolysis in liver and 50 percent from gluconeogenesis in the liver (Chandramouli et al., 1997; Landau et al., 1996).

The minimal amount of carbohydrate required, either from endogenous or exogenous sources, is determined by the brain's requirement for glucose. The brain is the only true carbohydrate-dependent organ in that it oxidizes glucose completely to carbon dioxide and water. Normally, the brain uses glucose almost exclusively for its energy needs. The endogenous glucose production rate in a postabsorptive state correlates very well with the estimated size of the brain from birth to adult life. However, not all of the glucose produced is utilized by the brain (Bier et al., 1977; Felig, 1973). The requirement for glucose has been reported to be approximately 110 to 140 g/d in adults (Cahill et al., 1968).

Nevertheless, even the brain can adapt to a carbohydrate-free, energy-sufficient diet, or to starvation, by utilizing ketoacids for part of its fuel requirements. When glucose production or availability decreases below that required for the complete energy requirements for the brain, there is a rise in ketoacid production in the liver in order to provide the brain with an alternative fuel. This has been referred to as "ketosis." Generally, this occurs in a starving person only after glycogen stores in the liver are reduced to a low concentration and the contribution of hepatic glycogenolysis is greatly reduced or absent (Cahill et al., 1968). It is associated with approximately a 20 to 50 percent decrease in circulating glucose and insulin concentration (Carlson et al., 1994; Owen et al., 1998; Streja et al., 1977). These are signals for adipose cells to increase lipolysis and release nonesterified fatty acids and glycerol into the circulation. The signal also is reinforced by an increase in circulating epinephrine, norepinephrine, glucagon, and growth hormone concentration (Carlson et al., 1994). The nonesterified fatty acids are removed by the liver and converted into ketoacids, which then diffuse out of the liver into the circulation. The increase in nonesterified fatty acids results in a concentration-dependent exponential increase in ketoacids (Hanson et al., 1965); glucagon facilitates this process (Mackrell and Sokal, 1969).

In an overnight fasted person, the circulating ketoacid concentration is very low, but with prolonged starvation the concentration increases dramatically and may exceed the molar concentration of glucose (Cahill, 1970; Streja et al., 1977). In individuals fully adapted to starvation, ketoacid oxidation can account for approximately 80 percent of the brain's energy requirements (Cahill et al., 1973). Thus, only 22 to 28 g/d of glucose are required to fuel the brain. This is similar to the total glucose oxidation rate integrated over 24 hours determined by isotope-

81

dilution studies in these starving individuals (Carlson et al., 1994; Owen et al., 1998).

Overall, the key to the metabolic adaptation to extended starvation is the rise in circulating nonesterified fatty acid concentrations and the large increase in ketoacid production. The glycerol released from the hydrolysis of triacylglycerols stored in fat cells becomes a significant source of substrate for gluconeogenesis, but the conversion of amino acids derived from protein catabolism into glucose is also an important source. Interestingly, in people who consumed a protein-free diet, total nitrogen excretion was reported to be in the range of 2.5 to 3.5 g/d (35 to 50 mg/kg), or the equivalent of 16 to 22 g of catabolized protein in a 70-kg man (Raguso et al., 1999). Thus, it is similar to that in starving individuals (3.7 g/d) (Owen et al., 1998). Overall, this represents the minimal amount of protein oxidized through gluconeogenic pathways (Du Bois, 1928). This amount of protein is considerably less than the Recommended Dietary Allowance (RDA) of 0.8 g/kg/d for adults with a normal body mass index (Chapter 10). For a 70-kg lean male, this equals 56 g/d of protein, which is greater than the estimated obligate daily loss in body protein from the shedding of cells, secretions, and other miscellaneous functions (approximately 6 to 8 g/d for a 70-kg man; see Chapter 10) and has been assumed to be due to inefficient utilization of amino acids for synthesis of replacement proteins and other amino acid-derived products (Gannon and Nuttall, 1999). In part, it also may represent the technical difficulty in determining a minimal daily protein requirement (see Chapter 10).

If 56 g/d of dietary protein is required for protein homeostasis, but the actual daily loss of protein is only approximately 7 g, then presumably the remaining difference (49 g) is metabolized and may be utilized for new glucose production. It has been determined that for ingested animal protein, approximately 0.56 g of glucose can be derived from every 1 g of protein ingested (Janney, 1915). Thus, from the 49 g of protein not directly utilized to replace loss of endogenous protein or not used for other synthetic processes, approximately 27 g (0.56 × 49) of glucose may be produced. In people on a protein-free diet or who are starving, the 16 to 22 g of catabolized protein could provide 10 to 14 g of glucose.

If the starving individual's energy requirement is 1,800 kcal/d and 95 percent is supplied by fat oxidation either directly or indirectly through oxidation of ketoacids (Cahill et al., 1973), then fat oxidation represents 1,710 kcal/d, or 190 g based upon approximately 9 kcal/g fat. The glycerol content of a typical triacylglycerol is 10 percent by weight, or in this case 19 g of glycerol, which is equivalent to approximately 19 g of glucose. This, plus the amount of glucose potentially derived from protein, gives a total of approximately 30 to 34 g ([10 to 14] + 19). Thus, a combination of protein and fat utilization is required to supply the small amount of glucose still required by the brain in a person fully adapted to starvation. Presumably this also would be the obligatory glucose requirement in people adapted to a carbohydrate-free diet. Thus, the normal metabolic adaptation to a lack of dietary protein, as occurs in a starving person in whom the protein metabolized is in excess of that lost daily, is to provide the glucose required by the brain. Nevertheless, utilization of this amount of glucose by the brain is vitally important. Without it, function deteriorates dramatically, at least in the brain of rats (Sokoloff, 1973).

The required amount of glucose could be derived easily from ingested protein alone if the individual was ingesting a carbohydrate-free, but energy-adequate diet containing protein sufficient for nitrogen balance. However, ingested amounts of protein greater than 30 to 34 g/d would likely stimulate insulin secretion unless ingested in small amounts throughout a 24-hour period. For example, ingestion of 25 to 50 g of protein at a single time stimulates insulin secretion (Krezowski et al., 1986; Westphal et al., 1990), despite a lack of carbohydrate intake. This rise in insulin would result in a diminution in the release of fatty acids from adipose cells and as a consequence, reduce ketoacid formation and fatty acid oxidation. The ultimate effect would be to increase the requirement for glucose of the brain and other organs. Thus, the minimal amount of glucose irreversibly oxidized to carbon dioxide and water requires utilization of a finely balanced ratio of dietary fat and protein.

Azar and Bloom (1963) reported that 100 to 150 g/d of protein was necessary for maintenance of nitrogen balance. This amount of protein could typically provide amino acid substrate sufficient for the production of 56 to 84 g of glucose daily. However, daily infusion of 90 g of an amino acid mixture over 6 days to both postoperative and nonsurgical starving adults has been reported to reduce urinary nitrogen loss without a significant change in glucose or insulin concentration, but with a dramatic increase in ketoacids (Hoover et al., 1975). Thus, the issue becomes complex in nonstarving people."[113]

Let me repeat the words of Gary Taubes: "What the brain uses and what it requires are two different things. Without carbohydrates in the diet, the brain and central nervous system will run on ketone bodies, converted from dietary fat and from the fatty acids released by the adipose tissue; on glycerol, also released from the fat tissue with the breakdown of triglycerides into free fatty acids; and on glucose, converted from the protein in the diet. Since a carbohydrate-restricted diet, unrestricted in calories, will, by definition, include considerable fat and protein, there will be no shortage of fuel for the brain."[114]

There is no essential need for carbohydrates. Thus, any individual, group, or organization espousing the need for carbohydrates must be advancing their own agenda, or advancing the agenda of a third party, whether they know it—and benefit from it—or not. We'll delve into that subject a little more later; for now, let's complete the metaphors.

In a similar way, then, though created within a much shorter time span, the treatment—the galaxy—of diabetes has evolved around and upon the singularity of the DCCT, yes, our supermassive black hole.

We see the DCCT cited in nearly *every* reference book that advocates a specific diet available at the Santa Clara City Library. If I ever survey those 3,359 diabetes books at the Library of Congress, and publish my findings, I will be sure to include a section on reference books published after the DCCT concluded, at which time I will be able to say with certainty how many and what percentage cite the DCCT. My best guess from the evidence gathered to date—my hypothesis if you will—is that the number of reference books with specific sections detailing diabetes mellitus, advocating a low-fat diet, that cite the DCCT, approaches 100%.

The oldest reference book, with a section devoted to diabetes mellitus, in the reference section at Santa Clara City Library, which included a citation of the DCCT, was *Family Medicine Principles & Practice, Fifth Edition* (1998). That reference book states:

"One study showed, however, that early poor control despite later good control results in diabetes complications. The Diabetes Control and Complications Trial (DCCT) proved the profound impact of intensive therapy on reducing the risk of microvasular complications. Decades of questions about the glucose hypothesis are therefore finally answered, with the obvious recommendation that most individuals with type 1 diabetes mellitus be treated with intensive therapy."[115]

According to *Rudolph's Pediatrics 21st Edition* (2003):

"The goals of treatment of children with type 1 diabetes mellitus are as follows: 1. Stabilize blood level of glucose within a target range; 2. Avoid metabolic decompensation (diabetic ketoacidosis, severe hypoglycemia); 3. Ensure normal growth and development at both a physical and emotional level; 4. Prevent long-term complication of both hyperglycemia and hypoglycemia. The best means to achieve these goals have been established through several long-term studies involving adolescents and adults, most notably the Diabetes Control and Complications Trial (DCCT). This 9-year prospective multicenter trial compared outcomes among patients who underwent intensive treatment in an attempt to maintain euglycemia with outcomes among those treated in the conventional manner, in which the goal was clinical well-being. Patients in the intensive therapy group received three or more insulin injections per day or used an insulin pump; measured blood glucose several times a day; had monthly clinic visits with the health-care team and weekly follow-up telephone calls; and were encouraged to use a dynamic regimen with adjustments for variation in daily food intake and activities. Those in the conventional treatment group received one to two insulin injections per day, were seen in the clinic every several months, and followed a static daily insulin regimen. The study showed definitively that tighter glucose control reduces the risk of long-term complications of type 1 diabetes mellitus, decreases risk of development of microvascular complications, and slows progression of preexisting lesions 35 to 75%. The DCCT showed that any improvement in glucose control lowers the risk of long-term complications. Every 10% decrease in HbA1c is associated with a 40 to 45% lower risk of progression of retinopathy. Therefore, even if the stated target range is not achieved, any incremental decrease in blood glucose value decreases the risk of future microvascular disease."[116]

In *Cecil Textbook of Medicine 22nd Edition* (2004):

"The benefits achieved by intensive control in the DCCT were not without risk. Weight gain was more common, and most importantly, the frequency of severe hyperglycemia (including episodes in some patients) was three-fold higher in the intensive care group. In many cases, such episodes occurred without classic warning symptoms, often while the patient was asleep. Thus, in some patients, the risks of intensive therapy may outweigh the benefits; possibly included are patients with advanced complications, young children, and patients who are unable or unwilling to participate in their management (e.g., self-monitoring of blood glucose). Such individuals are likely to benefit from less aggressive therapy designed to moderately lower glucose levels without the risk of hypoglycemia. It is noteworthy that despite the higher rate of hypoglycemia, intensive therapy in the DCCT had no detectable long-term effects on cognitive function."[117]

In *Harrison's Principles of Internal Medicine, 17th Edition* (2008):

"The DCCT demonstrated that improvement of glycemic control reduced nonproliferative and proliferative retinopathy (47% reduction), microalbuminuria (39% reduction), clinical nephropathy (54% reduction), and neuropathy (60% reduction). Improved glycemic control also slowed the progression of early diabetic complications."[118]

In *Williams Textbook of Endocrinology, Tenth Edition* (2003):

"On the basis of these results, the authors of the study [the DCCT] recommended that most patients with type 1 diabetes be treated with an intensive treatment regimen under the close supervision of a health-care team consisting of a physician, nurses, nutritionist, and behavioral and exercise specialists as needed."[119]

Additionally, according to the *International Textbook of Diabetes Mellitus* (2004):

"It was not until 1993 that definitive proof for the value of good glycemic control was established. The landmark Diabetes Control and Complications Trial (DCCT) study showed that the microvascular complications of diabetes could be delayed or avoided by good glycemic control, which required intensive insulin therapy."[120]

This idea is again validated in *Joslin's Diabetes Mellitus* (2005):

"Joslin and his early associates became identified with the conservative viewpoint that "good" control delayed or prevented microvascular complications, particularly in type 1 diabetes. This position inaugurated an intense nationwide 30-year debate that only ended in 1993 with the publication of the results of the Diabetes Control and Complications Trial, which clearly supported Joslin's claim."[121]

In the most recent reference book, *Lange 2009 Current Medical Diagnosis & Treatment* (2009), after summarizing the DCCT, the writers conclude:

"The general consensus of the ADA is that intensive insulin therapy associated with comprehensive self-management training should become standard therapy in patients with type 1 diabetes mellitus after the age of puberty. Exceptions include those with advanced renal disease and the elderly, since in those groups the detrimental risks of hypoglycemia outweigh the benefits of tight glycemic control."[122]

The far-reaching influence of the DCCT puts it at the center of the diabetes treatment galaxy. Let's now take a closer look at the study and its design.

The Diabetes Control and Complications Trial was launched by the National Institute of Diabetes, Digestive and Kidney Diseases (NIDDK) in 1981 when requests for proposals were issued for clinical centers and a central Data Coordinating Center. In early 1982 the Biostatistics Center of the George Washington University was awarded the contract to serve as the Coordinating Center. In addition, 29 clinical centers in the United States and Canada, and 8 central laboratories and units participated in the trial. The Coordinating Center contract spanned the period 1982-1998. The complete study group is listed in the Appendix to the principal publication of study results in the *New England Journal of Medicine*.[123]

Since the discovery of insulin in 1921, the medical community debated the glucose hypothesis that the marked elevation of blood glucose, hyperglycemia, associated with diabetes mellitus, was responsible for the development and progression of the microvascular complications of type 1 diabetes: retinopathy leading to blindness, nephropathy leading to end-stage kidney disease, and neuropathy leading to loss of sensation, ulceration and amputation. The DCCT was designed to definitively answer whether a program of intensive therapy aimed at near normal levels of glycemia, when compared to conventional therapy aimed at maintenance of clinical well being, would affect the risk of onset and progression of these complications.[124]

During the period 1983-1989, 1441 subjects were enrolled in the study, half the subjects assigned at random to intensive therapy and half to conventional therapy. All subjects were scheduled to be followed until the fall of 1993. However, the dramatic beneficial results of the trial lead to its termination one year early. The results were presented at the June, 1993, meeting of the American Diabetes Association and the initial principal results paper appeared in the *New England Journal of Medicine* in September of that year.[125] The risks of the microvascular complications over the average of 6.5 years of follow-up were reduced by 26-63% with intensive versus conventional therapy. Intensive therapy, however, was associated with an excess weight gain of about 1 kg per year greater than that with conventional therapy, and a 3-fold greater risk of episodes of hypoglycemia where patients experience seizures and/or loss of consciousness, compared to conventional therapy.[126]

Subsequent extensive statistical epidemiologic investigations showed that the risk of development of microvascular complications was principally determined by the lifetime exposure to hyperglycemia.[127] However, the risk of hypoglycemia was weakly related to the level of glycemia, and more strongly related to intensive versus conventional therapy.[128] All totaled, 57 papers have been published that present the various methods and results of the DCCT. The complete DCCT bibliography has been included in Appendix D.

The Harvard Health Letter named the DCCT the number one advance in medicine during 1993. In 1994, the DCCT Research Group was awarded the Charles H. Best Medal for distinguished service in the cause for diabetes, named for the co-founder of insulin, given by the American Diabetes Association. The DCCT has been used to set standards of care for diabetes mellitus worldwide.[129]

After the close of the DCCT, the NIDDK launched the study of the Epidemiology of Diabetes Interventions and Complications (EDIC), for which the Biostatistics Center also serves as the Data Coordinating Center. Under the EDIC, the original DCCT cohort is being followed to assess the development of significant microvascular disease and the development of cardiovascular and other macrovascular diseases.[130]

A more detailed examination of the DCCT shows that the improvements in the intensive therapy group were found with only a modest reduction in hemoglobin A1c. The mean hemoglobin A1c for the intensive therapy group was 7.1%, corresponding to a mean serum glucose level of 155 mg/dL. The DCCT intensive therapy protocol included a daily carbohydrate intake of 230 grams, self-monitoring of glucose levels at least four times daily, four daily insulin injections, monthly clinical visits, and a diet and exercise plan. Despite the extensive monitoring effort, the intensive therapy cohort had a threefold increase of severe hypoglycemic events compared with the standard therapy cohort. Accordingly, subjects following the intensive therapy had a reduction in long-term complications, but this benefit was tempered by an increased risk of severe hypoglycemic reactions.[131]

In the minds of those that led, supported, financed, and judged the DCCT, not to mention those that decided to include it as the basis for treatment in fixed reference media, the DCCT proved that an intensive treatment of insulin is the best way to treat type 1 diabetes. Case closed.

But isn't there one important question left to consider? I think you can see where this is going.

What was the diet used in both the conventional and intensive treatments?

To answer that question, as we surely must, we have to take a look at a document explaining how the trial was designed. Such a document exists. We can answer the question of what diets were used by reading through "The Diabetes Control and Complications Trial (DCCT) Design and

Methodologic Considerations for the Feasibility Phase," first published in *Diabetes,* in 1986.

Here is the diet fed to those participants of the standard (also known as the conventional) treatment group:

> "A balanced diet containing sufficient calories and other nutrients to maintain weight at 90-120% of ideal and normal growth and development in adolescents. The diet consists of approximately 45-55% of the calories as carbohydrate, no more than 30% as fat, cholesterol content of <600 mg/day, and a P/S ratio of approximately 1.0 [P/S ratio is the ratio between polyunsaturated and saturated fatty acids]. An individual meal plan is provided for each subject that includes daily snacks and emphasizes consistency and regularity of caloric and carbohydrate intake." [132]

And here is the diet fed to those participants of the experimental (also known as the intensive) treatment:

> "A balanced diet as in the standard treatment group." [133]

Stop to think about that for a moment. The same diet of approximately 45-55% of the calories as carbohydrates were fed to both the control group and the intensively treated group. True, keeping diets similar to test the effects of an independent variable—in this case insulin—is an indicator of a closely controlled study; but, the conclusion reached—that is, complications and risk are reduced by intensive insulin treatment—assumes you're eating carbohydrates as a major potion of your diet. This study does not provide us with any new, actionable information, as we've known through observation for more than a *century* that diabetes is the relative inability of the body to effectively oxidize carbohydrates, albeit words such as "oxidize," and "carbohydrate," weren't always used. And that we need to normalize our glucose levels if we want to reduce the risk of complications and shortened lifespan. This study really reminds type 1s that if prescribed bolus insulin, due to their consumption of carbohydrates, they should take enough—follow their prescription—to keep their blood sugar within normal range. And this enlightenment came at the expense of mostly tax-payer dollars, at a price of about $169 million.[134]

Let me add an analogy here for clarification. Remember the old "Off!" TV commercials? "Off!" is a name-brand mosquito repellent, and in the TV commercial, they showed two bare arms, each connected to a live human, of course, being placed consecutively into a long, glass container full of hungry mosquitoes. The first arm, which can be thought of as the experimental arm, is sprayed with a generous amount of "Off!," and the second, which can be thought of as the control arm, has not been sprayed with anything. Not surprisingly, the first arm, the one sprayed with "Off!," suffered fewer, if any, mosquito bites than that of the bare arm. This analogy can be related to diabetes in that the mosquito bites represent the complications, and the "Off!" represents the insulin. Carbohydrates are equivalent to the actual sticking of the arm into the mosquito-filled glass container.

I'm sure you're ahead of my discussion here; clearly it would be ideal to simply not be sticking your arm into a container full of hungry mosquitoes. This solution seems even more obvious than extricating a truck from an overpass by deflating its tires. Yes, "Off!" would come in handy if you're hiking in the woods; an activity to be enjoyed while on vacation or a pretty weekend day, but it's not something done often. Similarly, doesn't it make sense to, at a minimum, reduce your intake of carbohydrates?

So, this study's result is simply a monumental example of inherent bias.[135] The study itself was done well, the statistics are correct, there was no bias during the literature review of the study question, during selection of the study sample, during measurement of exposure or outcome, during analysis of the data, during the interpretation of the analysis, or even during the publication of the analysis. There was no selection bias, information bias, or confounding bias.

Further, there was no bandwagon effect, base rate fallacy, bias blind spot, choice-supportive bias, confirmation bias, congruence bias, conservatism bias, contrast effect, distinction bias, endowment effect, expectation bias, extreme aversion, focusing effect, framing, hyperbolic discounting, illusion of control, impact bias, irrational escalation, loss aversion, mere exposure effect, moral credential effect, need for closure, neglect of probability, omission bias, outcome bias, planning fallacy, post-purchase rationalization, pseudocertainty effect, reactance, selective perception, Von Restorff effect, wishful thinking, or zero-risk bias. There were no biases in probability and belief, social biases or memory errors.[136]

No, what we have here is just good, old fashioned, simple bias. The study was set up to not include a group that didn't raise their blood sugar to begin with by not eating carbohydrates.*

The bias to not add a group of test subjects that simply didn't eat carbohydrates could be thought of as a strain of "not invented here," a sociological phenomenon manifested as an unwillingness to adopt an idea because it originates from another culture, i.e., the practice of natural medicine. Sociologically, it could also stem from a status-quo bias, the tendency for people to like things to stay relatively the same.

Again, it only makes sense to, at a minimum, reduce your intake of carbohydrates. And a growing number of physicians would agree, including Daniel F. O'Neill, Eric C. Westman, M.D., M.H.S., and Richard K. Bernstein, M.D. In "The Effects of a Low-Carbohydrate Regimen on Glycemic Control and Serum Lipids in Diabetes Mellitus," (2003), the above authors state:

---

* In addition to refraining from carbohydrate consumption, type 1s should inject an optimal amount of basal insulin, also known as long-acting insulin, once or twice in a 24 hour period, to keep blood sugar stable throughout the day and offset the inevitable rise in BG caused by the dawn phenomenon.

"These DCCT findings suggest that normal glycemic control (hemoglobin A1c of 4.0-6.0%) is not possible even with intensive treatment, unless there is some other way to improve glycemic control without increasing the risk of hypoglycemia. Recent preliminary studies have suggested that reduction of daily carbohydrate intake leads to improved glycemic control. One study over a 19-month period found that diabetics who increased their daily carbohydrate consumption from 38% (206.3 g/day) carbohydrate to 45.4% (241.4 g/day) carbohydrate had an increase in mean hemoglobin A1c from 9.4% to 11.2%.[137] Another study with a cross-over design involving 28 type II diabetics found an increase in hemoglobin A1c from 7.8% to 9.2% after increasing dietary carbohydrate from 25% to 55% of the daily intake.[138] A third clinical series including type II diabetics who reduced their daily carbohydrate consumption to 100 g/day obtained a mean hemoglobin A1c of 6.9%.[139] Therefore a growing number of studies suggest that carbohydrate restriction can lead to better glycemic control."[140]

Interestingly, the authors of the above study also noted that prior to the discovery of insulin, Elliot P. Joslin recommended a low-carbohydrate diet as a treatment for diabetes mellitus.[141]

In "Dietary Carbohydrate Restriction in Type 2 Diabetes Mellitus and Metabolic Syndrome: Time for a Critical Appraisal," (2008), written by a host of renowned doctors, researchers and diabetologists including Anthony Accurso, Richard K. Bernstein, Annika Dahlqvist, Boris Draznin, Richard D. Feinman, Eugene J. Fine, Amy Gleed, David B. Jacobs, Gabriel Larson, Robert H. Lustig, Anssi H. Manninen, Samy I. McFarlane, Katharine Morrison, Jørgen Vesti Nielsen, Uffe Ravnskov, Karl S. Roth, Ricardo Silvestre, James R. Sowers, Ralf Sundberg, Jeff S. Volek, Eric C. Westman, Richard J. Wood, Jay Wortman, and Mary C. Vernon, the authors state:

"Current nutritional approaches to metabolic syndrome and type 2 diabetes generally rely on reductions in dietary fat. The success of such approaches has been limited and therapy more generally relies on pharmacology. The argument is made that a re-evaluation of the role of carbohydrate restriction, the historical and intuitive approach to the problem, may provide an alternative and possibly superior dietary strategy. The rationale is that carbohydrate restriction improves glycemic control and reduces insulin fluctuations which are primary targets.

93

Experiments are summarized showing that carbohydrate-restricted diets are at least as effective for weight loss as low-fat diets and that substitution of fat for carbohydrate is generally beneficial for risk of cardiovascular disease. These beneficial effects of carbohydrate restriction do not require weight loss. Finally, the point is reiterated that carbohydrate restriction improves all of the features of metabolic syndrome." [142]

In the same article, the authors amplify their position:

"The epidemic of diabetes continues unabated, and impassioned calls for better treatment and prevention strategies are common features of scientific conferences. While it is generally acknowledged that total dietary carbohydrate is the major factor in glycemic control, strategies based on reduction of dietary carbohydrate have received little support. The American Diabetes Association, for example, has traditionally recommend against low carbohydrate diets (less than 130 g/day); while the most recent guidelines admit such diets as an alternative approach to weight loss, they continue to emphasize concerns and downplay benefits. Similarly, the Diabetes and Nutrition Study Group of the European Association for the Study of Diabetes reported "no justification for the recommendation of very low carbohydrate diets in persons with diabetes." We feel, however, that there is ample evidence to warrant an alternative perspective and that diets based on carbohydrate restriction should be re-evaluated in light of current understanding of the underlying biochemistry and available clinical data." [143]

If you're scratching your head at this point, you're not alone. At some point in nearly every type 1 diabetic's life, this thought—"Hmmm, I'm eating carbohydrates and taking bolus insulin, what would happen if I didn't eat carbohydrates? Could I stop taking insulin?"—permeates the brain. It did for me early in my treatment. So, why not just stop eating carbohydrates, and, more importantly, why is it that the DCCT is so influential, resulting in treatments throughout the globe based upon carbohydrates and insulin?

To answer these two important questions, we might start by trying to figure out who is most negatively affected by restricting carbohydrates in a diabetic's diet. Not the diabetic, ironically. No, if we stop eating carbohydrates, and thus reduce our intake of exogenous insulin, it is the pharmaceutical companies that will sell less insulin, diminishing demand for all the complimentary insulin goods such as insulin delivery devices (syringes, pumps & pens), lancets, test strips, blood sugar meters, batteries, test kit carrying cases, glucose tabs, ketone test strips, alcohol wipes, et al. And, of course, we'll visit our health-care providers less often. The myriad carbohydrate manufacturers and marketers will find reduced demand for their products too, though, they can manufacture and market something else in a capital driven economy.

Too, if we stop eating carbohydrates, reducing our intake of exogenous insulin, we may even live a little longer.

So why does the DCCT continue to influence health-care providers on a near-global basis?

One explanation is termed "déformation professionnelle," a French phrase, meaning a tendency to look at things from the point of view of one's own profession, forgetting the broader perspective. It is a pun on the expression "formation professionnelle," meaning "professional training." The implication is that all, or most, professional training results to some extent in a distortion of the way the professional views the world.

A better explanation is what Richard Dawkins terms a "meme."[144] "Dawkins himself used the analogy to illustrate how natural selection pertains to anything that can replicate, not just DNA," as Steven Pinker describes in *How the Mind Works*.[145] According to Dawkins:

> "I think that a new kind of replicator has recently emerged on this very planet. It is staring us in the face. It is still in its infancy, still drifting clumsily about in its primeval soup, but already it is achieving evolutionary change at a rate that leaves the old gene panting far behind.
>
> The new soup is the soup of human culture. We need a name for the new replicator, a noun that conveys the idea of a unit of cultural transmission, or a unit of *imitation*. 'Mimeme' comes from a suitable Greek root, but I want a monosyllable that sounds a bit like 'gene'. I hope my classicist friends will forgive

me if I abbreviate mimeme to *meme*. If it is any consolation, it could alternatively be thought of as being related to 'memory', or to the French word *même*. It should be pronounced to rhyme with 'cream'.

Examples of memes are tunes, ideas, catch-phrases, clothes fashions, ways of making pots or of building arches. Just as genes propagate themselves in the gene pool by leaping from body to body via sperm or eggs, so memes propagate themselves in the meme pool by leaping from brain to brain via a process which, in the broad sense, can be called imitation. If a scientist hears, or reads about, a good idea, he passes it on to his colleagues and students. He mentions it in his articles and his lectures. If the idea catches on, it can be said to propagate itself, spreading from brain to brain. As my colleague N. K. Humphrey neatly summed up an earlier draft of this chapter: '...memes should be regarded as living structures, not just metaphorically but technically. When you plant a fertile meme in my mind you literally parasitize my brain, turning it into a vehicle for the meme's propagation in just the way that a virus may parasitize the genetic mechanism of a host cell. And this isn't just a way of talking—the meme for, say, "belief in life after death" is actually realized physically, millions of times over, as a structure in the nervous systems of individual men the world over.'" [146]

Commenting on Dawkins and memes, Steven Pinker said:

"Richard Dawkins has drawn the clearest analogy between the selection of genes and the selection of bits of culture, which he dubbed memes. Memes such as tunes, ideas, and stories spread from brain to brain and sometimes mutate in the transmission. New features of a meme that make its recipients more likely to retain and disseminate it, such as being catchy, seductive, funny, or irrefutable, will lead to the meme's becoming more common in the meme pool. In subsequent rounds of retelling, the most spreadworthy memes will spread the most and will eventually take over the population. Ideas will therefore evolve to become better adapted to spreading themselves. Note that we are talking about *ideas* evolving to become more spreadable, not *people* evolving to become more knowledgeable." [147]

So we see carbohydrates, fiber, the DCCT, black holes, supermassive black holes, wearing a baseball cap backward, *et al.*, *ad infinitum*, all in a new light. These are all memes, all replicators, each fighting for their own permanence, through replication, in an otherwise impermanent universe. Viruses, bacterium, animals, plants, fungi, names, forms, ideas, melodies, processes, fashion, games, methods, madness: memes all.

Now, whether some of them are good, bad, or indifferent, who knows, depending, of course, on who or what is the protagonist. Well, pardon my speciesism, and kingdomism for that matter, but I do believe we are not here to serve the interests of carbohydrates, or those whose interests include carbohydrates. While we are not the center of the universe, it is in our own best interest to, well, work in our own best interest.

How we deal with some of these competing memes may pose a bit of a dilemma, something we will solve by book's end. For now, though, having learned how we came to be where we are, let's develop and implement our optimal solution.

THE WAY THINGS OUGHT TO BE
(PART I)

"Change in diet is important in a changing species over time as long as fifty million years. The earliest creatures in the sequence leading to man were nimble-eyed and delicate-fingered insect and fruit eaters like the lemurs. Early apes and hominids, from *Aegyptopithecus* and *Proconsul* to the heavy *Australiopithecus*, are thought to have spent their days rummaging mainly for vegetarian foods. But the light *Australopithecus* broke the ancient primate habit of vegetarianism.

The change from a vegetarian to an omnivorous diet, once made, persisted in *Homo erectus*, Neanderthal man and *Homo sapiens*. From the ancestral light *Australopithecus* onwards, the family of man ate some meat: small animals at first, larger ones later. Meat is a more concentrated protein than plant, and eating meat cuts down the bulk and the time spent in eating by two-thirds. The consequences for the evolution of man were far-reaching. He had more time free, and could spend it in more indirect ways, to get food from sources (such as large animals) which could not be tackled by hungry brute force. Evidently that helped to promote (by natural selection) the tendency of all primates to interpose an internal delay in the brain between stimulus and response, until it developed into the full human ability to postpone the gratification of desire.

But the most marked effect of an indirect strategy to enhance the food supply is, of course, to foster social action and communication. A slow creature like a man can stalk, pursue and corner a large savannah animal that is adapted for flight only by cooperation. Hunting requires conscious planning and organisation by means of language, as well as special weapons. Indeed, language as we use it has something of the character of a hunting plan, in that (unlike the animals) we instruct one another in sentences which are put together from movable units. The hunt is a communal undertaking of which the climax, but only the climax, is the kill.

Hunting cannot support a growing population in one place…The choice for the hunters was brutal: starve or move." [148]

"The largest single step in the ascent of man is the change from nomad to village agriculture. What made that possible? An act of will by men, surely; but with that, a strange and secret act of nature. In the burst of new vegetation at the end of the

Ice Age, a hybrid wheat appeared in the Middle East. It happened in many places: a typical one is the ancient oasis of Jericho.

Jericho is older than agriculture. The first people who came here and settled by the spring in this otherwise desolate ground were people who harvested wheat, but did not yet know how to plant it. We know this because they made tools for the wild harvest, and that is an extraordinary piece of foresight; John Garstang found them when he was digging here in the 1930s. The ancient sickle edge would have been set in a piece of gazelle horn, or bone.

There no longer survives, up on the hill or tel[149] and its slopes, the kind of wild wheat that the earliest inhabitants harvested. But the grasses that are still here must look very like the wheat that they found, that they gathered for the first time by the fistful, and cut with that sawing motion of the sickle that reapers have used for all the ten thousand years since then. That was the Natufian pre-agricultural civilization. And, of course, it could not last. It was on the brink of becoming agriculture. And that was the next thing that happened on the Jericho tel.

The turning point to the spread of agriculture in the Old World was almost certainly the occurrence of two forms of wheat with a large, full head of seeds. Before 8000 BC wheat was not the luxuriant plant it is today; it was merely one of many wild grasses that spread throughout the Middle East. By some genetic accident, the wild wheat crossed with a natural goat grass and formed a fertile hybrid. That accident must have happened many times in the springing vegetation that came up after the last Ice Age. In terms of the genetic machinery that directs growth, it combined with fourteen chromosomes of wild wheat with the fourteen chromosomes of goat grass, and produced Emmer with twenty-eight chromosomes. That is what makes Emmer so much plumper. The hybrid was able to spread naturally, because its seeds are attached to the husk in such a way that they scatter in the wind.

For such a hybrid to be fertile is rare but not unique among plants. But now the story of the rich plant life that followed the Ice Ages becomes more surprising. There was a second genetic accident, which may have come about because Emmer was already cultivated. Emmer crossed with another natural goat grass and produced a still larger hybrid with forty-two chromosomes, which is bread wheat. That was improbable enough in itself, and we know now that bread wheat would not have been fertile but for a specific genetic mutation on one chromosome.

Yet there is something even stranger. Now we have a beautiful ear of wheat, but one which will never spread in the wind because the ear is too tight to break up. And if I do break it up, why, then the chaff flies off and every grain falls exactly where it grew. Let me remind you, that is quite different from the wild wheats or from the first, primitive hybrid, Emmer. In those primitive forms the ear is much more open, and if the ear breaks up then you get quite a different effect—you get grains which will fly in the wind. The bread wheats have lost that ability. Suddenly, man and the plant have come together. Man has a wheat that he lives by, but the wheat also thinks that man was made for him because only so can it be propagated. For the bread wheats can only multiply with help; man must harvest the ears and scatter their seeds; and the life of each, man and the plant, depend on the other. It is a true fairy tale of genetics, as if the coming of civilization had been blessed in advance by the spirit of the abbot Gregor Mendel.

A happy conjunction of natural and human events created agriculture. In the Old World that happened about ten thousand years ago, and it happened in the Fertile Crescent of the Middle East. But it surely happened more than once. Almost certainly agriculture was invented again and independently in the New World—or so we believe on the evidence we now have that maize needed man like wheat. As for the Middle East, agriculture was spread here and there over its hilly slopes, of which the climb from the Dead Sea to Judea, the hinterland of Jericho, is at best a characteristic piece and no more. In a literal sense, agriculture is likely to have had several beginnings in the Fertile Crescent, some of them before Jericho."[150]

"Jericho is a microcosm of history. There will be other sites found in coming years (there are some important new ones already) which will change our picture of the beginnings of civilization. Yet the power of standing in this place, the vision backward along the ascent of modern man, is profound in thought and in emotion equally. When I was a young man, we all thought that mastery came from man's domination of his physical environment. Now we have learned that real mastery comes from understanding and molding the living environment. That is how man began in the Fertile Crescent when he put his hand on plant and animal and, in learning to live with them, changed the world to his needs."[151]

And so, from the humble beginnings of agriculture 10,000 years ago, elegantly described above by Jacob Bronowski[152] from *The Ascent of Man*, the unintended consequence of our social, technological and dietary progress exacerbates, and in many cases, causes, the evolving complex of metabolic derangements commonly referred to as the diabetes condition. But it doesn't have to be.

One day you receive news that you are diabetic—a member of the club—and your life is changed forever. You now have to manually adjust your blood sugar and test, test, test. All the social queues you receive in one form or another reinforce the need to consume complex carbohydrates with complimentary doses of insulin. If you do everything right, says the dogma, if you eat a low-fat, high-complex-carbohydrate diet, religiously measure and take your insulin, lose weight and exercise, you can win the battle against all of nature's blood-sugar-increasing opponents: the redundant and powerful insulin antagonists, life's stressors, low temperatures, high pressures, and inadequate sleep. All while competing in school prior to joining the workforce, then again while competing in the hyper-competitive global marketplace. Not to mention fulfilling the role of a son, daughter, father, mother, or grandparent. Plus all of life's other activities.

While I can see, understand, and appreciate the arguments in favor of eating carbohydrates and metabolizing them with the aid of matching doses of exogenous bolus insulin—carbohydrates taste good, may make one temporarily feel good, and the availability of synthetic insulin enables flexibility to eat a wider variety of food—I respectfully disagree. Not out of opinion or bias or because I have a new diabetes drug on the market to sell; rather, and lucidly, based upon a preponderance of the evidence.

In my first book, *Thrive With Diabetes, Lead an optimistic, Fun, Challenging, Fit, Tenacious, Enlightened, Innovative & Heroic Life,* I presented a current summary of diabetes, its definition, history, diagnosis, prognosis, and management. All the research and articles used to create it were from the current, relevant, and most credible institutions such as the American Diabetes Association, the World Health Organization, and many others. It represented a general consensus. While subtle, the important take-away from the first part was its compression:

The Way Things Ought To Be (Part I)

"Diabetes is the relative inability of the body to naturally and effectively oxidize carbohydrates, causing serious short- and long-term complications. There is no cure; its treatment includes diet, lifestyle changes, and medication."[153]

Let's revisit the book's discussion on compression, written by Dr. John Barrow:

"Scientists employ observations to gather information about the world and to test predictions about how things will react to new circumstances. This is nothing more than the transformation of lists of observational data into abbreviated form by the recognition of patterns. The recognition of such a pattern allows the information content of the observed sequence of events to be replaced by a shorthand formula which possesses the same, or almost the same, information content. In general, the shorter the possible representation of a string of numbers, the less random it is. If there is no abbreviated representation at all, then the string is random. Any string of symbols that can be given an abbreviated representation is called compressible.

In practice, the intelligibility of the world amounts to the fact that we find it to be algorithmically compressible. We can replace sequences of facts and observational data by abbreviated statements which contain the same informational content. These abbreviations we often call "laws of nature." If the world were not algorithmically compressible, then there would exist no simple laws of nature.

We know that the world is not totally algorithmically compressible. There exist particular chaotic processes that are not algorithmically compressible, just as there exist mathematical operations that are non-computable. And it is this glimpse of randomness that gives us some inkling of what a totally incompressible world would look like. Its scientists would be librarians rather than mathematicians, cataloguing fact after unrelated fact.

We see science as the search for algorithmic compressions of the world of experience and the search for a single all-encompassing Theory of Everything as the ultimate expression of some scientists' deeply held faith that the essential structure of the Universe as a whole can be algorithmically compressed. But we recognize that the human mind plays a non-trivial in this evaluation. Inextricably linked to the apparent algorithmic compressibility of the world is the ability of the human mind to carry out compressions. Our minds have evolved out of the elements of the physical world and have been honed, at least partially, towards their present state by the perpetual process of natural selection. Their effectiveness as sensors of the environment, and their survival value, are obviously related to their abilities as algorithmic compressors. The more efficiently they can store and codify an organism's experience of the natural world, so the more effectively can that organism counter the dangers that an otherwise unpredictable environment presents.

In our most recent phase of history as *Homo sapiens*, this ability has attained new levels of sophistication. We are able to think about thinking itself. Instead of merely learning from experience as part of the evolutionary process, we have sufficient mental capacity to be able to simulate or imagine the likely results of our actions. In this mode, our minds are generating simulations of past experience embedded in new situations. But to do this effectively requires the brain to be rather finely balanced. It is obvious that mental capacity must be above some threshold in order to achieve effective algorithmic compression."[154]

"Our brains are the outcome of some evolutionary history that has no preordained goal. But the most probable outcome of this history will be a mental apparatus for gathering, representing, and using information about the world in order to predict its future course, a representation that becomes more and more accurate in its reflection of the true underlying reality. A poor mental categorization of the physical world would have a low survival value in comparison with one that was accurate. Any creature that thought that here was there or before was after, who failed to recognize the process of cause and effect, would be less likely to survive and reproduce and so would become an increasingly minor contributor to the gene pool."[155]

"At root, all the necessary conditions for the intelligibility of the world that we have been discussing amount to conditions which enable us to make sense out of what would otherwise be an intractable chaos. Making sense of things amounts to cutting them down to size, ordering them, finding regularities, common factors, and simple recurrences which tell us why things are as they are and how they are going to be in the future. This we should now recognize as the quest for algorithmic compressibility."[156]

We can now use our understanding of compression as a tool to view diabetes accurately, both graphically and mathematically. There have been many models of the Glucose-Insulin system and many, many mathematical models of cell and body metabolism. One of the most accepted realizations of the input-output model of the Glucose-Insulin system is shown here:[157]

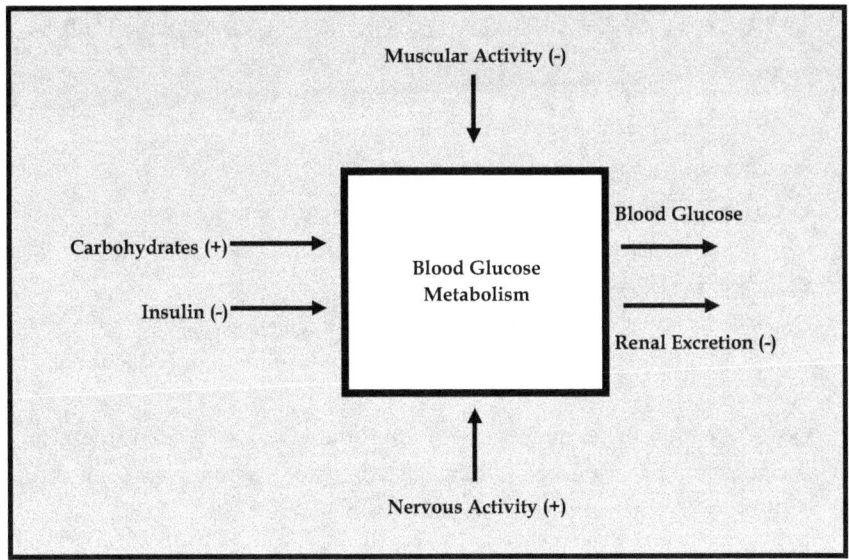

The above model simply presents blood glucose as a function of different inputs and outputs. Food, predominantly carbohydrates, affects blood glucose in a positive way; it raises blood sugar. Insulin, taken subcutaneously (injected under the skin), lowers blood glucose, by (1) signaling cells to accept some glucose for use as immediate energy, (2) storing some as glycogen in the muscle and liver, and (3) converting glucose to saturated fat and storing it in adipose tissue. Nervous activity, a general term for the realizations of all the insulin antagonists, muscular activity, and the amount of glucose taken out of the blood through the kidneys are also part of the system.

In building a mathematical model — an implementable compression — of the blood glucose system for a diabetic, although it is an ever-changing, dynamic process, we can say that blood glucose (BG) is a function of twelve highly influencing variables plus some negligibly influencing variables, combined as one, as presented in the following equation:

$$BG = f(Q_C, Q_{XI\text{-bolus}}, R_{GE}, E_{Renal}, Q_{Gly}, Q_{NI}, Q_{IA}, IS, Q_{XI\text{-basal}}, A, Q_{Sleep}, THP) + \alpha$$

Where:

Q_C = Quantity of digested carbohydrates

$Q_{XI\text{-bolus}}$ = Quantity of exogenous bolus insulin (fast-acting insulin)

R_{GE} = Rate of gastric emptying

E_{Renal} = Renal excretion of sugar

Q_{Gly} = Quantity of glucose converted from stored liver glycogen

Q_{NI} = Quantity of endogenous insulin (natural insulin produced internally by the pancreas)

Q_{IA} = Quantity of hormones that counter the effects of insulin (the insulin antagonists, e.g., glucagon, somatostatin, epinephrine, norepinephrine, cortisol, ACTH, growth hormone, & thyroxine)

IS = Insulin sensitivity, the inverse of insulin resistance[158]

$Q_{XI\text{-basal}}$ = Quantity of exogenous basal insulin (currently realized by insulin glargine and insulin detemir)[159]

A = Activity & heart rate[160]

Q_{Sleep} = Quantity of sleep[161]

THP = Temperature, humidity, & pressure

α = All other factors

This function states that blood glucose is the dynamic sum total of (1) the total quantity of carbohydrates ingested, regardless of being fast-, medium-, or slow-acting, (2) the quantity of injected fast-acting insulin used before meals, (3) the rate of gastric emptying, (4) excretion of sugar through the kidneys, (5) the quantity of glucose delivered to the blood converted from stored liver glycogen, (6) the quantity of endogenous insulin, if it's still produced, (7) the quantity of hormones that counter the effects of insulin, the insulin antagonists: glucagon, somatostatin, epinephrine, norepinephrine, cortisol, ACTH, growth hormone, & thyroxine, (8), insulin sensitivity, (9) the quantity of exogenous basal insulin (Insulin glargine or Insulin detemir), (10) the type and amount of exercise being undertaken, ideally, frequent light exercise, (11) the amount of sleep a subject obtains, as sleep duration and quality are significant predictors of HbA_{1c}, (12) the internal and external temperature, humidity, and pressure, and (13) all other factors which may have a negligible influence on blood sugar; these include the consumption of fat, protein, and other factors such as pH level of food, pH level of blood, the amount the intestinal wall is stretched, et al.

Although reputable sources diverge slightly on the end points of a normal blood glucose range,[162] consensus can be presumed to be as close to a range of 70–110 mg/dL as possible. Of course, blood sugars closer to the lower end point are better than those in the other direction.

Thus, diabetics taking both types of insulin (basal and bolus) seeking to keep their blood sugar stable are, mathematically speaking, optimizing the following model:

$$BG_{70} \leq f(Q_C, Q_{XI\text{-bolus}}, R_{GE}, E_{Renal}, Q_{Gly}, Q_{NI}, Q_{IA}, IS, Q_{XI\text{-basal}}, A, Q_{Sleep}, THP) + \alpha \leq BG_{110}$$

This simply states that all the inputs and outputs of glucose metabolism are kept within and including 70 to 110 mg/dL. Another way to read it is a blood sugar of 70 is less than or equal to the function of 12 variables plus α, which is less than or equal to a blood sugar of 110 mg/dL.

Note that this is the typical Heath Robinson advice given to insulin-dependent diabetics; namely, eat a balanced diet, count your carbohydrates, and take sufficient bolus insulin to cover such carbohydrate. If done methodically, says the dogma, one can achieve normal blood sugar.

The above model can be compressed much further.

Interestingly, all the literature containing mathematical models of the insulin-glucose system have food—especially carbohydrates—as an input. Some models are more detailed than others, but I have not found to date any article or book with a mathematical model that removes carbohydrates as an input. Well, what would happen to the model in this case? If a diabetic does not eat carbohydrates, then the first four variables (Q_C, $Q_{XI\text{-}bolus}$, R_{GE}, E_{Renal}) are dropped, leaving:

$$BG = f(Q_{Gly}, Q_{NI}, IS, Q_{IA}, Q_{XI\text{-}basal}, A, Q_{Sleep}, THP) + \alpha$$

We can also take out Q_{NI}, the quantity of endogenous insulin, because it too becomes at best negligible in a Type 1 diabetic,[*] which leaves:

$$BG = f(Q_{Gly}, IS, Q_{IA}, Q_{XI\text{-}basal}, A, Q_{Sleep}, THP) + \alpha$$

Optimized as:

$$BG_{70} \leq f(Q_{Gly}, IS, Q_{IA}, Q_{XI\text{-}basal}, A, Q_{Sleep}, THP) + \alpha \leq BG_{110}$$

Without carbohydrates, there's no need to take fast-acting insulin, and certainly no need to worry about the rate of gastric emptying, as it's the rate of carbohydrates being emptied into the small intestine and ultimately to the blood that's being calculated in that variable. The kidneys would not have to work at their capacity to excrete sugar through the urine either if BG does not rise significantly.

The following model accurately depicts the input-output model of the glucose-insulin system when carbohydrates are eliminated as an input:

---

[*] Note that in a Type 2 diabetic, $Q_{XI\text{-}basal}$, the quantity of exogenous basal insulin, is also removed from the function.

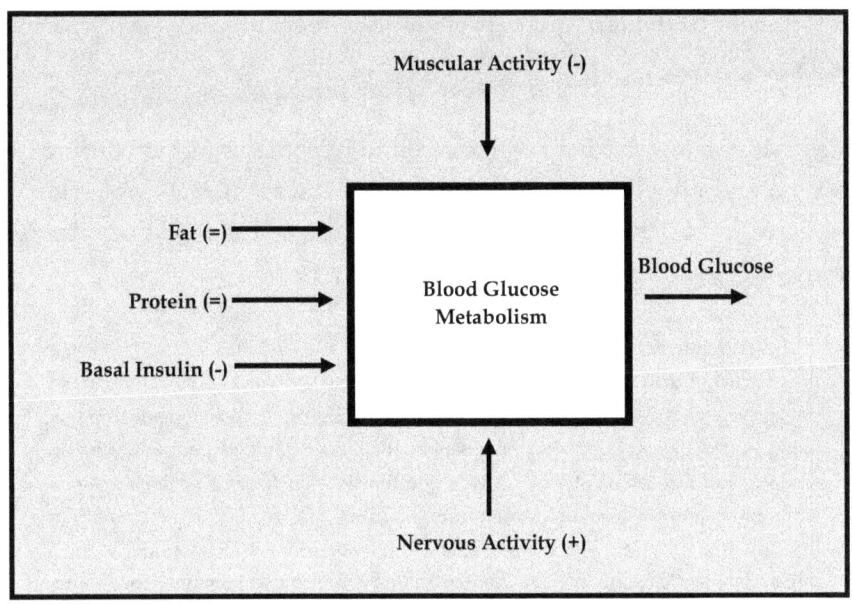

Both protein and fat have negligible effect upon blood glucose, however, protein will increase the stores of glycogen. Blood glucose is now simply a function of the glycogen released from the liver converting to glucose, the quantity of endogenous insulin produced by the pancreas, if any, the relative sensitivity to insulin, the quantity of insulin antagonists released into the circulating blood, the amount of long-acting insulin injected (basal insulin), the level of activity, the amount of sleep, and the ambient and body temperature, humidity, and pressure. All this can be achieved quite elegantly, and within normal blood sugar ranges, as if one didn't have diabetes.

Before delving into studies that support—primarily for diabetes, secondarily for weight control—at least a restricted carbohydrate diet, which would by necessity include a high percentage of fat and protein, it is worth noting the studies supporting a low-fat diet, with higher percentages of carbohydrates, to *best* control blood sugar.

Unfortunately, though quite profoundly, there are no such credible studies.

The basis of a low-fat diet revolves around hypotheses formed during the creation and growth of the Coronary Heart Disease (CHD) profession in the early to mid twentieth century.[163]   Renowned author Gary Taubes writes in "The Soft Science of Dietary Fat" (2001):

> "...an antifat movement evolved independently of science in the 1960s. It was fed by distrust of the establishment — in this case, both the medical establishment and the food industry — and by counterculture attacks on excessive consumption, whether manifested in gas-guzzling cars or the classic American cuisine of bacon and eggs and marbled steaks. And while the data on fat and health remained ambiguous and the scientific community polarized, the deadlock was broken not by any new science, but by politicians. It was Senator George McGovern's bipartisan, nonlegislative Select Committee on Nutrition and Human Needs — and, to be precise, a handful of McGovern's staff members — that almost single-handedly changed nutritional policy in this country and initiated the process of turning the dietary fat hypothesis into dogma..."[164]

The Framingham Heart Study is often cited as proof of the lipid hypothesis.[165] In 1948, the Framingham Heart Study — under the direction of the National Heart Institute (now known as the National Heart, Lung and Blood Institute or NHLBI) — embarked on an ambitious project in health research. At the time, little was known about the general causes of heart disease and stroke, but the death rates for CVD had been increasing steadily since the beginning of the century and had become an American epidemic. The Framingham Heart Study became a joint project of the National Heart, Lung and Blood Institute and Boston University.

The objective of the Framingham Heart Study was to identify the common factors or characteristics that contribute to CVD by following its development over a long period of time in a large group of participants who had not yet developed overt symptoms of CVD or suffered a heart attack or stroke.

The researchers recruited 5,209 men and women between the ages of 30 and 62 from the town of Framingham, Massachusetts, and began the first round of extensive physical examinations and lifestyle interviews that they would later analyze for common patterns related to CVD development. Since 1948, the subjects have continued to return to the study every two years for a detailed medical history, physical examination, and laboratory tests, and in 1971, the study enrolled a second generation—5,124 of the original participants' adult children and their spouses—to participate in similar examinations. In April, 2002, the Study entered a new phase: the enrollment of a third generation of participants, the grandchildren of the original cohort. Exam 1 of the Third Generation Study was completed in July, 2005, and involved 4,095 participants.[166]

According to Sally Fallon and Mary Enig, "After 40 years, the director of this study had to admit:

["In Framingham, Mass., the more saturated fat one ate, the more cholesterol one ate, the more calories one ate, the lower the person's serum cholesterol…we found that the people who ate the most cholesterol, ate the most saturated fat, ate the most calories, weighed the least and were the most physically active."[167]

"The study did show that those who weighed more and had abnormally high blood cholesterol levels were slightly more at risk for future heart disease, but weight gain and cholesterol levels had an inverse correlation with fat and cholesterol intake in the diet."[168]]"[169]

Dr. Mary Enig and Sally Fallon provide several examples dispelling the myth that a diet low in cholesterol and saturated fat actually reduces death from heart disease or in any way increase one's life span:

- "In a multi-year British study involving several thousand men, half were asked to reduce saturated fat and cholesterol in their diets, to stop smoking and to increase consumption of unsaturated oils such as margarine and vegetable oils. After one year, those on the "good" diet had 100 percent more deaths than those on the "bad" diet, in spite of the fact that those on the "bad" diet continued to smoke! But in describing the study, the author ignored these results in favor of a politically correct conclusion: "The implication for public health policy in the UK is that a preventative programme such as we evaluated in this trial is probably effective..."[170]

- "The Multiple Risk Factor Intervention Trial (MRFIT), sponsored by the National Heart, Lung and Blood Institute, compared mortality rates and eating habits of over 12,000 men. Those with "good" dietary habits (reduced saturated fat, reduced cholesterol and reduced smoking) showed a marginal reduction in total coronary heart disease, but their overall mortality from all causes was higher. Similar results have emerged in several other studies. The few trials that indicate a correlation between fat reduction and a decrease in coronary heart disease mortality also document a concurrent increase in deaths from cancer, brain hemorrhage, suicide, and violent death."[171]

- "The Lipid Research Clinics Coronary Primary Prevention Trial (LRC-CPPT), which cost 150 million dollars, is the study most often cited by the experts to justify lowfat diets. Actually, dietary cholesterol and saturated fat were not tested in this study as all subjects were given a low-cholesterol, low-saturated-fat diet. Instead, the study tested the effects of a cholesterol-lowering drug. Their statistical analysis of the results implied a 24 percent reduction in the rate of coronary heart disease in the group taking the drug compared with the placebo group; however, non-heart disease deaths in the drug group increased—deaths from cancer, stroke, violence and suicide.[172] Even the conclusion that lowering cholesterol reduces heart disease is suspect. Independent researchers who tabulated the results of this study found no significant statistical difference in coronary heart disease death rates between the two groups.[173] However, both the popular press and medical journals touted the LRC-CPPT as the long-sought proof that animal fats are the cause of heart disease, America's number-one killer."[174]

- "While it is true that researchers have induced heart disease in some animals by giving them extremely large doses of oxidized or rancid cholesterol— amounts ten times that found in the ordinary human diet—several population studies squarely contradict the cholesterol-heart disease connection. A survey of 1,700 patients with hardening of the arteries conducted by the famous heart surgeon Michael DeBakey, found no relationship between the level of cholesterol in the blood and the incidence of atherosclerosis.[175] A survey of South Carolina adults found no correlation of blood cholesterol levels with "bad" dietary habits, such as use of red meat, animal fats, fried foods, butter, eggs, whole milk, bacon, sausage and cheese. A Medical Research Council survey showed that men eating butter ran half the risk of developing heart disease compared to those using margarine."[176]

- "The relative good health of the Japanese, who have the longest life span of any nation in the world, is generally attributed to a low fat diet. Although the Japanese eat few dairy fats, the notion that their diet is low in fat is a myth; rather, it contains moderate amounts of animal fats from eggs, pork, chicken, beef, seafood and organ meats. With their fondness for shellfish and fish broth, eaten on a daily basis, the Japanese probably consume more cholesterol than most Americans. What they do not consume is a lot of vegetable oil, white flour or processed food (although they do eat white rice). The life span of the Japanese has increased since World War II along with an increase in animal fat and protein in the diet. Those who point to Japanese statistics to promote the low-fat diet fail to mention that the Swiss live almost as long on one of the fattiest diets in the world. Tied for third in the longevity stakes are Austria and Greece—both with high-fat diets."[177]

- "As a final example, let us consider the French. Anyone who has eaten his way across France has observed that the French diet is loaded with saturated fat in the form of butter, eggs, cheese, cream, liver, meats and rich patés. Yet the French have a lower rate of coronary heart disease than many other western countries. In the United States, 315 of every 100,000 middle-aged men die of heart attacks each year; in France the rate is 145 per 100,000. In the Gascony region, where goose and duck liver from a staple of the diet, this rate is a remarkably low 80 per 100,000.[178] This phenomenon has recently gained international attention and was dubbed the French Paradox. The French do suffer from many degenerative diseases, however. (They eat large amounts of sugar and white flour and in recent years have succumbed to the timesaving temptations of processed foods.)"[179]

Dr. Enig and Sally Fallon summarize conclusions based upon these studies in this way:

"Politically correct dietary gurus tell us that polyunsaturated oils are good for us and that saturated fats cause cancer and heart disease. Such misinformation about the relative virtues of saturated fats versus polyunsaturated oils has caused profound changes in western eating habits. At the turn of the century, most of the fatty acids in the diet were either saturated or mono-unsaturated, primarily from butter, lard, tallows, coconut oil and small amounts of olive oil. Today, most of the fats in the diet are polyunsaturated, primarily from vegetable oils derived from soy, as well as from corn, safflower and canola...

Excess consumption of polyunsaturated oils has been shown to contribute to a large number of disease conditions including increased cancer and heart disease, immune system dysfunction, damage to the liver, reproductive organs and lungs, digestive disorders, depressed learning ability, impaired growth, and weight gain...

The cause of heart disease is not animal fats and cholesterol but rather a number of factors inherent in modern diets, including excess consumption of vegetable oils and hydrogenated fats; excess consumption of refined carbohydrates in the form of sugar and white flour; mineral deficiencies, particularly low levels of protective magnesium and iodine; deficiencies of vitamins, particularly of Vitamin A, C and D, needed for the integrity of the blood vessel walls, and of antioxidants like selenium and Vitamin E, which protect us from free radicals; and, finally, the disappearance of antimicrobial fats from the food supply, namely, animal fats and tropical oil. These once protected us against the kinds of viruses and bacteria that have been associated with onset of pathogenic plaque leading to heart disease." [180]

Ancel Keys played a prominent role in the anti-fat movement and process, and was focused on researching the relationship between serum cholesterol and heart disease. [181] In his seminal work "Coronary Heart Disease among Minnesota Business and Professional Men Followed Fifteen Years," (1963) Ancel Keys wrote:

"Relative weight, body fatness (skinfold thickness), blood pressure, and serum cholesterol are reported from 281 Minnesota business and professional men, initially clinically healthy and aged 45 to 55, who were followed by annual examinations since the winter of 1947-48. In 15 elapsed years, coronary heart disease developed definitely in 32 men and possibly in 16 other men. The incidence of coronary heart disease tended to be higher among men above the median at first examination in relative weight, body fatness, systolic and diastolic blood pressure, and serum cholesterol concentration but these segregations were not statistically significant except with serum cholesterol. Comparison with similar follow-up data from Framingham, Massachusetts, Albany, New York, and Chicago, show a high degree of concordance. In all series relative weight had least significance and the incidence of coronary heart disease rose continuously with the serum cholesterol level." [182]

At the time, it was thought that the consumption of fat, particularly animal fat, thought of at the time as saturated fat,* was partially to blame for a higher incidence of serum cholesterol. Although somewhat divided even then, the majority of scientists believed that some fats were beneficial to serum cholesterol, i.e., that some fats decrease cholesterol, and others had a different fate once consumed.

Interestingly, in "Prevention of Coronary Heart Disease: Official Recommendations from Scandinavia," (1968) Ancel Keys wrote:

"While debate continues in the United States as to what to advise the public about dietary modification in efforts to prevent coronary heart disease, the medical Boards of Norway, Sweden and Finland have presented their conclusions in a collective recommendation released in Oslo, Stockholm, and Helsinki on May 3, 1968…

…First and foremost this re-arrangement should bring about a decrease in the consumption of foodstuffs containing a large quantity of fat and/or sugar. This would leave room for a higher consumption of foodstuffs rich in protein, mineral substances, and vitamins." [183]

But, he also wrote:

"The practical consequences of what has been said above mean:

The supply of calories in the diet should in many cases be reduced to prevent overweight. The total consumption of fat should be reduced from 40%–the present figure – to between 25% and 35% of the total calories. The use of saturated fat should be reduced and the consumption of polyunsaturated fats should be increased simultaneously. The consumption of sugar and products containing

---

* "The practice of calling animal fats "saturated" is not only misleading, it is just plain wrong. For example, beef fat is 54% unsaturated, lard is 60% unsaturated, and chicken fat is about 70% unsaturated. This makes these animal fats less than half saturated. Therefore, they really should be called unsaturated fats. These fats [animal fats] are called "saturated" because people have been misinformed and because they don't understand what the term saturated means when it is applied to edible fats and oils. Totally unsaturated oils are nonexistent in the natural foods." See Mary G. Enig, Ph.D. *Know Your Fats: The Complete Primer for Understanding the Nutrition of Fats, Oils, and Cholesterol.* Silver Spring, MD: Bethesda Press, 2000, pages 17-18.

sugar should be reduced. The consumption of vegetables, fruit, potatoes, skimmed milk, fish, lean meat and cereal products should be increased. From the medical and nutritional standpoint the importance of taking regular exercise from an early age for all those who have maintained sedentary occupations should also be emphasized."[184]

The statement closes with a request for cooperation in implementing these points by doctors, nutritionists, teachers, the food industry, the press, radio, and TV. All told, Ancel Keys provided good starting points, some of which have unfortunately been imprinted on many societies' collective minds as unquestioned tenets until recently.

- - - - - - -

Low-carbohydrate diets became a major weight loss and health maintenance trend during the late 1990s and early 2000s. While their popularity has waned recently from its peak, they still remain popular. This diet trend has stirred major controversies in the medical and nutritional sciences communities and, as yet, there is not a general consensus on their efficacy or safety. The majority of the medical community remains generally opposed to these diets for long term health despite several studies reporting positive results in both weight loss and improvement in health indicators.

It is worth noting that one of the fundamental criticisms of those who advocate low-carbohydrate diets has been the lack of long-term studies evaluating their health risks. This lack of long term studies is noted by Dr. Eric C. Westman of the Department of Medicine, Duke University Medical Center, even though he finds little evidence of the need to eat carbohydrates. In "Is Dietary Carbohydrate Essential for Human Nutrition?" (2002), Dr. Westman writes:

"…in exploring the risks and benefits of carbohydrate restriction, I was surprised to find little evidence that exogenous carbohydrate is needed for human function.

The Way Things Ought To Be (Part I)

The currently established human essential nutrients are water, energy, amino acids (histidine, isoleucine, leucine, lysine, methionine, phenylalanine, threonine, tryptophan, and valine), essential fatty acids (linoleic and α-linolenic acids), vitamin C (ascorbic acid), vitamin A, vitamin D, vitamin E, vitamin K, thiamine, riboflavin, niacin, vitamin B-6, pantothenic acid, folic acid, biotin, and vitamin B-12, minerals (calcium, phosphorus, magnesium, and iron), trace minerals (zinc, copper, manganese, iodine, selenium, molybdenum, and chromium), electrolytes (sodium, potassium, and chloride), and ultratrace minerals (Note the absence of specific carbohydrates from this list.).

Although one current recommended dietary carbohydrate intake for adults is 150 g/d, it is interesting to examine how this recommendation was determined at a recent international conference:[185]

"The theoretical minimal level of carbohydrate (CHO) intake is zero, but CHO is a universal fuel for all cells, the cheapest source of dietary energy, and also the source of plant fiber. In addition, the complete absence of dietary CHO entails the breakdown of fat to supply energy [glycerol as a gluconeogenic substrate, and ketone bodies as an alternative fuel for the central nervous system (CNS)], resulting in symptomatic ketosis. Data in childhood are unavailable, but ketosis in adults can be prevented by a daily CHO intake of about 50 g. This value appears to approximate the quantity of glucose required to satisfy minimal glucose needs of the CNS and during starvation. The Group therefore concluded that the theoretical minimum intake of zero should not be recommended as a practical minimum...about 100 g of glucose/d are irreversibly oxidized by the brain from the age of 3–4 y onward. However, this excludes recycled carbon, gluconeogenic carbon, for example from glycerol, and it does not account for glucose used by other non-CNS tissues. For example, in the adult, muscle and other non-CNS account for an additional 20–30 g of glucose daily. For this reason a safety margin of 50 g/d is arbitrarily added to the value of 100 g/d and the practical minimal CHO intake set at 150 g/d beyond the ages of 3–4 y."

Thus, although carbohydrate could theoretically be eliminated from the diet, the recommended intake of 150 g/d ensures an adequate supply of glucose for the CNS. However, it appears that during starvation (a condition in which the intakes of carbohydrate, protein, and fat are eliminated), an adequate amount of substrate for the CNS is provided through gluconeogenesis and ketogenesis.[186] The elimination of dietary carbohydrate did not diminish the energy supply to the CNS under the conditions of these experiments. Second, carbohydrate is recommended to avert symptomatic ketosis. In the largest published series on carbohydrate-restricted diets, ketosis was not typically symptomatic.[187]

The most direct way to determine whether carbohydrate is an essential nutrient is to eliminate it from the diet in controlled laboratory studies. In studies involving rats and chicks, the elimination of dietary carbohydrate caused no obvious problems.[188] It was only when carbohydrate restriction was combined with glycerol restriction (by substituting fatty acids for triacylglycerol) that chicks did not develop normally.[189] Thus, it appears that some minimum amount of a gluconeogenic precursor is essential–for example, glycerol obtained from fat (triacylglycerol) consumption. More subtle abnormalities from carbohydrate elimination might not have been observed in these studies. In addition, the essentiality of some nutrients is species-specific; therefore, these studies do not provide convincing evidence that elimination of dietary carbohydrate is safe in humans.[190]

The usual way to discover the essentiality of nutrients is through the identification of specific deficiency syndromes.[191] I found no evidence of a carbohydrate deficiency syndrome in humans. Protein deprivation leads to kwashiorkor, and energy deprivation leads to marasmus; however, there is no specific carbohydrate deficiency syndrome. Few contemporary human cultures eat low-carbohydrate diets, but the traditional Eskimo diet is very low (approx. 50 g/d) in carbohydrate.[192] It is possible that if more humans consumed diets severely restricted in carbohydrate, a carbohydrate deficiency syndrome might become apparent.

When carbohydrates are eliminated from the diet, there is a risk that intakes of vitamins, minerals, and perhaps yet unidentified beneficial nutrients provided by carbohydrate-rich foodstuffs (e.g., fiber) will be inadequate. There are case reports of extreme dieters who probably developed deficiencies. One dieter who only ate cheese, meat, and eggs (no vegetables) was reported to have developed thiamine-deficient optic neuropathy.[193] Another dieter may have developed a relapse of acute variegate porphyria.[194] However, most of the current low-carbohydrate, weight-reducing diets advocate the consumption of low-carbohydrate vegetables and vitamin supplements.

Although there is certainly no evidence from which to conclude that extreme restriction of dietary carbohydrate is harmless, I was surprised to find that there is similarly little evidence to conclude that extreme restriction of carbohydrate is harmful. In fact, the consequential breakdown of fat as a result of carbohydrate restriction may be beneficial in the treatment of obesity.[195] Perhaps it is time to carefully examine the issue of whether carbohydrate is an essential component of human nutrition."[196]

In 1863, William Banting, an obese English undertaker, published *Letter on Corpulence Addressed to the Public* in which he described a diet for weight control giving up bread, butter, milk, sugar, beer and potatoes. According to the Weston A. Price Foundation, his booklet was widely read, so much so that some people used the term "Banting" for the activity usually called "dieting."[197, 198]

In 1967, Dr. Irwin Stillman published *The Doctor's Quick Weight Loss Diet*. The "Stillman Diet" is a high-protein, low-carbohydrate and low-fat diet. It is regarded as one of the first low-carb diets to become popular in the US.[199] Other low-carbohydrate diets in the 1960's included *Air Force Diet*[200] and the *Drinking Man's Diet*.[201] Austrian physician Dr Wolfgang Lutz published his book *Leben Ohne Brot* (*Life Without Bread*) in 1967.[202] However, it was hardly noticed in the English speaking world.[203]

In 1972, Dr. Robert Atkins published *Dr. Atkins Diet Revolution* which advocated a low-carbohydrate diet he had successfully used in treating patients in the 1960s.[204] Like its predecessors the book met with some success but, because of research at that time suggesting risk factors associated with excess fat and protein, it was very widely criticized by the mainstream medical community as being dangerous and misleading, thereby limiting its appeal at the time. Among other things critics pointed out that Dr. Atkins had done little real research into his theories and based them mostly on anecdotal evidence. Dr. Atkins nevertheless continued to develop his theories and gain followers.[205]

The concept of the glycemic index was invented in 1981 by Dr. David Jenkins. This concept evaluates carbohydrates according to their insulin demand — with fast digesting simple carbohydrates having a high insulin demand and slower digesting complex carbohydrates such as grains having a lower insulin demand.[206]

In the 1990s Dr. Atkins published *Dr. Atkins New Diet Revolution* and other doctors began to publish books based on the same principles. This can be said to be the beginning of the "low carb craze."[207]

During the late 1990s and early 2000s low-carbohydrate diets became some of the most popular diets in the U.S. (by some accounts as much as 18% of the population was using a low-carbohydrate diet at its peak[208]) and spread to many countries. These were, in fact, noted by some food manufacturers and restaurant chains as substantially affecting their businesses. This was in spite of the fact that the mainstream medical community continued to vehemently denounce low-carbohydrate diets as being a dangerous trend.[209] It is, however, valuable to note that many of these same doctors and institutions at the same time quietly began altering their own advice to be closer to the low-carbohydrate recommendations (e.g., eating more protein, eating less starch, reducing consumption of juices by children).[210]

The low-carbohydrate advocates did some adjustments of their own increasingly advocating controlling fat and eliminating trans fat. It is also valuable to note that most of major medical groups have acknowledged at least that the low-carbohydrate diet is effective in the short-term. Many of the diet guides and gurus that appeared at this time intentionally distanced themselves from Atkins and the term *low carb* because of the controversies, even though their recommendations were based on largely the same principles, e.g., the Zone diet. As such it is often a matter of debate which diets are really low-carbohydrate and which are not. The 1990s and 2000s also saw the publication of an increased number of clinical studies regarding the effectiveness and safety, pro and con, of low-carbohydrate diets, notably a 2006 *NEJM* paper by Halton et al., describing a 20-year study. After 2004, the popularity of this diet trend began to wane significantly although it still remains quite popular.[211]

The term *low-carbohydrate diet* today is most strongly associated with the Atkins Diet. However, there is an array of other diets that share to varying degrees the same principles, e.g., the Zone Diet, the Protein Power Lifeplan, etc. Therefore, there is no widely accepted definition of what precisely constitutes a low-carbohydrate diet. For the purposes of this discussion, we focus on diets that reduce nutritive carbohydrate intake sufficiently to dramatically reduce or eliminate insulin production in the body and to encourage ketosis, production of ketones to be used as energy in place of glucose, but not ketoacidosis.[212]

Although originally low-carbohydrate diets were created based on anecdotal evidence of their effectiveness, today there is a much greater theoretical basis on which these diets rest. The key scientific principle which forms the basis for these diets is the relationship between consumption of carbohydrates and their effects on blood sugar, i.e., blood glucose, and hormone production. Blood sugar levels in the human body must be maintained in a fairly narrow range to maintain health. The two primary hormones related to regulating blood sugar levels, produced in the pancreas, are insulin, which lowers blood sugar levels, and glucagon, which raises blood sugar levels. In general, most western diets, and many others, are sufficiently high in nutritive carbohydrates that virtually every meal causes substantial insulin production and shuts down ketosis, thus causing excess energy in the diet to be stored as fat. By contrast, low-carbohydrate diets discourage insulin production and tend to cause ketosis. Some researchers suggest that this causes excess dietary energy and body fat to be eliminated from the body. Although these diets remain controversial there are clinical studies related to their effectiveness.[213, 214]

Low-carbohydrate diet advocates in general recommend reducing nutritive carbohydrates, commonly referred to as "net carbs," i.e., total carbohydrates reduced by the non-nutritive carbohydrates, to very low levels. This means sharply reducing consumption of desserts, breads, pastas, potatoes, rice, and other sweet or starchy foods. Some recommend levels as low as 20-30 grams of "net carbs" per day, at least in the early stages of dieting (for comparison, a single slice of white bread may contain 15-25 grams of carbohydrate, almost entirely starch). The diets often differ in the specific amount of carbohydrates allowed, whether certain types of foods are preferred, whether occasional exceptions are allowed, etc. Generally they all agree that processed sugar should be eliminated, or at the very least greatly reduced, and similarly generally discourage heavily processed grains, e.g., white bread.   They vary greatly in their recommendations as to the amount of fat allowed in the diet although the most popular versions today, including Atkins, generally recommend at most a moderate fat intake.[215]

As a related note, there is a set of diets known as low-glycemic-index diets (low-GI diets) or low-glycemic-load diets (low-GL diets). In reality, low-carbohydrate diets are, literally speaking, low-GL diets, and vice versa, in that they specifically limit what contributes to the glycemic load in foods. In practice, though, low-GI/low-GL diets differ from low-carbohydrate diets in the following ways:

- Low-carbohydrate diets treat all nutritive carbohydrates as having the same effect on metabolism and generally assume that their effect is independent of other nutrients in food. Low-GI/low-GL diets base their recommendations on the actual measured metabolic (glycemic) effects of the foods eaten.
- As a practical matter, low-GI/low-GL diets generally do not recommend diets with glycemic loads low enough to minimize insulin production and induce ketosis, whereas low-carbohydrate diets generally do.[216]

Another related diet type, the low-insulin-index diet, is very similar except that it is based on measurements of direct insulemic responses to food rather than glycemic response.   Although the diet recommendations mostly involve lowering nutritive carbohydrates, there are some low-carbohydrate foods that are discouraged as well, e.g., beef.[217, 218]

At the heart of the debate about most low-carbohydrate diets are fundamental questions about what a "normal" diet is and how the human body is supposed to operate.[219] These questions can be summarized as follows. Nutritive carbohydrates, i.e., starches and sugars, in the diet tend to break down very easily into glucose in the bloodstream when consumed. Glucose in the blood is used by the cells in the body for energy for their basic function. Excessive amounts of glucose in the blood are toxic to the human body, which is the reason that unchecked diabetes causes such serious health problems. In general, unless a meal is very low in starches and sugars the level of glucose will tend to rise to potentially dangerous levels. When this occurs, the pancreas automatically produces insulin to cause the liver to convert glucose into glycogen, called glycogenesis, and triglycerides, thus reducing the blood sugars to safe levels. Diets with a high starch and sugar content, therefore, cause sharp spikes in insulin production. As such the blood sugar levels are highly variable with every meal.[220]

By contrast, if the diet is very low in starches and sugars, as in low-carbohydrate diets, the blood sugar level can fall so low that there is insufficient glucose to fuel the cells in the body. This state causes the pancreas to produce glucagon. Glucagon causes the conversion of stored glycogen to glucose and, once the glycogen stores are exhausted, causes the liver to synthesize ketones, referred to as ketosis, and glucose, called gluconeogenesis, from fats and proteins, respectively. Most cells in the body can use ketones for energy instead of glucose and, since ketones are easier to produce, only a small amount of glucose is created. Because diets low in starches and sugars do not tend to directly affect blood sugar levels significantly, meals tend to have little direct effect on insulin levels, and so such diets tend to discourage insulin production in general.[221]

The diets of most people in modern, western nations, especially the United States, contain significant amounts of starches, and, frequently, significant amounts of sugars. As such, the metabolisms of most westerners tend to operate outside of ketosis and tend to involve significant insulin production. This has been regarded by medical science in the last century as being "normal." Ketosis has generally been regarded as a dangerous, potentially life-threatening, state which unnecessarily stresses the liver and causes destruction of muscle tissues. The view that has been developed is that getting energy more from protein than carbohydrates causes liver damage and that getting energy more from fats than carbohydrates causes heart disease. This view is still the view of the majority in the medical and nutritional science communities.[222]

Most advocates of low-carbohydrate diets, specifically those that recommend diets similar to the Atkins Diet, argue that this metabolic state, using primarily blood glucose for energy, is not normal at all and that the human body is, in fact, supposed to function primarily in ketosis. They argue that high insulin levels can, in fact, cause many health problems, most significantly, fat storage and weight gain. They argue that the purported dangers of ketosis are unsubstantiated, and, in fact, some of the arguments against ketosis result from confusion between ketosis and ketoacidosis which is a related but very different process. Further, whereas insulin in the bloodstream causes storage of food energy, when the body is in ketosis, excess ketones, which contain excess energy, are excreted in the urine and the breath.[223]

Some argue, on this basis, that the ketogenic low-carbohydrate diets offer a *metabolic advantage,* in that the body automatically eliminates food energy that it does not need even with a high-energy diet. This argument has not yet been demonstrated in clinical studies; one 2006 study failed to find such an advantage over non-ketogenic low-carb diets.[224, 225]

This debate is on-going and no consensus currently exists.

Although there has been some research done throughout the twentieth century, most directly relevant scientific studies have occurred in the 1990s, and early 2000s, and, as such, are relatively new. The difficulty rests with using human subjects for testing and devising suitable such tests.[226]

That said, one study found no correlation between a low-carbohydrate, high fat/protein diet and coronary heart disease in women, and a moderate reduction in risk if the fat and protein were primarily from plant rather than animal sources.[227] Other studies have found possible benefits to individuals with diabetes,[228] renal cancer[229] and autism.[230] The Johns Hopkins diet, with 90% of energy from fat and much of the remaining from protein, has also been used for more than 80 years to treat epilepsy, though generally it has been superseded by medication.

A study conducted in 1965 at the Oakland (California) Naval Hospital used a diet of 1000 kilocalories per day, high in fat and limiting carbohydrates to 10 grams (40 kilocalories) daily. Over a ten-day period, subjects on this diet lost more body fat than did a group who fasted completely.[231] Some advocates of low-carbohydrate diets have termed this the *metabolic advantage* of such diets.

In "Effect of Body Composition and other Parameters in Obese Young Men of Carbohydrate Level of Reduction Diet," (1971), which focused upon weight loss, the authors concluded:

> "Weight loss, fat loss, and percent weight loss as fat appeared to be inversely related to the level of carbohydrate in the isocaloric, isoprotein diets."[232]

In "Effects of Varying Carbohydrate Content of Diet in Patients with Non-Insulin-Dependent Diabetes Mellitus," (1994), the authors concluded:

"In NIDDM patients, high-carbohydrate diets compared with high-mono-unsaturated-fat diets caused persistent deterioration of glycemic control and accentuation of hyperinsulinemia, as well as increased plasma triglyceride and very-low-density lipoprotein cholesterol levels, which may not be desirable."[233]

In "Deleterious Metabolic Effects of High-Carbohydrate, Sucrose-Containing Diets in Patients with Non-Insulin-Dependent Diabetes Mellitus," (1987), the effects of variations in dietary carbohydrate and fat intake on various aspects of carbohydrate and lipid metabolism were studied in patients with non-insulin-dependent diabetes mellitus (NIDDM). Two test diets were utilized, and they were consumed in random order over two 15-day periods. One diet was low in fat and high in carbohydrate, and corresponded closely to recent recommendations made by the American Diabetes Association (ADA), containing (as percent of total calories) 20% protein, 20% fat, and 60% carbohydrate, with 10% of total calories as sucrose. The other diet contained 20% protein, 40% fat, and 40% carbohydrate, with sucrose accounting for 3% of total calories. Here are the conclusions of that study:

"These results document that low-fat, high-carbohydrate diets, containing moderate amounts of sucrose, similar in composition to the recommendations of the ADA, have deleterious metabolic effects when consumed by patients with NIDDM for 15 days. Until it can be shown that these untoward effects are evanescent, and that long-term ingestion of similar diets will result in beneficial metabolic changes, it seems prudent to avoid the use of low-fat, high-carbohydrate diets containing moderate amounts of sucrose in patients with NIDDM."[234]

The results of studies from Stanford University[235] (2007), and Duke University[236] (2005), favored low-carbohydrate diets for both weight loss and health indicators.

In "Efficacy and Safety of Low-Carbohydrate Diets," (2003), the authors conducted a literature search study of low-carbohydrate diet studies conducted between 1966 and 2003. The paper concluded:

"There is insufficient evidence to make recommendations for or against the use of low-carbohydrate diets, particularly among participants older than age 50 years, for use longer than 90 days, or for diets of 20 grams per day or less of carbohydrates. Among the published studies, participant weight loss while using low-carbohydrate diets was principally associated with decreased caloric intake and increased diet duration but not with reduced carbohydrate content."[237]

The investigators of "The Effects of Low-Carbohydrate versus Conventional Weight Loss Diets in Severely Obese Adults: One-Year Follow-up of a Randomized Trial," (2004), conducted a one-year study of 132 obese adults. The authors concluded the following:

"Participants on a low-carbohydrate diet had more favorable overall outcomes at 1 year than did those on a conventional diet. Weight loss was similar between groups, but effects on atherogenic dyslipidemia and glycemic control were still more favorable with a low-carbohydrate diet after adjustment for differences in weight loss."[238]

In "A Low-Carbohydrate, Ketogenic Diet to Treat Type 2 Diabetes," (2005), the authors concluded that:

"The low-carbohydrate, ketogenic diet (LCKD) may be effective for improving glycemia and reducing medications in patients with Type 2 diabetes. The LCKD had positive effects on body weight, waist measurement, serum triglycerides, and glycemic control in a cohort of 21 participants with Type 2 diabetes. Most impressive is that improvement in hemoglobin A_{1c} was observed despite a small sample size and short duration of follow-up, and this improvement in glycemic control occurred while diabetes medications were reduced substantially in many participants."[239]

In "Low-Carbohydrate Nutrition and Metabolism," (2007), the authors concluded that:

"...under conditions of carbohydrate restriction, fuel sources shift from glucose and fatty acids to fatty acids and ketones, and that ad libitum-fed carbohydrate-restricted diets lead to appetite reduction, weight loss, and improvement in surrogate markers of cardiovascular disease."[240]

The benefits of a restrictive carbohydrate diet are nicely summarized in "Comparison of Low Fat and Low Carbohydrate Diets on Circulating Fatty Acid Composition and Markers of Inflammation," (2007), this way:

> *"In summary, a very low carbohydrate diet resulted in profound alterations in fatty acid composition and reduced inflammation compared to a low fat diet."* [241]

Meta-analysis is a method to succinctly summarize and combine the results from multiple individual studies.

In "Restricted-Carbohydrate Diets in Patients with Type 2 Diabetes: A Meta-Analysis," (2007), the investigators searched for articles published in English between 1980, and April, 2006, regarding carbohydrate-restricted diets that included and reported separate results for adult, nonpregnant patients with Type 2 diabetes.[242] Articles were limited to studies completed in the United States and Canada. Available data on study design, carbohydrate composition of diet, duration of diet, and the outcomes of weight, lipid levels (total, low-density lipoprotein and high-density lipoprotein cholesterol, and triglycerides), hemoglobin A1c percent and/or fasting glucose were extracted. A total of 56 studies or reviews were evaluated. Thirteen studies met their inclusion criteria. Meta-regression analyses show that hemoglobin A1c, fasting glucose, and some lipid fractions (triglycerides) improved with lower carbohydrate content diets. Here is the main conclusion from this article:

> "This meta-analysis indicates that lower-carbohydrate diets can be beneficial in treating Type 2 diabetes, not only because of improved glycemic control, but also because of potential salutary changes in the lipid profile. Improvements in fasting glucose, HbA$_{1c}$, and triglycerides appear to result from even moderate decreases in carbohydrate intake.
>
> Diabetes mellitus is, in part, a disorder of carbohydrate metabolism that results in hyperglycemia. Carbohydrates are the component of the diet that exerts the greatest influence on postprandial blood glucose. Thus, it is logical that diets lower in carbohydrates would result in less hyperglycemia." [243]

The challenges of this article, echoed by a majority of studies whose data supports the use of a ketogenic diet, were that there is an absence of a standard definition of low-carbohydrate diet and that long-term studies of the efficacy of that diet have yet to be undertaken and analyzed.

A meta-analysis of randomized controlled trials by the Cochrane Collaboration in 2002, concluded that fat-restricted diets are no better than calorie restricted diets in achieving long term weight loss in overweight or obese people.[244]

A more recent meta-analysis that included randomized controlled trials published after the Cochrane review[245] found that "...low-carbohydrate, non-energy-restricted diets appear to be at least as effective as low-fat, energy-restricted diets in inducing weight loss for up to 1 year. However, potential favorable changes in triglyceride and high-density lipoprotein cholesterol values should be weighed against potential unfavorable changes in low-density lipoprotein cholesterol values when low-carbohydrate diets to induce weight loss are considered."[246] Although studies from Stanford University and Duke University were not meta-analytic, their results favored the low-carbohydrate approach,[247] as opposed to the aforementioned study which questions which is better.

In "Effect of Low Fat-High Carbohydrate Diets in Hypertensive Patients with Non-Insulin-Dependent Diabetes Mellitus," (1990), by Fuh MM, Lee MM, Jeng CY, Ma F, Chen YD, and Reaven GM, the authors found that:

"Plasma glucose and insulin concentrations were significantly (P less than .001) elevated throughout the day when patients consumed the 60% carbohydrate diet. Fasting plasma total and very-low-density lipoprotein (VLDL) and triglyceride (TG) concentrations increased by 30% (P less than .001) after 15 days on the 60% carbohydrate diet. Total plasma cholesterol concentrations were similar on both diets, as were low-density lipoprotein (LDL) and high-density lipoprotein (HDL) cholesterol concentrations."[248]

In "A Low-Carbohydrate Diet May Prevent End-Stage Renal Failure in Type 2 Diabetes. A Case Report," (2006), by Jørgen Vesti Nielsen, Per Westerlund, and Per Bygren, the authors introduce us to the problem:

"Insulin treatment in type 2 diabetes patients usually leads to weight increase which may cause further injury to the kidney. Although other unknown metabolic mechanisms cannot be excluded, it is likely that the obesity caused by the combination of high-carbohydrate diet and insulin in this case contributed to the patient's deteriorating kidney function. In such patients, where control of bodyweight and hyperglycemia is vital, a trial with a low-carbohydrate diet may be appropriate to avoid the risk of adding obesity-associated renal failure to already failing kidneys.

In Sweden the number of patients with type 2 diabetes accompanied by end-stage renal failure has increased by 80% since 1991. Control of blood glucose is crucial because of the proven link between HbA_{1c} and the rate of decline of the kidney function in diabetic nephropathy. Metabolic control in such patients is, however, difficult because the recommended low-fat diet with its high content of carbohydrates usually leads to a vicious cycle: hyperglycemia caused by the high-carbohydrate diet necessitates the use of insulin; efforts to normalise the blood glucose with insulin leads to increase of appetite and bodyweight; the rise of bodyweight exposes the patient to the risk of obesity-associated renal failure. A low-carbohydrate diet, however, is a potent antihyperglycemic remedy and may at the same time lead to weight loss."[249]

Here was the study's focus:

"An obese patient with type 2 diabetes whose diet was changed from the recommended high-carbohydrate, low-fat type to a low-carbohydrate diet showed a significant reduction in bodyweight, improved glycemic control and a reversal of a six year long decline of renal function. The reversal of the renal function was likely caused by both improved glycemic control and elimination of the patient's obesity."[250]

And the conclusion:

"We report here a significant reduction in body weight, improved glycemic control and reversal of a six year long decline of renal function in a patient with type 2 diabetes, whose diet we changed from the usually recommended high-carbohydrate, low-fat type to the opposite.

The present case report shows that a low-carbohydrate, high-fat diet improves glycemic control, reduces body weight and may prevent the development of end-stage renal failure in an overweight patient with type-2 diabetes. Furthermore, it raises the concern that the obesity caused by the combination of a high-carbohydrate diet and insulin may have contributed to the patient's failing kidney function."[251]

In a retrospective follow-up of previously studied subjects on a low carbohydrate diet, "Low-Carbohydrate Diet in Type 2 Diabetes. Stable Improvement of Bodyweight and Glycemic Control During 22 Months Follow-Up," (2006), by Jørgen Vesti Nielsen and Eva Joensson, the authors stated that:

"We previously reported that a 20% carbohydrate diet was significantly superior to a 55–60% carbohydrate diet with regard to bodyweight and glycemic control in 2 non-randomised groups of obese diabetes patients observed closely over 6 months. The effect beyond 6 months of reduced carbohydrate has not been previously reported. The objective of the present study, therefore, was to determine to what degree the changes among the 16 patients in the low-carbohydrate diet group at 6-months were preserved or changed 22 months after start, even without close follow-up. In addition, we report that, after the 6 month observation period, two thirds of the patients in the high-carbohydrate changed their diet. This group also showed improvement in bodyweight and glycemic control."[252]

The authors further stated that:

"Low-carbohydrate diets in the management of obese patients with type 2 diabetes seem intuitively attractive due to their potent antihyperglycemic effect."[253]

And concluded:

"Advice on a 20% carbohydrate diet with some caloric restriction to obese patients with type 2 diabetes has lasting effect on bodyweight and glycemic control."[254]

These are but a few of the recent research studies available on point. There are many, many more. For reviews of recent books on the subject of low-carbohydrate diets, see "Individual Reviews of a Dozen Books on

Low-Carb Diets," in *Malignant Medical Myths: Why Medical Treatment Causes 200,000 Deaths in the USA Each Year, and How to Protect Yourself*, by Joel M. Kauffman, Ph.D. (West Conshohocken, PA: Infinity, 2006).[255]

To conduct your own research, it will prove helpful to access the PubMed database, a service of the US National Library of Medicine and the National Institutes of Health, at the following web site: http://www.ncbi.nlm.nih.gov/sites/entrez?db=pubmed. Some of the articles you may be interested in reviewing that are available on the PubMed database have been provided in Appendix C, which lists low-carbohydrate related articles in descending order by year back to 1948.

And the last article from this book's Appendix C, written in 1948, "Control of Dental Caries by a Low Carbohydrate Diet,"[256] segues nicely to a fascinating article I reviewed as this book was getting ready to go to print.

In "Dietary Carbohydrates and Dental-Systemic Diseases," (2009), the author, Dr. Philippe Hujoel, describes the two competing hypotheses of dental-systemic health associations. From the abstract:

"Two contradictory hypotheses on the role of dietary carbohydrates in health and disease shape how dental-systemic associations are regarded. On one side, Cleave and Yudkin postulated that excessive dietary fermentable carbohydrate intake led—in the absence of dental interventions such as fluorides—*first* to dental diseases and *then* to systemic diseases. Under this hypothesis, dental and systemic diseases shared—as a common cause—a diet of excess fermentable carbohydrates. Dental diseases were regarded as an alarm bell for future systemic diseases, and restricting carbohydrate intake prevented both dental and systemic diseases. On the opposite side, Keys postulated the lipid hypothesis: that excessive dietary lipid intake caused systemic diseases. Keys advocated a diet high in fermentable carbohydrate for the benefit of general health, and dental diseases became regarded as local dietary side effects. Because general health takes precedence over dental health when it comes to dietary recommendations, dental diseases became viewed as local infections; interventions such as fluorides, sealants, oral hygiene, antimicrobials, and dental fillings became synonymous with maintaining dental health, and carbohydrates were no longer considered as a common cause for dental-systemic diseases. These opposing dietary hypotheses have increasingly been put to the test in clinical trials. The emerging trial results favor Cleave-Yudkin's hypothesis and may affect preventive approaches for dental and systemic diseases." [257]

And from body of the article, the author describes cause and effect:

"Fermentable carbohydrates are recognized as a necessary cause of dental caries. The United States' National Research Council, while advocating increased fermentable carbohydrate consumption for systemic health, reported that 'dental caries does not develop in the absence of fermentable carbohydrates' (NRC, 1989). The deceivingly simple rule 'no carbohydrates, no caries' appears to be strong not because of the presence of unequivocal randomized controlled trial evidence, but because of the inability to refute the hypothesis in a wide variety of research settings. For instance, in the Vipeholm study, it was reported that a "low carbohydrate, high fat diet depressed caries activity to practically nil" (Gustafsson *et al.*, 1954). The carbohydrate-caries connection has been documented in five continents, in humans and other animals, and as far back in time as archeology allows us to go.

Tribes who lived on an almost exclusively carnivorous diet rarely developed caries. The advent of agriculture and the development of staple crops that are high in carbohydrates increased caries prevalence (Hillson, 1996). For instance, around the Arabian Gulf, tribes living on an exclusively marine diet had virtually no caries, much like the Eskimos, whereas tribes consuming a mixture of the marine diet with carbohydrates had increased caries rates (Littleton and Frohlich, 1993). In another striking example, unprecedented high caries rates were observed in ancient Chileans upon the introduction of sticky fruit into the diet (Kelley and Larsen, 1991). The "no carbohydrates, no caries" dictum applies equally to animals. Gorillas eat less fruit than chimpanzees and also have less caries (Hillson, 1996)." [258]

I bring especially Dr. Hujoel's important article to your attention because the latest work on the correlation between carbohydrates, dental caries, and systemic health serves as a concise re-formulation of the first tome on the subject. The one book that should have changed the world of nutrition for good, often cited, denigrated by powerful interests of the carbohydrate-promoting industry, was written by a dentist, Weston A. Price, D.D.S., (1870-1948), in 1939. That book is *Nutrition and Physical Degeneration* (La Mesa, California: Price-Pottenger Nutrition Foundation,

2008), now in it's 18th printing, which details a series of ethnographic nutritional studies performed by Dr. Price across diverse cultures.

Price traveled the world over in order to study isolated human groups, including sequestered villages in Switzerland, Gaelic communities in the Outer Hebrides, Eskimos and Indians of North America, Melanesian and Polynesian South Sea Islanders, African tribes, Australian Aborigines, New Zealand Maori and the Indians of South America. Wherever he went, Dr. Price found that beautiful straight teeth, freedom from decay, stalwart bodies, resistance to disease and fine characters were typical of primitives on their traditional diets, rich in essential food factors.[259]

In his studies he found that plagues of modern civilization, including headaches, general muscle fatigue, dental caries, impacted molars, tooth crowding, allergies, heart disease, asthma, diabetes, and degenerative diseases such as tuberculosis and cancer, were not present in those cultures sustained by indigenous diets. However, within a single generation these same cultures experienced all the above listed ailments with the inclusion of Western foods in their diet: refined sugars, refined flours, canned goods, etc.[260]

And a major feature of native diets that Price found was that they were rich in fat. Whether from coconuts, insects, eggs, fish, game animals, or domesticated herds, primitive peoples knew that they would get sick if they did not consume enough fat. Dr. Price's research proved that dental decay is caused primarily by nutritional deficiencies, and that those conditions that promote decay also promote disease.

THE WAY THINGS OUGHT TO BE
(PART II)

So where do carbohydrates come in? According to one of the pre-eminent doctors studying diabetes and treating diabetics, Dr. Ron Rosedale, "they don't." What is the minimum daily requirement for carbohydrates? "Zero."

"I didn't say you can't have any carbs, I said fiber is good. Vegetables are great; I want you to eat vegetables. The practical aspect of it is that you are going to get carbs, but there is no essential need. The traditional Eskimo subsists on almost no vegetables at all, but they get their vitamins from organ meats and things like eyeball, which are a delicacy, or were.

So, you don't really need it, but sure, vegetables are good for you and you should eat them. They are part of the diet that I would recommend, and that is where you'll get your vitamin C. I recommend Vitamin C supplements, I don't have anything against taking supplements, I use a lot of them.

Fruit is a mixed blessing. You can divide food on a continuum. There are some foods that I really can't say anything good about and the other end of the spectrum are foods that are totally essential, like omega-3 fatty acids for instance, which most people are very deficient in, and even those have a detriment because they are highly oxidizable, so you had better have the antioxidant capacity. So if you are going to supplement with cod liver oil you should supplement with Vitamin E too or it will actually do you more harm than good.

Most foods fall somewhere in the middle of the continuum. For example, with strawberries you are going to get a lot of sugar, but you are also going to get a food that is the second or third highest in antioxidant potential of any food known, the first being garlic, the second either being strawberries or blueberries. I will let some patients put strawberries in, let's say, a protein smoothie in the morning. But if they are a hard core diabetic, strawberries are out.

It doesn't take much, any type I diabetic who is not producing any insulin can tell you what foods do to their blood sugar. It doesn't take much. What is very surprising to these people once they really measure is what little carbohydrate it takes to cause your blood sugar to skyrocket.

One saltine cracker will take the blood sugar to over 100, and in many people it will cause the blood sugar to go to 150 for a variety of reasons, not just the sugar in it.

We only have one hormone that lowers sugar, and that's insulin. Its primary use was never to lower sugar. We've got a bunch of hormones that raise sugar, cortisone being one and growth hormone another, and epinephrine and glucagon.

Our primary evolutionary problem was to raise blood sugar to give your brain and your nerves enough as well as, primarily, red blood cells, which require glucose. So from an evolutionary sense if something is important we have redundant mechanisms. The fact that we only have one hormone that lowers sugar tells us that it was never something important in the past.

So you get this rush of sugar and your body panics, your pancreas panics and it stores, when it is healthy, insulin in these granules that is ready to be released. It lets these granules out and it pours out a bunch of insulin to deal with this onslaught of sugar and what does that do?

Well the pancreas generally overcompensates, and it causes your sugar to go down, and just as I mentioned, you have got a bunch of hormones then to raise your blood sugar, they are then released, including cortisone. The biggest stress on your body is eating a big glucose load.

Then epinephrine is released too, so it makes you nervous, and it also stimulates your brain to crave carbohydrates, to seek out some sugar. So you are craving carbohydrates, so you eat a bowl of cheerios or a big piece of fruit so that after your sugar goes low, and with the hormone release, your sugars go way up again, which causes your pancreas to release more insulin and then it goes way down.

Now you are in to this sinusoidal wave of blood sugar, which causes insulin resistance. Your body can't stand that for very long so you are constantly putting out cortisone."[261]

So, according to Dr. Rosedale, most carbohydrates are out. This paradigm begs the question, "what's left to eat?"

> "I think you should be using fat as your primary energy source, and fat is kind of neutral when it comes to acidifying or alkalinizing. In general, over 50 percent of the calories should come from fat..."[262]

Dr. Rosedale adds that insulin is not the only cause of disease:

> "There are other considerations in disease, such as iron. We know that high iron levels are bad for you. If a person's ferritin is high, red meat is out for a while until the level goes down.
>
> There is a great deal of difference between a non-grain-fed cow and a grain-fed cow. Non-grain fed will have only 10 percent or less saturated fat. Grain-fed can have over 50 percent.
>
> Also, a non-grain-fed cow will actually be high in omega-3 oils. Plants have a pretty high percentage of omega-3, and if you accumulate it by eating it all day, every day for most of your life, your fat gets a pretty high proportion of omega-3. I would try for 50 percent oleic fat, and the other fats would depend on the individual, but about 25 percent of the other two.
>
> In a heavy diabetic I would probably go down on the saturated fat and go 60 percent oleic, and 1 to 1 on the omega-6 to 3 ratio—that would be therapeutic. The maintenance ratio would be about 2.5 to 1 for the omega-6 to 3 ratio. I would try to do most of this through diet. There are some practicalities involved. I would ask the person if they like fish and if they practically puke in front of me they are going on a tablespoon of cod liver oil, the best brand is made by Carlson, which doesn't taste fishy at all.
>
> Most people end up going on a supplement of omega-3 oils because they are not going to eat enough fish to get an adequate amount. It is a little hard to get that much entirely from diet.
>
> Sardines are a very good therapeutic food. They are baby fish so they haven't had time to accumulate a bunch of metal. They are smoked so they are not cooked and the oil is not spoiled in them. You have to eat the whole thing, not the boneless and skinless. You need to eat all the organs as they are high in vitamins and magnesium."[263]

Fat, protein, minimal carbohydrates, and supplements. That, according to Dr. Ron Rosedale, is the key to help prevent—except in the autoimmunal type I case—and by adding basal insulin to offset the Dawn Phenomenon[264] and provide long-acting control, treat diabetes.

From Dr. Ron Rosedale, we move to Richard K. Bernstein, M.D., whom I propose should be a future Nobel Laureate.[265,266]

Richard K. Bernstein, M.D., is a physician and an advocate for "normal blood sugars" through tight blood sugar control for diabetics to reduce risks and complications. Bernstein himself suffers from type 1 diabetes. His private medical practice in Mamaroneck, New York is devoted solely to diabetes and prediabetic conditions. He is a fellow of the American College of Nutrition and of the American College of Endocrinology and is a Diplomate of the American Academy of Wound Management. He is the author of four books on diabetes and normalizing blood sugars.[267]

In 1946, at the age of twelve, Richard Bernstein developed type 1 diabetes, and for more than two decades, Bernstein was what he calls, "an ordinary diabetic"—one who dutifully followed doctor's orders. Despite his diligence with maintaining the disease, the complications from his diabetes worsened over the years, and like many diabetics in similar circumstances, he faced death at a very early age as well as poor quality of life. By the time Bernstein reached his thirties, many of his body's systems began to deteriorate.

In October 1969, Dr. Bernstein came across an advertisement in the trade journal Lab World. It was for a new blood sugar meter that would give a reading in 1 minute, using a single drop of blood. The device was intended for emergency staff at hospitals to distinguish an unconscious diabetic and an unconscious drunk. The instrument weighed three pounds, cost $650, and was only available to certified physicians and hospitals. Determined to take control of his situation, Bernstein asked his wife, a doctor, to order the instrument for him.

Bernstein began to measure his blood sugar about 5 times each day, and soon realized that the levels fluctuated significantly throughout the day. To even out his blood sugars, he adjusted his insulin regimen from one injection per day to two, and experimented with his diet, notably by reducing his consumption of carbohydrates. Three years after Bernstein began monitoring his own blood sugar levels, his complications were still progressing and he began researching scientific articles about the disease. He discovered that complications from diabetes had repeatedly been prevented, and even reversed, in animals through normalizing blood sugars. This is in contrast to the then extant treatment of diabetes which focused on low-fat diets, preventing hypoglycemia, and ketoacidosis.

Bernstein set out to achieve normal blood sugars, and within a year had refined his insulin and diet to the point that they were normal throughout the day. After years of chronic fatigue and complications, Bernstein felt healthy and energized. His serum cholesterol and triglyceride levels were now in the normal ranges, and friends commented that his complexion was no longer gray. He is believed to be the first individual to self-monitor his blood sugar and was an early advocate for such monitoring by diabetics.

Bernstein believed that the same technique could be used to assist diabetics whose quality of life could vastly improve if they followed a similar lifestyle. Despite its effectiveness in treating his own condition, as a layperson he had difficulty gaining the necessary attention of the medical field to change the standard treatment of diabetics. Bernstein wrote a paper describing his technique and attempted to get it published in many major medical journals, but none would accept it, in part because he was not an MD. In 1977, he decided to give up his job and become a physician—"I couldn't beat 'em, so I had to join 'em."

At 45 years old, Richard Bernstein entered the Albert Einstein College of Medicine. In 1983 he opened his own medical practice near his home in Mamaroneck, New York.

In 2007, at 72 years of age, Bernstein has surpassed the life expectancy of type 1 diabetics at the time of his diagnosis. He attributes his longevity to the low-carbohydrate dietary approach and lifestyle changes he developed for diabetics.

Dr Bernstein's program for treating diabetes is highly regarded amongst his patients and achieves great blood sugar control, which reduces some or most of the complications associated with diabetes. The tradeoff is compliance with a very restricted diet and in cases of poor control, frequent testing and insulin shots. Dr. Bernstein strongly opposes the dietary guidelines from the American Diabetes Association (ADA) for both type I and type II diabetics.[268]

According to Dr. Bernstein in *The Diabetes Diet:*

> "The reason that a low-carb diet can help you become or remain slim is tightly linked to the hormone insulin, which is the principal fat-building hormone. The process works like this: the lower the amount of fast-acting or concentrated carbohydrate you eat, the less significant is the increase of your blood sugar. The less significant the effect on your blood sugar, the less of the fat-building hormone insulin you will need (either injected or made by your body) to stabilize blood sugar. With less insulin at large in your bloodstream, fats you eat will not be stored but metabolized (you will literally pee them away as water or breathe them away as carbon dioxide). In addition, as blood sugars decrease, the efficiency of insulin increases, further minimizing insulin levels in your body, with the result that existing body fat will start to metabolize as well—it will, as they say, just melt away."[269]

In *Dr. Bernstein's Diabetes Solution: The Complete Guide to Achieving Normal Blood Sugars*, Dr. Bernstein shares diet guidelines essential to the treatment of all diabetics:

"Research into creating replacement cells for burned-out insulin producing pancreatic beta cells is so promising that it's tempting to think of a "cure" not in terms of if but when. The reality is, however, less rosy. There may one day be a cure, but to put off normalizing your blood sugars until then is simply to ignore the reality of your situation. If you're going to control your diabetes and get on with a normal life, you will have to change your diet, and the when is now. No matter how mild or severe your diabetes, the key aspect of all treatment plans for normalizing blood sugars and preventing or reversing complications of diabetes is diet. In the terms of the Laws of Small Numbers, the single largest "input" you can control is what you eat." [270]

Dr. Bernstein discusses each of the macronutrients quite nicely in *The Diabetes Diet* and *Dr. Bernstein's Diabetes Solution: The Complete Guide to Achieving Normal Blood Sugars*. These books also contain information describing which foods to avoid and which foods to include in the diet, and also presents other foods that the reader may prefer to try such as toasted nori and frozen diet soda pops. Although he states that items such as nuts should be avoided, nut oil, highly recommended by Dr. Rosedale, should be included. Alcoholic beverages are also thoroughly discussed, as are strategies for mitigating blood sugar rises during illness and hospitalization.

And, of course, Dr. Bernstein is famous for his lipid profile. He states the following:

"Dare your physician. Ask him or her if his or her lipid profile on a low-fat diet can remotely compare to mine, on a high-fat, low carbohydrate diet:

LDL – the "bad" cholesterol – 63 (below 130 is considered normal)
HDL – the "good" cholesterol – 116 (above 30 is considered normal)
Triglycerides – 45 (below 150 is considered normal)
Lipoprotein(a) – undetectable (below 30 is considered normal)

Contrary to popular myth, fat is not a demon. It's the body's way of storing energy and maintaining essential organs such as the brain. Without essential fatty acids, your body would cease to function." [271]

The 100+ pages of recipes added at the end of Dr. Bernstein's *The Diabetic Diet* are innovative, delicious, and a great resource for anyone, diabetic or not, looking for healthy alternatives. You are encouraged to supplement Dr. Bernstein's advice with the remarkable book *Know Your Fats: The Complete Primer for Understanding the Nutrition of Fats, Oils, and Cholesterol,* by Mary G. Enig, Ph.D., which contains a survey of all the available oils and fats, their analysis, and in-depth discussions.[272]

As I wrote in my first book, the food pyramid presented by the USDA (http://www.mypyramid.gov/) is quite a good guide for diabetics, *if you turn it upside down.* And if you forgo fruits, whole grains, starches, and fat-free milk products. As a function of energy, each meal should be comprised of 50%-65% fat, 25%-35% protein, with as little carbohydrates as can be achieved. Please do perform your own search for information, and consult with your doctor, about supplement use to include aspirin,[*] chromium, vitamin D, fiber, niacin, vitamin B, vanadium, vitamin C, fish oil (EPA & DHA), cod liver oil, & others.[273]

The following figure, then, depicts what the food pyramid would look like when it incorporates all the research from this book:

---

[*] For a particularly good, brief history and discussion providing light on how the daily use of aspirin is unwarranted, see the chapter entitled "Myth 1: Taking an Aspirin a Day Forever Will Make You Live Longer," in *Malignant Medical Myths: Why Medical Treatment Causes 200,000 Deaths in the USA Each Year, and How to Protect Yourself,* by Joel M. Kauffman, Ph.D. West Conshohocken, PA: Infinity, 2006, pages 16-44.

Dr. Kauffman also provides a good overview of vitamin D: "Where there is inadequate daily sun exposure, oral doses of 1,000-2,000 IU/d are now considered routine, with much higher doses (up to 50,000 IU) for rapid repletion now considered safe." See "Benefits of Vitamin D Supplementation," by Joel M. Kauffman, Ph.D. *Journal of American Physicians and Surgeons,* Volume 14, Number 2, Summer, 2009. Available online at http://www.jpands.org/vol14no2/kauffman.pdf. Retrieved on 6/29/09.

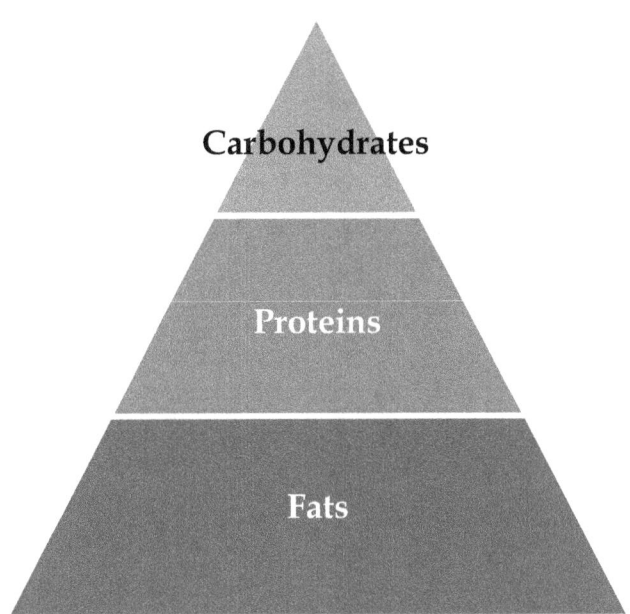

The Food Pyramid for People with Diabetes

Fats* and oils to include in your diet should include those consisting primarily of saturated fat, such as coconut oil and real cheese;[274] mono-unsaturated fat, such as macadamia nut oil and olive oil; and, in much smaller amounts, polyunsaturated oil, such as fish oil and flaxseed oil.

Speaking to the problems of polyunsaturated vegetable oils, Barry Groves in *Trick and Treat: How 'Healthy Eating' is Making us Ill*, states:

> "Of course the real problem with all vegetable oils is that they are not extracted by pressing; heats and solvents are used. Few fatty acids will stand up to that. Olive oil is only healthy because it comes from a super oily seed and can be produced in

---

* Note that all fats are part mono-unsaturated, part poly-unsaturated, & part saturated; do not use if partially or fully hydrogenated. For the best source of information about fats, see Mary G. Enig, Ph.D. *Know Your Fats: The Complete Primer for Understanding the Nutrition of Fats, Oils, and Cholesterol.* Silver Spring, MD: Bethesda Press, 2000.

a healthy manner; squashing fruits under a heavy object at ambient temperature. Olive oil — or any oil — that is extracted with heat and solvents can be expected to be as full of contaminants as the 2003 study shows canola oil to be."[275]

Other mostly saturated fats that could be used in the diet include cream, tallow, butter, cocoa butter, nutmeg butter and palm oil.[276] Other mostly mono-unsaturated fats include pecan oil, almond oil, avocado oil, sesame oil, chicken fat, duck fat, goose fat, turkey fat, peanut oil, lard, & canola oil;[277] and other mostly polyunsaturated oils include, black currant oil, borage oil, primrose oil, krill oil, cod liver oil & walnut oil.

In Dr. Mary Enig's seminal work — all her books are — *Eat Fat, Lose Fat,* she espouses the use of coconut oil* in every meal, as a snack, and in your tea. I'll take you through a few of her insights.

- "The body can use coconut oil for energy more rapidly and efficiently than any other fat source. Special fats in coconut (called medium-chain fatty acids, MCFAs) are not normally stored in your body as fat. Instead, they're quickly converted to energy, making coconut ideal for weight loss.
- Small amounts of the MCFAs in coconut oil are used in the complex processes that enable cells to communicate with each other.
- Coconut improves thyroid function in people with hypothyroid disease.
- People in countries where coconut is an important part of the diet have lower rates of heart disease and cancer than Americans. For example, a 1996 report by the National Cancer Institute lists Thailand (with the highest coconut consumption of any country in the world) as having the lowest cancer rates for both men and women out of the 50 countries studied. (No other coconut-eating countries were included in the survey.) Inhabitants of the Philippines have some of the lowest rates of heart disease in the world, according to a study published in the *Philippine journal of Internal Medicine,* 1992.
- Coconut oil is currently used in infant formulas and hospital invalid foods because it confers special health benefits. It's also used in sports drinks to help athletes produce lean body mass.
- The fats in coconut help fight infections of all kinds."[278]

---

* "There are no side effects from adding coconut oil products to your diet unless you are allergic to coconut. Even if you are, you can still probably take coconut oil, because the allergenic components of coconut are protein compounds found in the meat of the coconut, not in the oil." See Enig, Mary, and Fallon, Sally. *Eat Fat, Lose Fat*. New York: Penguin Group, First Plume Printing, 2006, page 16.

"Experts who promote the lipid hypotheses point to studies in which feeding coconut raised cholesterol levels in animals. However, the coconut oil used in these experiments was fully hydrogenated, that is, fully saturated with hydrogen, which turns all the fatty acids into saturated fats. (Partial hydrogenation creates mostly trans fatty acids, not all saturated fats.) The researchers were investigating the effects of essential fatty acid deficiency on the test animals, and full hydrogenation to eliminate all the essential fatty acids in the coconut oil. They used coconut oil because it is the only fat that can be fully hydrogenated and still be soft enough to eat.

As expected, the cholesterol levels in the animals went up, confirming other studies showing that essential fatty acid deficiency raises cholesterol levels. Yet, many commentators have pointed to this study as proof that coconut oil raises cholesterol levels, without mentioning that the researchers were not using natural coconut oil, but fully hydrogenated coconut oil that *created* the deficiency.

Other studies comparing various fats and oils found that coconut oil promoted the assimilation and storage of essential fatty acids, therefore *preventing* essential fatty acid deficiency. So it's the lack of essential fatty acids that created the health risk, not the coconut oil itself. And in these studies, an increase in cholesterol levels was simply a marker for another condition—not the *cause* of health problems." [279]

"Among saturated fats, coconut is queen because of its special properties," says Dr. Enig. "Coconut contains abundant medium-chain fatty acids (MCFAs), contains high amounts of lauric acid, and is synergistic with essential fatty acids." Dr. Enig concludes her discussion of coconut oil with the following written inset:

"How do lauric acid and monolaurin boost your immunity? They have antimicrobial properties and will help your body fight disease organisms, including:

- Viruses, such as herpes virus, measles virus, and HIV;
- Bacteria, such as listeria (which causes food poisoning), staphylococcus, and streptococcus;
- Protozoa (parasites), such as giardia lamblia (which causes gastro-enteritus)." [280]

For quite credible insight on the use of saturated fat specifically for those with diabetes, let's return to the review entitled "Dietary Carbohydrate Restriction in Type 2 Diabetes Mellitus and Metabolic Syndrome: Time for a Critical Appraisal," (2008), cited in the last chapter, written by a host of renowned doctors, researchers and diabetologists. Here the authors state:

> "A primary goal of current recommendations is to put limits on dietary saturated fat but published results are inconsistent. Several critical reviews have pointed up the general failure to meet the kind of unambiguous outcomes that would justify blanket condemnation of saturated fat, *per se*. Notably, during the obesity and diabetes epidemic, the proportion of dietary saturated fat decreased. In men, the *absolute* amount decreased by 14%. Similarly, the WHI revealed no difference in CVD incidence for people who consumed <10% saturated fat or those whose consumption was >14%. Dreon, et al., showed that increased saturated fat lead to a *decrease* in small, dense LDL.[281] Perhaps most remarkable was a study by Mozaffarian [et al.] which showed that greater intake of saturated fat was associated with *reduced* progression of coronary atherosclerosis; greater carbohydrate intake was linked to increased progression."[282, 283]

Since using cold-pressed coconut oil instead of macadamia nut oil—saturated fat instead of mono-unsaturated fat—as the predominant fat in my diet in 2008, all else nearly equal, at that time my VLDL level decreased from 26 to 15 mg/dL (a 38% decrease), my HDL level increased from 46 to 61 mg/dL (an increase of 33%), my LDL level was relatively unchanged, and my triglyceride level decreased from 132 to 81 mg/dL (a decrease of 39%). But, the real question is: does lowering LDL or raising HDL have anything to do with health? Does any of this business reduce the risk of heart disease?

In Uffe Ravnskov's brief response to an article on hypercholesterolemia and its management entitled *"Hypercholesterolaemia:* Should Medical Science Ignore the Past?" he provides support for his stance that revision of the cholesterol campaign by scientists without links to the food or drug industry are needed, and in so doing, provides a good summary of the arguments in favor of a diet high in fat:

- "No association between cholesterol and degree of atherosclerosis has been found in postmortem studies of unselected individuals.
- High cholesterol is not a risk factor for women, patients with renal failure, diabetic patients, or old people.[284]
- Old people with high cholesterol live longer than those with low cholesterol.[285]
- In cohorts of people with familial hypercholesterolaemia, cholesterol is not associated with the incidence or prevalence of cardiovascular disease, and their average life span is similar to other peoples'.
- No randomised, controlled, unifactorial, dietary, cholesterol lowering trial has ever succeeded in lowering coronary or total mortality.[286]
- No clinical or angiographic trial has found exposure-response between individual degree of cholesterol lowering and outcome.[287]
- More than 20 cohort studies found that patients with coronary heart disease ate the same amount of saturated fat as did healthy controls.[288]
- Seven of 10 cohort studies found that patients with stroke ate less saturated fat than did healthy controls.
- The concentration of short chain fatty acids in adipose tissue, the most reliable reflection of saturated fat intake, is similar or lower in patients with coronary heart disease compared with healthy individuals in five case-control studies.
- The effect of statin treatment is grossly overstated and is not due to cholesterol lowering.[289] Only a small percentage gain benefit—and then only if they are men at high risk—and the benefit is easily outweighed by side effects that are more common and more serious than reported in the statin trials, if reported at all.[290"][291]

I cannot possibly do the subject of cholesterol and heart disease justice. There are, however, many great, recent books on the subject that I can point you to that provide a good discussion of both. What they all have in common, as de Lorgeril and Salan have recently pointed out, is that the risk of sudden coronary death is independent of total cholesterol and LDL, and sudden coronary death accounts for over 50% of all cardiac mortality. In fact, careful analysis of the available data, including randomised trials, indicates that, contrary to a widespread opinion, cholesterol lowering does not appear to be a very effective way of reducing cardiac and overall mortality in the general population.[292]

Ischemic heart disease is *not* developed from plaque made up of particles of fat and cholesterol that stick to the artery walls like sewage inside a pipe; rather, it is arterial muscle tissue, white blood cells, collagen, calcium, blood platelets, and more, that gets trapped as boils within the first and second layers of the arterial wall that serves as the genesis of atherosclerosis.[293] Subsequent clot formation after the contents of the plaque — better described as a boil — bursts through the arterial wall is the most likely cause of a coronary event.

For an accessibly written tome attributing ischemic heart disease to anergy,* bacteria, prothrombin, homocysteine, and increased iron — that the vulnerable atherosclerotic plaque, better called a boil, is produced by neutrophil leucocytes — and not by cholesterol *per se*, you are encouraged to read *Fat and Cholesterol are Good for You! What Really Causes Heart Disease*, by Uffe Ravnskov, MD, PhD (Sweden: GB Publishing, 2009).[294]

Kilmer S. McCully, MD, is recognized as the first person to discover and propose the homocysteine theory of heart disease in 1969. His book, *The Heart Revolution: The Extraordinary Discovery That Finally Laid the Cholesterol Myth to Rest* (New York: Perennial, 1999), is simply fascinating, albeit his diet includes a large percentage of carbohydrates. Not to worry; we can easily incorporate his advice without adhering to his diet. According to Dr. McCully:

> "When there is too much homocysteine in the blood, arteries are damaged and plaques form. The result is arteriosclerosis and heart disease. This happens when we don't get enough of certain vitamins — namely B6, B12, and folic acid. These B vitamins are missing in our diets because processing and refining foods (think white flour, sugar, and canning) destroys these sensitive vitamins."[295]

Incidentally, Kilmer S. McCully and Uffe Ravnskov collaborated on a paper in 2009, specifically identifying the mechanism by which heart

---

* Anergy is defined by Dr. Ravnskov as a condition where the immune system is functioning poorly; people who have anergy are therefore at high risk of infectious diseases. See Ravnskov, Uffe. *Fat and Cholesterol are Good for You.* Sweden: GP Publishing, 2009, page 24.

disease is developed, something that has never been done in the alternative lipid-heart hypothesis of heart disease.[296]

Another good, recent book on cholesterol is *The Great Cholesterol Con: The Truth About What Really Causes Heart Disease and How to Avoid It*, by Dr. Malcolm Kendrick (London, England: John Blake Publishing, Ltd., 2008). See also *Trick and Treat: How 'Healthy Eating' is Making us Ill*, by Barry Groves (London, UK: Hammersmith Press Limited, 2008). And see Anthony Colpo's *The Great Cholesterol Con: Why Everything You've Been Told About Cholesterol, Diet and Heart Disease is Wrong!* (Distributed by Lulu, 2006). Mr. Colpo's book is especially focused and informative, presenting and analyzing all the relevant medical studies. In addition, he highlights the terribly negative effects of high blood sugar in the formation of free radicals, which, unlike cholesterol, are a causal, not secondary, factor in the development of cardiovascular disease. However, he writes:

> "In the Diabetes Control and Complications Trial, early and intensive treatment to keep blood sugar levels close to normal in type I diabetics slashed the risk of cardiovascular disease by forty-two percent, and cut the risk of heart attack and stroke by fifty-seven percent—far better results than those achieved by any cholesterol or blood pressure drug."[297]

I doubt he realized that this result was achieved through a diet of 45%-55% carbohydrates, plus intensive treatment of insulin, with significant risk of hypoglycemia. Had he known this information, he most likely would not have included the reference, attesting to the power of the DCCT meme.

And, for a particularly good, in-depth discussion of VLDLs, HDLs, IDLs, and LDLs, see *Good Calories, Bad Calories*, by Gary Taubes (New York: Anchor Books, 2008, pages 153-177).

One fervent proponent of the very low-fat diet is Dean Ornish, though his arguments are defeated by Sally Fallon and Mary Enig, Ph.D., in *Eat Fat Lose Fat*:

"...Nor, sadly, did Ornish find any real evidence that this diet [a very low-fat diet] lives up to its claim to protect you from heart disease. The study that launched the Ornish program, published in *The Lancet* in 1990, did not actually look at the long-term outcome of a severely fat-restricted diet. Instead, the researchers used a diagnostic technique called angiography to measure the diameter of the coronary arteries in a small group of patients (22 in the experimental group and 19 in the control group). They found that those on the low-fat diet had slightly more widening of the arteries. But no conclusions can be drawn from this finding because as arteries begin to get clogged [within the endothelial layers per Colpo, Ravnskov, Groves, Kendrick, et al.] they actually widen a bit. It's only after the clogging becomes serious that the arteries narrow. Thus, the slight widening that the Ornish researchers measured could have resulted from the arteries becoming more clogged, not less!

Patients in the treatment group did at first report lessened angina (chest pain), but after five years there was no difference between the two groups in the frequency or amount of angina. Nor did the researchers follow up to see how the study group fared in the long term.

Another flaw of this study was that very few people could be persuaded to stay on the diet. Of the 53 initially selected for the experimental group, only 28 agreed to participate after the program was explained to them. Subsequently, a few more dropped out, and one died during heavy exercise. As a result, so few were left in the experimental group that the researchers could not draw any valid conclusions."[298]

Returning to our discussion of macronutrients, protein sources include all varieties of fish, sashimi,[299] beef, pork, fowl, whey, fermented soy,[300] and eggs.[301] Remember that some carbohydrates and fat are present in animal muscle; seek non-grain fed animal products.

Vegetables are the recommended carbohydrates to consume and should be eaten raw, which tends to raise blood sugar much slower than cooked vegetables. Acceptable vegetables include artichoke hearts, asparagus,[302] bamboo shoots, beet greens, bell peppers, bok choy, broccoli, Brussels sprouts, cabbage, celery, collard greens, daikon radish, dandelion greens, eggplant, endive, escarole, hearts of palm, kohlrabi, mushrooms, mustard greens, okra, pumpkin, radicchio, rhubarb, sauerkraut, scallions, snow peas, spinach, string beans, squash, turnip greens, turnips, water chestnuts, watercress, and zucchini.

You may be familiar with these lines from T. S. Eliot's poem *The Little Gidding*:

> "We shall not cease from exploration
> And the end of all our exploring
> Will be to arrive where we started
> And know the place for the first time." [303]

These lines sum up the sentiments of coming full circle. Arriving back where we started, we seek new answers to old questions, and pose new questions to old answers. We thus find this place anew; possibly, we find ourselves renewed. Review the diet described above again—fat, mostly saturated including coconut oil; beef, seafood, and eggs, called protein today; and restricted carbohydrates. Does it not look surprisingly similar to the diet described by John Rollo, Charles Purdy, and Richard Thomas Williamson more than a century ago?

- - - - - - -

Most of our lives we are caught up in the moment. Let us now take a moment to look at diabetes from 10,000 feet up, where we can see clear patterns and insight emerge from the fog of hypoglycemia, and its opposite, hyperglycemia. If we plot carbohydrate consumption from low to high on the y-axis, and injected, fast acting (bolus) insulin from low to high on the x-axis, we can see all possible combinations of expected results on the following matrix:

	Low	Medium	High
High	Eats carbohydrates at will; Hyperglycemia; Ketoacidosis; A1c > 7%; Polyuria; Polydipsia; Polyphagia; Glycosuria; DKA; Dementia	Hyperglycemia	Hypo-Hyperglycemic rollercoaster ride
Medium	Hyperglycemia	Eats balanced meals; Injects both basal & bolus insulin; Attains A1c < 7% with great effort; Blood pressure increasing over time; Weight increasing over time; Moderate exercise	Hypoglycemia
Low	Eats fat, protein, & minimal carbohydrates; Injects optimimal amount of basal Insulin & zero bolus insulin; Maintains A1c < 7% effortlessly; Frequent light exercise	Hypoglycemia	Hypoglycemia

Carbohydrate Consumption (vertical axis)

Injected Bolus Insulin (horizontal axis)

When injected bolus insulin is low or zero, and carbohydrate consumption is high, we are presented with the classical triad of diabetes symptoms: polyuria, polydipsia, and polyphagia: respectively, frequent urination, increased thirst and consequent increased fluid intake, and increased appetite. Other manifestations will include weight loss (despite normal or increased eating), irreducible fatigue, and changes in the shape of the lenses of the eyes, resulting in vision changes.

When the glucose concentration in the blood is raised beyond the renal threshold, reabsorption of glucose in the proximal renal tubuli is incomplete, and part of the glucose remains in the urine (glycosuria).

Patients may also present with diabetic ketoacidosis (DKA), an extreme state of metabolic dysregulation characterized by the smell of acetone on the patient's breath; a rapid, deep breathing known as Kussmaul breathing; nausea; vomiting and abdominal pain; and any altered states of consciousness or arousal such as hostility and mania or, equally, confusion and lethargy. In severe DKA, coma may follow, progressing to death.

Surrounding this cell on the matrix is hyperglycemia, both to the right, when carbohydrates consumed are high and injected insulin is moderate, but not enough to cover the load, and below, when a decrease in carbohydrates is consumed, but still not offset enough by injected insulin.

In the middle of the chart, where one eats a moderate amount of carbohydrates and injects a moderate amount of bolus insulin, lies the typical diabetes treatment. Remember, however, that we defined a moderate intake of carbohydrates in the first chapter as 30%-40% of calories; anything more than that could very well be considered high. "Eat a balanced diet and learn to adjust your insulin accordingly" is the principal treatment that is followed here. It is possible to attain near-normal A1c levels with this approach, i.e., with great effort, however, normal bodyweight may prove unreachable.

Furthermore, this area of the table is fraught with negative consequences at nearly all adjacent and opposite borders. Not enough insulin puts one in hyperglycemia territory both to the left and above. Not enough carbohydrates, and one finds themselves hypoglycemic to the right and below.

At the other extreme, when injected insulin is high, and carbohydrates consumed are too low, severe hypoglycemia could result, necessitating a visit from the local paramedics when subsequent low blood glucose causes unconsciousness. If not attended to quickly, coma and death could occur.

Too, if carbohydrates and insulin injected are high, the result is a hyper-hypo-glycemic swing—a rollercoaster ride if you will—of great magnitude, where the patient is constantly adjusting carbohydrate and insulin loads to offset their blood sugar.

But look what happens when both carbohydrates consumed and insulin injected are as low as possible. At the far lower-left cell of the matrix, one doesn't eat a great many carbohydrates, and, subsequently, does not need to inject much insulin as a result. In this case, one can achieve a stable, normal blood sugar concentration and enjoy the benefits of a healthy, happy life including a stable or decreasing weight, and less anxiety not having to think about whether one has injected the right amount of bolus insulin or eaten the right amount of carbohydrates several times daily. And testing can be reduced to once a day, in the morning, to validate your successful basal insulin dosing, i.e., whether or not your morning BG is in the 70-110 mg/dL range. This home base is where thriving begins.

At the zero bolus-insulin and near-zero carbohydrate home, you may thrive for a long, long time. There are three major centenarian studies going on around the world.[*] According to Dr. Ron Rosedale:

> "They are trying to find the variable that would confer longevity among this group of people who live to be 100 years old. Why do centenarians become centenarians? Why are they so lucky? Is it because they have low cholesterol, exercise a lot and live a healthy, clean life?

> What researchers are finding from these major centenarian studies is that there is hardly anything in common among these people. They have high cholesterol and low cholesterol, some exercise and some don't, some smoke, some don't. Some are nasty as can be, some nice and calm and some are ornery. But, they all have relatively low sugar for their age, and they all have low triglycerides for their age. And, they all have relatively low insulin...The way to treat virtually all of the so-called chronic diseases of aging is to treat insulin itself." [304]

---

[*] See the New England Centenarian Study online at http://www.bumc.bu.edu/Dept/Home.aspx?departmentid=361, the Georgia Centenarian Study online at http://www.geron.uga.edu/research/centenarianstudy.php, and the Okinawa Centenarian Study online at http://www.okicent.org/.

Although the use of exogenous bolus insulin as a treatment to mitigate the effects of carbohydrate consumption was innovative, exciting, and promising nearly a century ago, its use has become — save on the acutely serious hyperglycemic — obsolete with the development of synthetic basal insulin, and the knowledge that carbohydrates are non-essential.

A remarkable picture develops when you take those three highlighted cells from the previous figure and place them on two different axes, one a continuum of complexity from low to high, and the other, a continuum of knowledge, skill, efficiency, and effectiveness, again, from low to high.

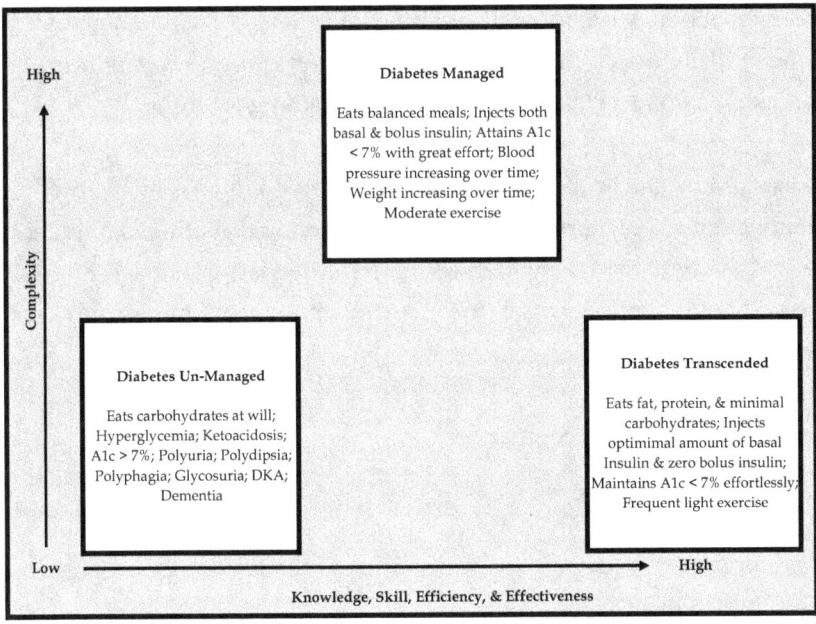

The y-axis, complexity, relates to the treatment — medication & nutrition — and lifestyle a person implements or recommends. Regarding the x-axis, knowledge, skill, efficiency, and effectiveness, it could be looked at from two perspectives; one, from a diabetic's perspective, where the focus is on their knowledge & skill as it relates to implementing advice from a third-party or self-directed behavior, and another, from the perspective of a third-party's knowledge & skill, be it friend, relative, caregiver, nutritionist, nurse, or doctor. Treatment efficiency and effectiveness in either case is also measured.

The lowest complexity matched with the lowest skill & knowledge, will result in a diabetic on the brink. It is quite easy for them to eat carbohydrates at will and develop the hyperglycemic symptoms of full-blown diabetes: polyuria, glycosuria, polydipsia, polyphagia, ketoacidosis, weight loss, etc., culminating in shortened life span. Knowledge for the patient about diabetes may be non-existent, and they will likely seek out medical attention for help, though, unfortunately, some don't or for many reasons even if they do, helpful advice is not available. Acquaintances will also most likely notice the change in persona or appearance, and they too will make it a point to tell the person that something is wrong.

"Diabetes Managed" represents a diabetic trying to follow the instructions and advice of his or her general practitioner, though both are influenced by a wide variety of stakeholders with oftentimes divergent self-interests. A majority of the influencers in the medical advice providing supply chain include:

- Pharmaceutical companies
- Researchers
- Doctors
- Endocrinologists[305]
- Nutritionists
- Educators
- American Diabetes Association
- World Health Organization
- Medical schools
- Nurses
- Reference media such as *the Physician's Desk Reference*[306]

- Food manufacturers
- Food marketers
- Popular internet sites, print media & the news
- Friends, family, co-workers & acquaintances

By default, advocates of each group act in their own perceived best interest, based upon their knowledge and skill, which may in turn be based upon the state of information available at their time of training or education. Many of the above stakeholders, with the exception of the end users themselves — the people with diabetes — have significant power. In fact, some have a near-absolute advantage in the marketplace — the ability to influence behavior without question or pause — leaving the buyer of an optimal diabetes treatment treating their diabetes sub-optimally, i.e., carbohydrate & bolus-insulin intensive.

And the results? Perhaps an HbA$_{1c}$ at or below 7%, weight gain, increasing blood pressure, too much time spent counting carbohydrates and measuring insulin doses, anxiety caused by constantly wondering whether or not too much or too little carbohydrates were eaten or insulin dosed, the ever present chance of hypo- or hyper-glycemia, constant blood sugar testing, and the list goes on. "Diabetes Managed" may not achieve optimal results for the end user, but, for the other stakeholders, it brings and keeps customers longer.

Although the science behind the drugs that either limit the amount of glycogen released from the liver or that bind and carry glucose from the blood to the receptors that transport it across cell membranes is remarkable, it is based upon two assumptions: (I) that carbohydrates are an essential majority part of the diet, and/or (II) that through education, a patient cannot, will not, or should not keep from consuming them. Remove those key assumptions, and the house of cards from which that remarkable science is based comes toppling down.

Caveat emptor. "Diabetes Managed" may be the first natural step for diabetics to enter — a complex medical-advice-providing system — in progression of their self-treatment, but it doesn't have to be.

As knowledge about diabetes increases, trusted advisers and patients alike will choose a less-complex method, one that transcends diabetes by avoiding the root cause of symptoms and complications — carbohydrates — and, instead, consuming fat & protein only, resulting in benefits such as healthy weight loss, satiety, reduced mTOR activity,[307] normal blood pressure, etc.; in short, leading to a longer, happier,[308] healthier life.

To transcend diabetes requires reduced carbohydrate consumption to near zero, with emphasis on a combination of fat and protein. It is orders of magnitude less complex, less worrisome, and less risky than counting carbohydrates and matching it with doses of bolus insulin. It is simple.[*] The above becomes quite easy to optimize in the following model discussed previously:

$$BG_{70} \leq f(Q_{Gly}, IS, Q_{IA}, Q_{XI\text{-basal}}, A, Q_{Sleep}, THP) + \alpha \leq BG_{110}$$

When the blood sugar function is optimized this way, then, a new, refreshing meaning to the words of Frederick G. Banting, largely credited for the idea behind the work which led to the discovery of insulin, becomes evident:

> "...with the relief of the symptoms of the disease...the pessimistic, melancholy diabetic becomes optimistic and cheerful."[309]

---

[*] According to Occam's razor, all other things being equal, the simplest theory is the most likely to be true — hence the importance of the concept of simplicity in epistemology. Simplicity is a meta-scientific criterion by which to evaluate competing theories. The similar concept of Parsimony is also used in philosophy of science, that is the explanation of a phenomenon which is the least involved is held to have superior value to a more involved one. The definition provided by Stanford Encyclopedia of Philosophy is that "Other things being equal, simpler theories are better."

DILEMMAS

"No one in this world, so far as I know, has ever lost money by underestimating the intelligence of the great masses of the plain people."

H.L. MENCKEN, *Chicago Tribune*, September 19, 1926

This book was written in the conviction that an optimal solution to diabetes once presented a great mystery, but that it is a mystery no longer because it is solved.[310]   Dr. Richard Bernstein solved the problem by experimenting with his diet, notably by reducing his consumption of carbohydrates. In so doing, Dr. Bernstein validated the work done nearly a century before him by Richard Thomas Williamson, Charles Purdy, and many others, who, of course, validated John Rollo's solution recommended 100 years before them. We have added, and shall continue to add, footnotes to the optimal solution, such as developing the insulins glargine & detemir that enable us type 1s to achieve a normal, stable blood sugar level in our sleep, upon awakening, and throughout the day.

Too, I wrote this book because I continue to be surprised and dismayed that so many people seem not only unaware of the elegant and beautiful *dietary* solution to our problem; but, incredibly, actually many are unaware what the problem is in the first place!

There are two problems, really. First, diabetes mellitus manifests itself in our bodies as ineffective carbohydrate processing due to an insulin function disturbance; we produce too much, too little, or none at all. And second, the optimal solution espoused by would-be health-providers may be optimal for their needs, not ours. Humbly, though passionately, I hope that my books — and the citations therein — have removed all sane doubt as to the veracity of the first problem and its solution. Explaining, proving then solving the second problem is the focus of this chapter.

So to present this material, let me briefly introduce an effective framework for understanding relationships between people with opposing interests, the basis of all dilemmas. We will then apply this device to a couple of real-world scenarios. "Game theory" is thus our topic, William Poundstone our teacher, *Prisoner's Dilemma* our textbook, and the decision strategy of a couple of imprisoned gang members our subject.

Two members of a criminal gang are arrested and imprisoned. Each prisoner is in solitary confinement with no means of speaking to or exchanging messages with the other. The police admit they don't have enough evidence to convict the pair on the principal charge. They plan to sentence both to a year in prison on a lesser charge. Simultaneously, the police offer each prisoner a Faustian bargain. If he testifies against his partner, he will go free while the partner will get three years in prison on the main charge. Oh, yes, there is a catch. If *both* prisoners testify against each other, both will be sentenced to two years in jail.[311]

The prisoners are given little time to think this over, but in no case may either learn what the other has decided until he has irrevocably made his decision. Each is informed that the other prisoner is being offered the very same deal. Each prisoner is concerned only with his own welfare—with minimizing his own prison sentence. The below 2x2 matrix graphically depicts the scenario. Note that the first number in each cell is the payoff in terms of jail time for the row player, "A," and the second number in each cell is the payoff in terms of jail time for the column player, "B."

	B refuses deal	B turns state's evidence
A refuses deal	1 year, 1 year	3 years, 0 years
A turns state's evidence	0 years, 3 years	2 years, 2 years

The prisoners can reason as follows: "Suppose I testify and the other prisoner doesn't. Then I get off scot-free, rather than spending a year in jail. Suppose I testify and the other prisoner does too. Then I get two years, rather than three. Either way I'm better off turning state's evidence. *Testifying takes a year off my sentence, no matter what the other guy does.*"

The trouble is, the other prisoner can and will come to the very same conclusion. If both parties are rational, both will testify and both will get two years in jail. If only they had both refused to testify, they would have got just a year each!

And so ends this short but prophetic tale. For a great primer on game theory, you are encouraged to read William Poundstone's classic book *Prisoner's Dilemma: John Von Neumann, Game Theory, and the Puzzle of the Bomb* (New York: Doubleday, 1992). Here we will move from theoretical games to the actual challenge, for that is where we — fellow members of the club — find ourselves.

You go to your health-provider(s) with the classical triad of symptoms of polyuria, polydipsia, and polyphagia — respectively, frequent urination, increased thirst and consequent increased fluid intake, and increased appetite — with the hope that they are more knowledgeable than you and will help you find an optimal solution. But therein lies the dilemma: your health-provider(s) may not be fully vested in your interests alone.

Much has been written on the subject. In "Conflict of Interest in Clinical Practice," (2007), first published in *Chest*, the author Mark R. Tonelli, M.D., M.A., FCCP, provides some background:

> "The inherent tension built into remuneration for the healing arts has been recognized as far back as Plato, who devoted a small part of *The Republic*[312] to the issue.[313] In a classic fee-for-service arrangement, physicians benefit financially from the provision of more interventions, with patients and the market poorly positioned to make judgments regarding the necessity of these services.[314]

Historically, a physician's service largely equated with the physician's presence, but systemic conflicts of interest could still arise, such as agreements for fee splitting from referrals or commissions from pharmacies. As the number and kinds of medical services have exploded over the last half-century, so has the potential for clinicians to profit from the profligate use of these services. The practice of medicine now provides the entrepreneurial physician with ample opportunities to develop ancillary business interests, such as owning radiology and other diagnostic or therapeutic centers or equipment, even entire hospitals.[315] Clearly, the attendant financial gain in "self-referring" a patient for testing or intervention under such circumstances creates a conflict of interest as, logically, only a subset of patients will be likely to benefit from the additional procedures, whereas all patients (at least all those with the ability to pay) sent for testing or intervention would financially benefit the physician-owner. Empiric evidence amply demonstrates that such circumstances lead not simply to a perceived conflict of interest, but to a marked increase in utilization of services when compared to financially disinterested clinicians."[316,317]

We're primarily concerned with the ongoing treatment of diabetes, so, admittedly, there's little to worry that your general practitioner will recommend visiting a radiologist in exchange for a small referral fee when presented with your potential blood sugar surges. There are, however, other ancillary service providers in the supply chain that would be happy to pay a small referral fee for a new customer, e.g., an endocrinologist, dietician, exercise trainer, laboratory technician. The predominant source of referrals, better stated, gifts, as the authors of the article suggest, are the pharmaceutical and medical device providers.

"Over the last several years, particular professional and public attention has been focused on conflicts of interest that arise from various relationships between the pharmaceutical and medical device industries and clinicians.[318] Businesses that happen to make drugs or medical devices have interests that are no different than those of other businesses: maximizing shareholder value, generally by increasing sales.[319] The profession of medicine, in general, and individual practitioners, in particular, continue to embrace a primary goal of improving and maintaining the health and well-being of individual patients. A conflict of interest develops when interactions with industry create circumstances in which the individual physician's interest coincides with that of business, not patients. Beyond appearances, such conflicts have demonstrated the potential to alter physician practice in a manner that favors the pharmaceutical industry at the expense of the patient. Multiple specific interactions between industry and clinicians, including gift giving, consultancy arrangements, support of CME and guideline development, create conflicts of interest that vary in terms of effect, but each acts to bias the clinician away from patients and toward the interests of industry." [320,321]

And, in case you wondering about the percentage of doctors receiving these gifts, there was a study performed recently that provides that information. In "A National Survey of Physician-Industry Relationship," (2007), the authors surveyed physicians to collect information about their financial associations with industry and the factors that predict those associations. They conducted a national survey of 3,167 physicians in six specialties (anesthesiology, cardiology, family practice, general surgery, internal medicine, and pediatrics) in late 2003 and early 2004. The raw response rate for this probability sample was 52%. Here are the results:

"Most physicians (94%) reported some type of relationship with the pharmaceutical industry, and most of these relationships involved receiving food in the workplace (83%) or receiving drug samples (78%). More than one third of the respondents (35%) received reimbursement for costs associated with professional meetings or continuing medical education, and more than one quarter (28%) received payments for consulting, giving lectures, or enrolling patients in trials. Cardiologists were more than twice as likely as family practitioners to receive payments. Family practitioners met more frequently with industry representatives than did physicians in other specialties, and physicians in solo, two-person, or group practices met more frequently with industry representatives than did physicians practicing in hospitals and clinics." [322]

The results of this national survey indicate that relationships between physicians and industry are common and underscore the variation among such relationships according to specialty, practice type, and professional activities.

And as you delve deeper into the literature, specifically on the results of medical practice, the information can leave you feeling quite pessimistic. According to Dr. Joseph Mercola, in his popular natural health website:

"The traditional medical paradigm contains fatal flaws that have led to this startling statistic: doctors are the third leading cause of death in this country killing a quarter million people a year. Cancer and heart disease are the only two causes that have killed more people. Drugs, surgeries and hospitals are rarely the answer to chronic health problems. Diet, exercise, and lifestyle are the key components to staying healthy."[323]

Hard to believe; but, if there was nothing to the theory of good doctors doing what they were trained to do with poor results, then surely if there were periods in recent memory without available doctors, we would see sickness and/or death rates *increasing*. Alas, the evidence points in the opposite direction. According to Barry Groves in *Trick and Treat: How 'Healthy Eating' is Making us Ill*, Israel, Canada, the US, and Columbia share a common occurrence:

"Doctors don't often go on strike, but it has happened sufficiently often for a disturbing trend to be noticed. During the rare times that they have gone on strike — in several countries — the death rate has always gone down."[324]

Once again, you're probably a step ahead of this writing, so, yes, a read of *Do We Still Need Doctors* by John D. Lantos, MD, may be indicated here.[325] Although it is an interesting book, the issues involved in the disintermediation of an entire channel from the marketplace are a bit overwhelming, so I won't discuss here whether or not we need doctors other than to say that more likely than not — outside of acute emergency medical situations, and to prescribe basal insulin and delivery devices — as we will see, they probably need you more. The plain and simple fact is: we *will* see a doctor.

Whatever it is that doctors do — primarily consult with patients — potential customers have the perception that doctors may provide hope; they know or can at least access information and products that patients do not know or cannot access without the aid and support of, yes, doctors. We call this phenomenon "information asymmetry," and sufficient demand for doctors is all the driving force necessary to incentivize a supply for them in the marketplace. Vice-versa, a supply of doctors in the marketplace will induce demand. When tastes, preferences, and population are held constant, the only true, measurable variables are the price paid for by patients, received by doctors, based upon the *quantity* of services exchanged between them. Service *quality* may be an assumption by those on the demand side, but aside from government- and industry-mandated requirements, not much else enters into the equation.

So let us now return to discuss this specific, real-life diabetic's dilemma. There are two cases here: 1) you are not prepared with any information, or 2) you have done your homework. Let's take a look first at those that are not prepared and, instead, will rely on their doctor to give the optimal treatment with the intent on following it.

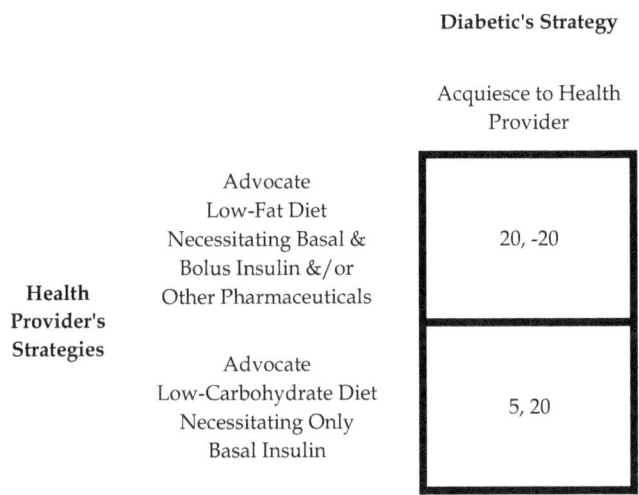

		Diabetic's Strategy
		Acquiesce to Health Provider
Health Provider's Strategies	Advocate Low-Fat Diet Necessitating Basal & Bolus Insulin &/or Other Pharmaceuticals	20, -20
	Advocate Low-Carbohydrate Diet Necessitating Only Basal Insulin	5, 20

The above table shows the asymmetrical relationship. Note that the real power comes from the health-provider's strategy, as they ultimately decide which treatment the diabetic will follow, and, subsequently, the payoffs. Although the payoffs noted in the table are assertions, those assertions are based upon the evidence presented in the previous chapter. Recall that the first number is the payoff for the row player, the health-provider, and the second number is the payoff for the column player, the diabetic. The numbers themselves are somewhat arbitrary, however, they are used here for illustrative purposes; namely, that a low-fat diet, with corresponding necessity for a high consumption of carbohydrates, will lead to an increase in free radicals and oxidative stress in the body, and, if bolus insulin is taken, the risk of hypoglycemia is ever-present. When the health-provider recommends, and the diabetic follows, the low-fat diet, utilizing both basal and bolus insulin, and perhaps other drugs too, the diabetic's payoff is -20.

"Health-provider" is a deliberately general title, as it may include all those influencers noted in the previous chapter and more, including pharmaceutical companies, pharmacists, researchers, doctors, endocrinologists, nutritionists, educators, the American Diabetes Association, the World Health Organization, medical schools, nurses, reference media such as *the Physician's Desk Reference*, food manufacturers, food marketers, popular internet sites, print media, the news, friends, family, co-workers & acquaintances.

Moreover, the payoff at this point for the diabetic is -20 because the diabetic now returns again and again for checkups, providing a fee to the clinic each time; some of the stated health-providers, doctors especially, are in the business of patient management. This system keeps the dutiful patient coming back for regular doctor appointments, while at the same time keeping the pharmacist busy refilling prescriptions. And medical insurance coverage becomes an absolute necessity. Of course, the health-provider's payoff is +20, because they're the ones being paid. They espouse party-line mis-information due to the constraints of their clinical practice guidelines; and, given the perceived information asymmetry, most patients will believe them. The final irony is the report that physicians frequently choose low-carbohydrate diets for themselves while recommending low-fat for their patients.[326]

Now let's imagine the case of a symmetrical relationship between health-providers and diabetics. In the next table, we'll enable the diabetic with power of his/her own: the ability to make an informed choice regarding their treatment, based upon the insight imparted by cited authors.

		Diabetic's Strategies	
		Acquiesce to Health Provider	Insist on a Low-Carbohydrate Diet
Health Provider's Strategies	Advocate Low-Fat Diet Necessitating Basal & Bolus Insulin &/or Other Pharmaceuticals	20, -20	**5, 20**
	Advocate Low-Carbohydrate Diet Necessitating Only Basal Insulin	5, 20	5, 20

In *Prisoner's Dilemma*, William Poundstone described how Dr. John Nash[327] proved that every two-person finite game has at least one equilibrium point, but that there are a few catches. These equilibrium points can have "strange and undesirable properties." In fact, sometimes Nash equilibriums appear to be distinctly irrational.

The best solution for our diabetic is to always "insist on a low-carbohydrate diet." This strategy earns, on average, 20 "points," whereas, acquiescing to the health-provider earns, on average, zero. But contrast that to the health-provider's strategies. On average, they receive 5 "points" for doing the right thing, whereas, if they always preach party-line, that is, advocate a low-fat diet with basal and bolus insulin, and perhaps other drugs, they will earn on average 12.5 "points."

Is that not a strange and undesirable property? The client-health-provider relationship is now on its head. The payoff "incentivizes" all health-providers to advocate the deleterious diet plus ample meds. We—the patients—are now responsible for teaching and training them. And we pay the health-providers for the opportunity to do so.

Whether or not they *can* be trained is another matter entirely. We've seen that it is in their best interest to always choose the "advocate low-fat diet" strategy, and this is the diet based upon certain standards of care. Those standards of care, at least in North American and European societies, are called Clinical Practice Guidelines (CPGs), and they are intended to present a synthesis of current evidence and recommendations preformed by expert clinicians and may affect the practice of large numbers of physicians. As a result, any influence that the authors of CPGs experience from their interactions with pharmaceutical companies may be transmitted many times over to the readers of CPGs. Consequently, if individual authors have relationships that pose a potential conflict of interest, readers of these CPGs may wish to know about them to evaluate the merit of those guidelines.

In 2002, Niteesh K. Choudhry, M.D., Henry Thomas Stelfox, M.D., and Allan S. Detsky, M.D., Ph.D., surveyed authors of CPGs throughout North America and Europe to find out the extent to which the authors of CPGs interact with the pharmaceutical industry. They were seeking to provide empirical evidence concerning this issue to improve the process of CPG development in the future. Here are the conclusions from that study:

> "Eighty-seven percent of authors had some form of interaction with the pharmaceutical industry. Fifty-eight percent had received financial support to perform research and 38% had served as employees or consultants for a pharmaceutical company. On average, CPG authors interacted with 10.5 different companies. Overall, an average of 81% (95% confidence interval, 70%-92%) of authors per CPG had interactions. Similarly, all of the CPGs for 7 of the 10 diseases included in our study had at least 1 author who had some interaction. Fifty-nine percent had relationships with companies whose drugs were considered in the

guideline they authored, and of these authors, 96% had relationships that predated the guideline creation process. Fifty-five percent of respondents indicated that the guideline process with which they were involved had no formal process for declaring these relationships. In published versions of the CPGs, specific declarations regarding the personal financial interactions of individual authors with the pharmaceutical industry were made in only 2 cases. Seven percent thought that their own relationships with the pharmaceutical industry influenced the recommendations and 19% thought that their coauthors' recommendations were influenced by their relationships."[328]

Although the survey's response rate was low,[329] there appears to be considerable interaction between CPG authors and the pharmaceutical industry.

The most interesting, and perhaps regrettable, part of the discussion on clinical practice guidelines, is that there isn't one, universally accepted guideline for diabetes. There is one universally established way of looking at gravitation & gravity — gravitation is a general term describing the phenomenon by which bodies with mass are attracted to one another, while gravity refers specifically to the net force exerted by the Earth on objects in its vicinity as well as by other factors, such as the Earth's rotation — but, like politics, there are many diabetes treatment paradigms.

There are guidelines written for type 1 and 2 diabetes from the American Association of Clinical Endocrinologists, the American Academy of Family Physicians, the American Geriatrics Society, the Canadian Diabetes Association, the Institute for Clinical Systems Improvement, the National Institute for Health and Clinical Excellence, the Scottish Intercollegiate Guidelines Network, and the Veterans Health Administration. In fact, each independent health-provider, or health-providing group may have their own clinical practice guidelines. Utilizing GOOGLE for a quick internet search of "Clinical Practice Guidelines Diabetes" returned 1,500,000 hits, where I found the 2009 Clinical Practice Guidelines for Malaysia, which, by the way, and, of course, encouraged a balanced diet consisting of 50-60% energy from carbohydrate, 15-20% energy from protein and 25-30% energy from fats, not to mention a high fibre diet.[330]

But one organization, the American Diabetes Association, provides the most commonly cited and adopted guidelines in the US, and, perhaps, throughout the world.

According to their website:

> "The Association funds research to prevent, cure and manage diabetes; delivers services to hundreds of communities; provides objective and credible information; and gives voice to those denied their rights because of diabetes. Founded in 1940, our mission is to prevent and cure diabetes and to improve the lives of all people affected by diabetes."[331]

Quite a noble mission. In fact, they do allocate millions of dollars per year toward research; in 2008, it was approximately $43 million.[332] But our focus here is not the relative good that they do in the world, for surely a person with type 1 diabetes that eats carbohydrates and undergoes an intensive insulin regimen is far better off than one that solely eats carbohydrates at will, given that their body's cells lack an effective glucose uptake mechanism. Rather, it is the inherent conflict between the ADA's conclusions promulgated through guidelines, and who supports that platform, that is of particular concern.

Cutting to the chase, the ADA works in its own best interest as evidenced by the following, taken directly from their conflict of interest policy:

> "The American Diabetes Association and its subsidiaries (collectively, the Association) requires all members of the Board of Directors, members of Board-appointed committees and staff to act solely in the best interest of the Association without regard to their personal or business interests."[333]

The ADA isn't as altruistic as one would like to believe. They don't act primarily in the interest of diabetics; but, instead, in their own best interest, and, at least in appearance, based upon their guidelines — as we will shortly see — in the interest of their main stakeholders. But just who are their main stakeholders? According to the ADA's strategic plan, the folks that have the deepest pockets from which the ADA will base their growth upon are the corporate and pharmaceutical organizations, for whom the following strategy applies:

> "Maximize corporate, pharmaceutical and foundation contributions to achieve revenue of $42 million, which reflects an annual compound growth rate of 9.1%."[334]

Nothing at first can appear more difficult to believe than that the American Diabetes Association, a credible, long-standing institution in the community, does not necessarily act in the best interest of those most negatively affected by the complications of diabetes. The truth of the following assertion, however, cannot be disputed: the only way to get pharmaceutical companies to contribute at that level, i.e., $42,000,000 per year, and at that growth rate, i.e., 9.1%, is to serve their interests; the only way to effect that is to directly or indirectly support the use of their products, which, of course, are the many insulins and their compliments. And the only way to support that endeavor is to espouse carbohydrates as an essential source of energy. *A* source of energy; yes, exogenous carbohydrates are that. An *essential* source of energy? No. *Homo sapiens* can manufacture their own glucose in the liver after the ingestion and digestion of exogenous fat and protein.[335]

So let's now look a little more closely at the ADA's Guidelines. I'll call this story "The Tale of the Tell."

As late as 2006 and 2007, the ADA's position, promulgated sedulously through their guidelines, was that "Low-carbohydrate diets (restricting total carbohydrate to <130 g/day) are not recommended in the management of diabetes," and that "Saturated fat intake should be <7% of total calories."[336] The ADA in 2006 wrote:

"Low-carbohydrate diets are not recommended in the management of diabetes. Although dietary carbohydrate is the major contributor to postprandial glucose concentration, it is an important source of energy, water-soluble vitamins and minerals, and fiber. Thus, in agreement with the National Academy of Sciences-Food and Nutrition Board, a recommended range of carbohydrate intake is 45–65% of total calories. In addition, because the brain and central nervous system have an absolute requirement for glucose as an energy source, restricting total carbohydrate to <130 g/day is not recommended."[337]

They went on to state:

"Similar to the general population, people with diabetes are encouraged to choose a variety of fiber-containing foods, such as legumes, fiber-rich cereals (≥5 g fiber/serving), as well as fruits, vegetables, and whole-grain products because they provide vitamins, minerals, fiber, and other substances important for good health."[338]

And, of course, the Guidelines were based upon the DCCT:

"The DCCT clearly showed that intensive insulin therapy (three or more injections per day of insulin or continuous subcutaneous insulin infusion (CSII, or insulin pump therapy) was a key part of improved glycemia and better outcomes. At the time of the study, therapy was carried out with short- and intermediate-acting human insulins. Despite better microvascular outcomes, intensive insulin therapy was associated with a marked increase in severe hypoglycemia (62 episodes per 100 patient-years of therapy). Since the time of the DCCT, a number of rapid-acting and long-acting insulin analogs have been developed. These analogs were designed to be more "physiological" in their pharmacokinetics and pharmacodynamics and are associated with less hypoglycemia with equal A1C lowering in type 1 diabetes.

Therefore, recommended therapy for type 1 diabetes consists of the following components: 1) use of multiple dose insulin injections (3–4 injections per day of basal and prandial insulin) or CSII therapy; 2) matching of prandial insulin to carbohydrate intake, premeal blood glucose, and anticipated activity; and 3) for many patients (especially if hypoglycemia is a problem), use of insulin analogs. There are excellent reviews available that guide the initiation and management of insulin therapy to achieve desired glycemic goals."[339]

And in 2007, not much had changed:

> Low-carbohydrate diets (restricting total carbohydrate to <130 g/day) are not recommended in the treatment of overweight/obesity [or in diabetes]. The long-term effects of these diets are unknown, and although such diets produce short-term weight loss, maintenance of weight loss is similar to that from low-fat diets and the impact on CVD risk profile is uncertain.[340]

But then in 2008, what seems like a sea-change occurred in the ADA's Guidelines. For the first time, the ADA added the following:

> "For weight loss, either low-carbohydrate or low-fat calorie-restricted diets may be effective in the short term (up to 1 year)."[341]

Though a subtle caveat was placed on the low-carbohydrate diet:

> "For patients on low-carbohydrate diets, monitor lipid profiles, renal function, and protein intake (in those with nephropathy), and adjust hypoglycemic therapy as needed."[342]

And although I have been able to find *hundreds* of studies concluding then espousing the efficacy of low-carbohydrate diets, the ADA justified their position with only three:

> "The optimal macronutrient distribution of weight loss diets has not been established. Although low-fat diets have traditionally been promoted for weight loss, several randomized controlled trials found that subjects on low-carbohydrate diets (<130 g/day of carbohydrate) lost more weight at 6 months than subjects on low-fat diets; however, at 1 year, the difference in weight loss between the low-carbohydrate and low-fat diets was not significant and weight loss was modest with both diets. Another study of overweight women randomized to one of four diets showed significantly more weight loss at 12 months with the Atkins low-carbohydrate diet than with higher-carbohydrate diets. Changes in serum triglyceride and HDL cholesterol were more favorable with the low-carbohydrate diets. In one study, those subjects with type 2 diabetes demonstrated a greater decrease in A1C with a low-carbohydrate diet than with a low-fat diet. A recent meta-analysis showed that at 6 months, low-carbohydrate diets were associated with greater improvements in triglyceride and HDL cholesterol concentrations

than low-fat diets; however, LDL cholesterol was significantly higher on the low-carbohydrate diets."[343]

Still, the ADA, in 2008, remained firmly planted in making sure folks ingest their 130 grams of carbohydrates per day:

"The recommended dietary allowance (RDA) for digestible carbohydrate is 130 g/day and is based on providing adequate glucose as the required fuel for the central nervous system without reliance on glucose production from ingested protein or fat. Although brain fuel needs can be met on lower-carbohydrate diets, long-term metabolic effects of very-low-carbohydrate diets are unclear, and such diets eliminate many foods that are important sources of energy, fiber, vitamins, and minerals and are important in dietary palatability."[344]

And the DCCT continued to be cited as the holy grail:

"Glycemic control is fundamental to the management of diabetes. The DCCT, a prospective, randomized, controlled trial of intensive versus standard glycemic control in type 1 diabetes, showed definitively that improved glycemic control is associated with sustained decreased rates of microvascular (retinopathy and nephropathy) as well as neuropathic complications. Follow up of the DCCT cohorts in the Epidemiology of Diabetes Interventions and Complications (EDIC) study has shown persistence of this effect in previously intensively treated subjects, even though their glycemic control has been equivalent to that of previous standard arm subjects during follow-up. In addition, EDIC has shown a significant reduction of the rate of cardiovascular outcomes in the previous intensive arm.

The DCCT clearly showed that intensive insulin therapy (three or more injections per day of insulin or continuous subcutaneous insulin infusion [CSII, or insulin pump therapy]) was a key part of improved glycemia and better outcomes. At the time of the study, therapy was carried out with short- and intermediate-acting human insulins. Despite better microvascular outcomes, intensive insulin therapy was associated with a marked increase in severe hypoglycemia (62 episodes per 100 patient-years of therapy). Since the time of the DCCT, a number of rapid-acting and long-acting insulin analogs have been developed. These analogs were designed to be more "physiological" in their pharmacokinetics and pharmacodynamics, and are associated with less hypoglycemia with equal A1C lowering in type 1 diabetes.

Therefore, recommended therapy for type 1 diabetes consists of the following components: 1) use of multiple dose insulin injections (3-4 injections per day of basal and prandial insulin) or CSII therapy; 2) matching of prandial insulin to carbohydrate intake, premeal blood glucose, and anticipated activity; and 3) for many patients (especially if hypoglycemia is a problem), use of insulin analogs. There are excellent reviews available that guide the initiation and management of insulin therapy to achieve desired glycemic goals."[345]

The 2009 ADA Guidelines are replicated from those of 2008. The DCCT continues to serve as the foundation of their Guidelines—the foundation to a house of cards—as it "clearly showed that intensive insulin therapy was a key part of improved glycemia and better outcomes." Yet I, and countless others, who simply don't eat many carbohydrates, and therefore haven't a need for an intensive insulin treatment, able to keep our glucose levels within a normal range, simply, effectively, and efficiently, wonder not who holds the extreme, unsupported view.

William Poundstone stated at the end of his book that "The only satisfying solution to the prisoner's dilemma is to avoid prisoner's dilemmas."[346] Options in applying that to our situation are rather limited. Clearly, not getting diabetes is the ideal. Not sure how to accomplish that with any level of confidence, so let's move on to something a little more promising. A vaccine—two such vaccines in the works are GAD-alum and BCMA— might be a little late for type 1s without any remaining beta function, but if they can save the beta cells of anyone, then I'm all for it.[347]

One could simply live in a state of denial, eating carbohydrates at will, not checking their BG, too, not seeing any health providers. Yes, it is a simple option, though, not very effective or efficient.

We're really left with one simple, inexpensive, non-time consuming, effective, efficient option. It is both the way to solve and the way to avoid the prisoner's dilemma. And we've known about it, sans the basal insulin, for more than two centuries.

Essential Diabetes Leadership

EPILOGUE

Diabetes is the relative inability of the body to naturally and effectively process carbohydrates due to an insulin function disturbance; either our bodies are resistant to our own insulin and perhaps we produce too much, or, in the case of type 1s, we do not produce enough, or any. We can buy different types of analog insulin — with a prescription — and take basal plus bolus insulin, consume a balanced diet including 45%-55% carbohydrates, and live with the ever-present chance of hyper- and hypo-glycemia. Or we can forgo the bolus insulin and carbohydrates, and eat just fat and protein. The logical question to then ask is: "Are carbohydrates essential to human life?" If yes, then our hypothesis — forgo the bolus insulin and carbohydrates, and eat just fat and protein to live a healthy, long life — falls on its face. If no, then the simple solution, the trivial solution, the optimal solution, the solution left unharmed sitting atop Occam's razor is basal insulin, fat and protein, sans bolus insulin and carbohydrates. The ample evidence presented points to the latter.

If carbohydrates are not essential, then, and our diet is based upon fat — and saturated fat at that — will our arteries clog and our destiny manifest itself in heart disease? If yes, then, once again, our hypothesis is moot. If no, then basal plus bolus insulin plus carbohydrates descends down

Ocamm's razor and basal insulin, fat, and protein remain safely perched on top. The overwhelming evidence presented by authors such as Dr. Uffe Ravnskov, Dr. Barry Groves, Dr. Malcolm Kendrick, Dr. Kilmer S. McCully, Gary Taubes, et al., points again to the latter.

And what about a cure? Can type 2's go under anesthesia and a knife to have a gastric bypass? Yes. Is there a day in the not too distant future when type 1s can have stem cells effectively and efficiently grown to replace our atrophied beta cells? The answer, again, is yes.

And those two treatments simply scratch the surface. There are many other interventions being investigated from metabolic control, i.e., developing an artificial pancreas, to regenerating insulin producing cells, to replacing beta cells with functioning ones from a donor, to artificial preventative treatments, i.e., stopping or reversing the immune system response that causes diabetes.

But, especially in type 1s, then what? Eat normal, balanced meals, burn out the replacement beta cells, and then go in for a refill? Does anyone think that, for example, stem cells implanted in a recipient's pancreas will somehow not be subjected to the same influencers in the environment that originally triggered the condition, and, overtime, fail too?

I do not know why some people stay slim and healthy throughout life and others develop a deranged metabolism given the same carbohydrate load. When doctors don't understand a metabolic process, they call it "genetics," when ethologists can't pinpoint a reason for an animal's behavior, they call it "instinct." You too probably know a slim, healthy person that eats far more than their fair share of cereal with milk in the morning, sandwiches on white bread with potato chips for lunch, ice cream for dessert, and a thousand more calories for dinner made up of those same carbohydrates and a variety more, plus acidic, caffeinated, carbonated, sugar water, and still manage to look good at the beach.

Epilogue

Although I must say that I'm happy for them—yes, it all sounds so delicious—it is a disappointment.

But far more disappointing are the health-professionals, health-based organizations, figureheads, and speakers, whether knowledgeable on the subject of diabetes or not, that recommend, prescribe or otherwise espouse the role of carbohydrates as the basis of our diet and treatment. My disappointment culminated when a former favorite author of mine, and, through his books, mentor, Stephen R. Covey, partnered with the American Association of Diabetes Educators, and Bayer Diabetes Care, to write for and distribute free of charge a pamphlet entitled *The 7 Habits of Highly Effective People with Diabetes* in 2007. Discussing his second habit, "Begin with the end in mind," he wrote to "Choose one behavior and set a small goal," and here is one proposed goal:

"For Healthy Eating, *I will switch from whole milk to skim milk* [my italics]."[349]

Milk—whole, 2%, 1%, low-fat, skimmed, or skim—contains a considerable amount of the simple sugar lactose and will rapidly raise blood sugar once consumed. Skim milk contains the most lactose per ounce. By his suggestion, Dr. Covey displays support for the "fat antagonizes diabetes" dogma—a diabetic should reduce their consumption of fat, and, instead, increase the amount of carbohydrate. He espouses a dogma on the same par as that of health benefits to lungs from five to ten minute sessions of repeatedly inhaling and exhaling the smoke of burning, rolled-up, dried tobacco particulate.

Recall that memes propagate themselves in the meme pool by leaping from brain to brain via a process which, in the broad sense, can be called imitation. When a credible, respected member of human society helps to spread an idea, from the idea's perspective it is the idea evolving to become better adapted at spreading itself. So another way to look at it is that Dr. Covey's well intended but misguided effort is the result of being infected with an evolved strain of the "fat antagonizes diabetes" virus, which may be better stated as the "eat carbohydrates" virus. He too spreads it, but as you read these words now, and those of the preceding chapters, be hopeful that it can be countered by the "don't eat carbohydrates" meme, of which I am a proud and purposeful carrier.

And there are other noble meme's to spread.

The Millennium Development Goals[350] (MDGs) are eight goals commissioned by the UN Secretary General and supported by the UN Development Group to be achieved by 2015, that respond to the world's main development challenges. The MDGs are drawn from the actions and targets contained in the Millennium Declaration[351] that was adopted by 189 nations-and signed by 147 heads of state and governments during the UN Millennium Summit in September, 2000. Here are the eight goals:

- Eradicate extreme poverty and hunger.[352]
- Achieve universal primary education.
- Promote gender equality and empower women.
- Reduce child mortality.
- Improve maternal health.
- Combat HIV/AIDS, malaria and other diseases.
- Ensure environmental sustainability. Integrate the principles of sustainable development into country policies and programs and reverse the loss of environmental resources.
- Develop a Global Partnership for Development. Develop further an open, rule-based, predictable, nondiscriminatory trading and financial system, which includes a commitment to good governance, development, and poverty reduction, both nationally and internationally.

Complementing these eight Millennium Development Goals are the 14 Grand Challenges for Engineering in the 21st Century, sponsored by the

National Science Foundation.[353] Here are the 14 Grand Challenges for Engineering in the 21st Century:

- Make solar energy affordable
- Provide energy from fusion
- Develop carbon sequestration methods[354]
- Manage the nitrogen cycle
- Provide access to clean water
- Restore and improve urban infrastructure
- Advance health informatics
- Engineer better medicines
- Reverse-engineer the brain
- Prevent nuclear terror
- Secure cyberspace
- Enhance virtual reality
- Advance personalized learning
- Engineer the tools for scientific discovery

I never could find answers to life's questions — nor an optimal solution to our diabetes dilemma, which I had wanted to find first — at, or working my way to, the bottom of a bottle, glass, or can of beer. Although, yes, I have tried. In seeking an optimal solution via paradigms in physics, astronomy, mathematics, cosmology, medicine, ethology, geology, or simple trial and error, I've found that the best lens to view the problem comes from Charles Darwin.[355] As it has been said, nothing in biology makes sense except in the light of evolution.

"Nothing in Biology Makes Sense Except in the Light of Evolution"[356] is a 1973 essay by the evolutionary biologist and Russian Orthodox Christian Theodosius Dobzhansky,[357] criticizing anti-evolution creationism and espousing theistic evolution. The essay was first published in the *American Biology Teacher*.[358]

Dobzhansky first published the title statement, in a slight variation, in a 1964 article in *American Zoologist*, "Biology, Molecular and Organismic," to assert the importance of organismic biology in response to the challenge of the rising field of molecular biology. The term "light of evolution" — or *sub specie evolutionis* — had been used earlier by biologist Julian Huxley.

Dobzhansky starts with a *reductio ad absurdum* of the alleged geocentrism of an Arab cleric (identical to or namesake of Shaikh Abdulaziz bin Baz, later the Grand Mufti of Saudi Arabia) who believes the Sun revolves around the Earth because of scripture. Dobzhansky asserts his own belief that scripture and science do not contradict each other. He criticizes creationists for implying that God is deceitful and asserts that this is blasphemous.

Dobzhansky then goes on to describe the diversity of life on Earth, and that the diversity of species cannot be best explained by a creation myth because of the ecological interactions between them. He uses examples of evidence for evolution: the genetic sequence of cytochrome C to show evidence for common descent (citing the work of Emanuel Margoliash & Walter M. Fitch); embryology; and his own work on fruit flies in Hawaii. Dobzhansky concludes that scripture and science are two different things: "It is a blunder to mistake the Holy Scriptures for elementary textbooks of astronomy, geology, biology, and anthropology."

The central issue of the essay is the need to teach biological evolution in the context of debate about creation and evolution in public education in the United States. The fact that evolution occurs explains the interrelatedness of the various facts of biology, and so makes biology make sense. The concept has become firmly established as a unifying idea in biology education.

The notion of the "light of evolution" came originally from the Jesuit priest Pierre Teilhard de Chardin, whom Dobzhansky much admired. In the last paragraph of the article, de Chardin is quoted as having written the following:

> *"(Evolution) is a general postulate to which all theories, all hypotheses, all systems must henceforward bow and which they must satisfy in order to be thinkable and true. Evolution is a light which illuminates all facts, a trajectory which all lines of thought must follow — this is what evolution is."*

The phrase "nothing in biology makes sense except in the light of evolution" has come into common use by those opposing creationism or its variant called intelligent design. While the essay argues that Christianity and evolutionary biology are compatible, a position described as *evolutionary creationism* or *theistic evolution*, the phrase is also used by those who consider that "in biology" includes anthropology, and those who consider a creator to be unnecessary, such as Richard Dawkins who published *The Selfish Gene* just three years later.[359]

And it is Richard Dawkins, one of my favorite authors, that provides answer upon answer to some of life's greatest questions, e.g., "why are people?"[360] It is only after understanding the answer to that question that we can begin to grasp the answer to "why is diabetes?"

All his books are seminal in their own right, but most remarkable is *The Ancestor's Tale: A Pilgrimage to the Dawn of Evolution* (New York: Houghton Mifflin Company, 2005). In this treatise, Richard Dawkins creatively, eloquently utilizes backward chronology to search out ancestors to "sensibly aim towards a single distant target." On opposite ends of a small log, he serves as gentle, factual storyteller, bringing us "back to the universal progenitor of all surviving organisms, probably resembling some kind of bacterium." His lexicon includes "rendezvous," "confluence," and, most notably, "concestor."

> "In a backward chronology, the ancestors of any set of species must eventually meet at a particular geological moment. Their point of rendezvous is the last common ancestor that they all share, what I shall call their 'Concestor': the focal

rodent or the focal mammal or the focal vertebrate, say. The oldest concestor is the grand ancestor of all surviving life." [361]

And the oldest concestor, according to Dawkins, before animals and plants, before multicellularity, is the single cell progenitor bacteria.

"The analogy of insect colony to human body is often made, and it is not a bad one. The majority of our cells subjugate their individuality, devoting themselves to assisting the reproduction of the minority that are capable of it: 'germ-line' cells in the testes or ovaries, whose genes are destined to travel, via sperm or eggs, into the distant future. But genetic relatedness is not the only basis for subjugation of individuality in fruitful division of labor. Any sort of mutual assistance, where each side corrects a deficiency in the other, can be favored by natural selection on both." [362]

In answering our diabetes conundrum, it makes sense to see what, if anything, benefits from diabetes. I'm sure that sounds strange, after all, how could anything benefit from our decline? Well, our environment consists of living things that are themselves adapted to profit at our expense. Although all the evidence isn't in just yet, it seems that cancer is one example of a beneficiary.

In "Diabetes and Cancer. Epidemiological Evidence and Molecular Links," (2008), the authors highlighted the following findings:

"...cancer cells growing under hyperglycemic conditions with elevated levels of insulin and other glucose-regulating hormones do have an advantage compared to healthy cells and even over the same cancer cells in a non-diabetic setting." [363]

"Numerous studies revealed a direct link between hyperglycemia, high insulin levels and high concentrations of insulin-like growth factor (IGF) and an increased risk of various types of cancer." [364]

"Many studies revealed that dietary patterns that accelerate insulin resistance or secretion, including high consumption of sucrose, various sources of starch, a high glycemic index and high saturated fatty acid intake [sic], are associated with a higher risk of colon cancer." [365]

Epilogue

"...we discovered that most cancer cell lines display enhanced features of tumor progression when cultured under diabetic conditions. Not only the established stimulus for cell proliferation—insulin—increased the activity of tumor cells, but also hyperglycemic glucose concentrations per se enhanced proliferation and migratory activity of tumor cells." [366]

In "The Relationship Between Diabetes and Cancer," authors Dion Smyth and Theresa Smyth point out the following:

- Insulin and insulin-like growth factor-1 (IGF-1) have been shown to act as growth-promoting hormones that foster cell proliferation and inhibit apoptosis. [367]
- High circulating levels of IGF-1 increase the risk of breast cancer in premenopausal women. [368]
- High levels of IGF-1 are also associated with an increased risk of prostate cancer. [369]
- Various studies have shown that adults with impaired glucose tolerance have a greater risk of cancer mortality. [370]
- Type 2 diabetes is a risk factor for endometrial cancer. [371]
- Data from the long-running US Nurses Health Study suggest a slight but significant increased risk of breast cancer in post-menopausal women with type 2 diabetes. [372]
- Recent reports have suggested that diabetes and high blood glucose levels appear to increase the risk of cancer independent of obesity. [373]
- A prospective cohort study of almost 1.3 million Koreans, who are typically leaner than their Western counterparts, found that increased levels of fasting serum glucose were strongly linked with an increased risk of pancreatic cancer and significantly associated with an increased risk of cancers of the gullet, liver and colorectum in men and the cervix and liver in women. [374]
- The Khaw, et al. (2004), study suggested that high blood glucose levels—even levels below those diagnostic of diabetes—could be linked to bowel cancer and people with diabetes could be up to 3 times more likely to get colorectal cancer. [375]
- The role of medication such as exogenous insulin (that is, the use of therapeutic insulin injections) in the development of cancer has been reported on. The US National Cancer Institute (NCI) highlighted research

presented at the most recent American Association for Cancer Research Annual Meeting that men who had diabetes and took medication are at 4 times the risk of developing liver cancer and 2.5 times the risk of developing pancreatic cancer of men who did not have diabetes.[376]

- Continuous use of insulin for a period of more than 3 years was associated with a significant risk of developing colorectal cancer.[377]

Validated from another source, patients diagnosed with cancer who have preexisting diabetes are at increased risk for long-term, all-cause mortality compared with those without diabetes.[378]

In "Abnormal Glucose Tolerance and the Risk of Cancer Death in the United States," by Saydah SH, Loria CM, Eberhardt MS, and Brancati FL, the authors first stated that "…Although abnormal glucose tolerance is a well-established risk factor for cardiovascular disease, its relation to cancer risk is less certain." After performing their study, they concluded that "…in the United States, impaired glucose tolerance is an independent predictor for cancer mortality."[379]

In "Diabetes Mellitus as a Predictor of Cancer Mortality in a Large Cohort of US Adults," by S. Coughlin, E. Calle, L. Teras, J. Petrelli, and M. Thun, one of the largest prospective studies worldwide, enrolling 467,922 men and 588,321 women who had no reported history of cancer at the time of enrollment, revealed after 16 years of follow up that:

> "…diabetes was significantly associated with fatal colon cancer in men and women, and with prostate cancer in men, and significantly associated with liver cancer and bladder cancer. In addition, diabetes was significantly associated with breast cancer in women. These findings strongly suggest that diabetes is an independent predictor of mortality from these cancer entities."[380]

The Västerbotten Intervention Project is a subcohort of the Northern Sweden Health and Disease Cohort, and, in brief, all residents in the county of Västerbotten in northern Sweden were invited to a health survey, in the years in which they became 40, 50, or 60 years old since

1985. The results are detailed in "Prospective Study of Hyperglycemia and Cancer Risk," (2007), where the authors stated:

> "In conclusion, our finding of a statistically significant association of hyperglycemia with overall cancer risk in women and an increase in risk of cancer at many sites in women and men is essentially in accordance with the observations in some other large cohort studies, suggesting that abnormal glucose metabolism is a general risk factor for cancer development. Although the proportion of subjects with hyperglycemia was highest among obese subjects, the absolute numbers of subjects with hyperglycemia were larger among women and men who were overweight or had normal body weight, and plasma glucose levels remained associated with cancer risk after adjustment for BMI. This observation may have considerable implications for public health strategies, as key determinants of hyperglycemia are known and modifiable. A lifestyle that decreases plasma glucose levels may reduce overall cancer risk not only among overweight or obese subjects but most likely also among subjects with normal body weight. At the same time, current evidence suggests that such a strategy also would contribute to the prevention of diabetes and cardiovascular disease."[381]

Cancer, according to the National Cancer Institute, US National Institutes of Health (www.cancer.gov), is a term used for diseases in which abnormal cells divide without control and are able to invade other tissues. Cancer cells can spread to other parts of the body through the blood and lymph systems.[382] Cancer is a class of diseases in which a group of cells display *uncontrolled growth* (division beyond the normal limits), *invasion* (intrusion on and destruction of adjacent tissues), and sometimes *metastasis* (spread to other locations in the body via lymph or blood). These three malignant properties of cancers differentiate them from benign tumors, which are self-limited, and do not invade or metastasize. Most cancers form a tumor but some, like leukemia, do not. Leukemia is a cancer of the blood or bone marrow and is characterized by an abnormal proliferation of blood cells, usually white blood cells (leukocytes).[383]

In short, cancer is the abnormal proliferation of cells.

With our above discussion on diabetes, cancer and that specific definition of cancer in mind, then, at best, diabetes enables cancer. If we relax the above definition, however, from "abnormal proliferation of *cells*," to "abnormal proliferation of *cells or substances* (e.g., hormones)," and we recall the essence of untreated diabetes, that it is:

- the abnormal proliferation of insulin (type 2)
- the abnormal proliferation of glucose
- the abnormal proliferation of glycosylated hemoglobin
- the abnormal proliferation of triglycerides
- the abnormal proliferation of complications

then we see that, at worst, diabetes *is* cancer. Sans any tumor(s).

Just as Copernicus showed that the universe does not revolve around the earth, Darwin showed that the natural world does not revolve around humans; we are no more unique than any other species. In his own words:

> "I view all beings not as special creations, but as the lineal descendants of some few beings which lived long before the first bed of the Silurian system was deposited, they seem to me to become ennobled."[384]

And all species—all memes—struggle to survive, reproductively, at the level of the individual.[385]

Nothing is alone in the universe. The possibilities for organisms, cells, organelles, proteins, etc., to interact in the universe, include, and are on a continuum of, altruism to exploitation, antagonism to synergism, attraction to repulsion, catabolism to anabolism, catalyst to anti-catalyst, stimulator to repressor, and mutualism through commensalism to parasitism; with specific roles, whether one to one, one to many, or many to many, such as brother to sister, cell wall to environment, enzyme to reactant, friend to friend, husband to wife, manipulator to submitter, master to slave, parasite to host, parent to child, predator to prey, signaler to receiver, et al. And in the rivalrous, predator-prey and parasite-host relationships, arms races explain the relative increasing strength of sides in the struggle for fitness.[386]

Cancer does not appreciate any of our discoveries or advancements, whether we can travel to or populate distant stars and ocean depths, or whether our deep thinking scientists are working to tie—let alone succeed in tying—the forces of gravity, weak, strong, and electromagnetic into a theory of everything. It does not care about our civilization, our cultures, our libraries, languages, Betts or Cassavetti Stradivarii. It does not sit in awe listening to Dufay, Palestrina, de Prez, Gesualdo, Monteverdi, Bach, Albinoni, Handel, Haydn, Mozart, Beethoven, Paganini, Schubert, Berlioz, Mendelssohn, Chopin, Schumann, Liszt, Verdi, Wagner, Bruckner, Brahms, Saint-Saëns, Bizet, Mussorgsky, Tchaikovsky, Dvořák, Grieg, Rimsky-Korsakov, Puccini, Mahler, Debussy, Strauss, Sibelius, Rachmaninoff, Schoenberg, Ravel, Bartók, Stravinsky, Webern, Berg, Villa-Lobos, Prokofiev, Orff, Gershwin, Copland, Khachaturian, Shostakovich, Messiaen, Barber, Cage, Britten, Bernstein, Xenakis, Ligeti, Penderecki, Glass, and many, many more. It, better stated, *they*, are content siphoning our blood, glucose, and, eventually, our lives.[387]

Once cancer manifests itself in daughter cells that further divide, it may not even care about itself. It certainly doesn't care about its host. Cancer works toward its own end, an unintended yet deeply troubling double entendre, emphasizing the difficulty we humans have placing it in the universal schema. And killing it before it kills us is the central problem in cancer treatment:

> "The mutations that benefit the survival and reproduction of cells in a tumor are the things that drive it towards malignancy. Evolution is also driving therapeutic resistance. When you apply chemotherapy to a population of tumor cells, you're quite likely to have a resistant mutant somewhere in that population of billions or even trillions of cells. This is the central problem in oncology. The reason we haven't been able to cure cancer is that we're selecting for resistant tumor cells. When we spray a field with pesticide, we select for resistant pests. It's the same idea."[388]

Returning to the question that started this discussion, why is diabetes? Well, having lived with it for so many years, I can answer that question first by saying that it is certainly not here to benefit us, unless a prompt leading to self-development and enlightenment can be thought of as a benefit. Yes, diabetes is related to stress—stress from injury, surgery, infection, pregnancy, mental anguish and the like—or it could be a natural consequence of aging. It may simply be attributed to metabolic error or miscommunication between cells, imposed on a random selection of unlucky individuals in the human population, though that doesn't explain why some populations have a higher incidence than others.[389] Nor does it explain why other substances or cells are able to thrive in its environment. Obesity, inflammation, and immunosuppression can lead to a myriad of complications, not the least of which is diabetes; but, we're left wondering why some with the former conditions do not develop the latter.[390]

Diabetes may exist due to faulty genes, though that doesn't explain why some with the "genes for diabetes" don't express the disease and some do.[391] It may exist for the benefit of health-providers, though that is hopefully a tenuous explanation for a disease that has been around longer than a profession. It could be that its purpose is to benefit itself, i.e., that diabetes is its own meme, and that it too is struggling for lineage-based reproductive survival against the odds of a solitary, poor, nasty, brutish, and short existence.[392] The Coxsackie B4 virus is strongly associated with the development of insulin dependent diabetes mellitus.[393] Conversely, it appears that bacterial phyla normally present in the human gut may provide protection against developing diabetes.[394]

There are cases of chemicals, environmental toxicants and drugs causing temporary or permanent type 1 or type 2 diabetes documented in the medical literature. High serum selenium concentrations are associated with higher prevalence of diabetes.[395] The atypical antipsychotic drugs clozapine, olanzapin, risperidone, quetiapine and ziprasidone are known to induce insulin resistance, hyperglycemia, and even diabetic ketoacidosis (DKA).[396] The biologic plausibility of a diabetogenic effect of exposure to persistent organic pollutants, e.g., dioxins, polychlorinated biphenyls, and organophosphate insecticides, e.g., chlordane, is supported by numerous studies.[397] Alloxan, synthesized by the oxidation of uric acid by nitric acid, and the antibiotic streptozocin, produced by the soil fungus *Streptomyces achromogenes*, are two of the best known toxins capable of damaging the pancreatic beta cells.[398] Vacor, a rat poison derived from the waste product urea, also has been reported to cause insulin dependent diabetes in humans who survived the exposure.[399]

The existence of naturally occurring toxins produced by many species of fungi capable of causing diabetes is also deeply troubling. Fungi are living things in our environment adapted to profit at our expense, though other microorganisms are probably the "intended" victims.[400] According to A.V. Costantini, M.D., Head (retired) of the World Health Organization Collaborating Center For Mycotoxins In Food:

> "Fungi are masters at producing a wide array of biologically active substances which serve the producing fungus extremely well. These biological metabolites are anti-predatory, i.e., territory-protective, and exist to ensure that the fungus will survive as long as possible in this quite hostile world. These metabolites are anti-viral, anti-bacterial, anti-protozoan, anti-insect, anti-animal and, of course, anti-human. These metabolites are referred to as mycotoxins. The term is derived from the Greek *mykes*, meaning fungus, and *toxicum*, meaning toxin or poison. Fungi and mycotoxins are present in variable amounts in the food products of Western civilization such as the stored grains, particularly corn, fat-ladened meat of stored grain-fed animals, yeast-fermented beer, wine, bread, cheeses, coffee, and cured (fermented) meats and tobacco leaf."[401]

Others too, such as Doug Hoffman and David Holland, M.D.,[402] and Laurens Maas,[403] each extensively drawing from Dr. Costantini's works, emphasize, perhaps better stated as reiterate, that the link between diabetes and fungi is not entirely from the "utterly rotten fabric of guess and speculation."[404] Although I agree that it is disconcerting to think that we are mere fodder for some other form, these authors do make a strong case.

What I do know with much certainty is that eliminating carbohydrates from the diet halts the abnormal proliferation of all five of the aforementioned items: insulin, glucose, glycosylated hemoglobin, triglycerides, and complications. If the relaxed definition makes sense to you, and you prefer to collectively call those five items cancer, then carbohydrate consumption is the proximate cause and ingesting near-zero of the same is the cure.[405]

Diabetes manifests itself in the body as ineffective carbohydrate processing; the corollary is that diabetes is a disease of insulin derangement. Too much insulin ought to be treated with too few carbohydrates. Not enough, or any, insulin ought to be treated similarly, with the addition of just enough exogenous, long-acting, basal insulin. Fat and protein only, as diet for both.

No, it's not easy; nothing worthwhile ever is. But it is simple. And it works without enabling ischemic heart disease, cancer, or any other parasitoid, from any biota or mineralia, more, from any category — kingdom, chemical, compound, name, form, or idea — providing the great escape from our prisoner's dilemma.

POSTSCRIPT

"Why in this stultifying and needless conflict between reason and tradition, it should be so easy to believe the incredible and so difficult to accept the obvious, is a riddle which is not flattering to contemplate."[406]

F. J. COLE, 1944

In this book, the hypotheses and proof that a ketogenic—high fat, medium protein, low-carbohydrate—diet for diabetics, as part of an overall BG optimization model, supports a long, happy, healthy life in general, I included specifics from six of the twelve total systems: the (1) circulatory, (2) digestive, (3) endocrine, (4) excretory, (5) nervous, (6a) skeletal (teeth), and (7a) integumentary (gingiva: the gums).[407]

Regarding the (5) nervous system, which includes the sense organs and vestibular system, the last endnote of the "Epilogue" provided supporting evidence for the use of a ketogenic diet in the successful treatment of epilepsy. Since there's more to the nervous system, and to the diseases of, than forty different kinds of epilepsy, this "Postscript" suggests a couple other information sources.

Reminiscent of Dr. Weston Price, we find a brave treatise written by another dentist. First published in 2001, then condensed in 2005, *Alzheimer's Solved*, by Dr. Henry Lorin, proffers a thoroughly researched theorem—his book references over 2,500 scientific articles—that better explains the data and observations than any other work on the subject: "It is indeed possible for a person to have blood cholesterol levels that are too low."[408] Reading through his manuscript, that conclusion is inescapable.

From aging to xanthomas, Dr. Lorin's theorem in *Alzheimer's Solved* unifies seemingly diverse conditions such as AIDS, Alzheimer's disease, brain surgery, Cushing's disease, dementia, depression, Down syndrome, epilepsy, head injury, HIV, osteoporosis, Parkinson's disease, vasculitis, and others, with his remarkably simple deduction that amyloid — beta amyloid plaques — "is the body's temporary substitute for cholesterol molecules. Amyloid is to be used as a short-term 'bandage' for cell membranes until more cholesterol is provided."[409] Should that cholesterol, for whatever reason, be withheld, nearly all the aforementioned diseases inevitably become terminal. Dr. Lorin summarizes his diet — beyond important micronutrients such as vitamin D — quite eloquently in one sentence: "The easiest and most natural way to do this [preventing and treating most of the described diseases] is by eating foods that contain cholesterol, while minimizing the consumption of foods that are primarily carbohydrates (starches)."[410]

You may also be interested in reading *The Brain Trust Program* (2007), by Larry McCleary, MD, which accessibly describes the important component parts of the nervous system, then delivers a striking contrast to all the also-ran diet-brain books published on how to best support them through diet. Although he doesn't outright advocate a low-carbohydrate diet, his 7-day menu plan sure does resemble one.[411] A person with diabetes would simply need to skimp further on the fruit and minimal multigrain bread and crackers mentioned.

Here I could discuss the (8) muscular system in detail, but so much data exists on low-carbohydrate diets and exercise physiology, overlapping some with the (9) respiratory system — and I reprinted with permission much of the material written by Professor Emeritus Robert S. Horn on the subject in my first book — that, although tempting, I shall not rehearse the subject here, other than to say that Stephen D. Phinney provides great additional insight.

In "Ketogenic Diets and Physical Performance," which contains many good sources for further reading, Dr. Phinney states in the Abstract that "impaired physical performance is a common but not obligate result of a low carbohydrate diet. Lessons from traditional Inuit culture indicate that time for adaptation, optimized sodium and potassium nutriture, and constraint of protein to 15–25 % of daily energy expenditure allow unimpaired endurance performance despite nutritional ketosis."[412]

And he concludes:

> "Both observational and prospectively designed studies support the conclusion that submaximal endurance performance can be sustained despite the virtual exclusion of carbohydrate from the human diet. Clearly this result does not automatically follow the casual implementation of dietary carbohydrate restriction, however, as careful attention to time for keto-adaptation, mineral nutriture, and constraint of the daily protein dose is required. Contradictory results in the scientific literature can be explained by the lack of attention to these lessons learned (and for the most part now forgotten) by the cultures that traditionally lived by hunting. Therapeutic use of ketogenic diets should not require constraint of most forms of physical labor or recreational activity, with the one caveat that anaerobic (i.e., weight lifting or sprint) performance is limited by the low muscle glycogen levels induced by a ketogenic diet, and this would strongly discourage its use under most conditions of competitive athletics."[413]

Based upon Dr. Phinney's work, my blood glucose model, of which I proudly presented in the chapter entitled "The Way Things Ought To Be (Part I)," recommended frequent, light exercise.

If you were thinking that I would now go over each of remaining five human organ systems (five because I'm including the skeletal system proper, the bones, and the integumentary system proper, the skin, hair and nails), I have a shocker for you: the medical literature world is predominantly data- and theorem-light—more, ignorant—about how macronutrients, not just vitamins and minerals, but how macronutrients— fats, proteins, and carbohydrates—and, specifically, a low-carbohydrate, medium-protein, high-fat diet, affect all but one of the remaining systems.

True, we know how the use of sugar *per se* affects nearly every organ system; two accessible books on the subject that you may find interesting are *Lick the Sugar Habit* (2001) and *Suicide by Sugar* (2009), both by Nancy Appleton, PhD.[414] By the way, these books remind me of an experiment on dogs performed by an ex-physician about two hundred years ago. Let me share this brief story.

> "In 1816, in an attempt to understand the biological value of certain foodstuffs, Francois Magendie—a child of revolutionary Paris and a former physician—set out to observe the effects of a restricted diet. He was particularly interested in what role nitrogen has to play in digestion. The answer he got back, after ten years of painstaking work was none at all: 'As so often in research,' Magendie wrote, with what bitterness we may imagine, 'unexpected results had contradicted every reasonable expectation.' But in the pursuit of this knowledge, Magendie had stumbled upon a striking, if unpleasant discovery: he had found that he was able to starve his experimental dogs to death on diets that should, on the face of it, have given them all the energy they needed for life.
>
> By his own account, Magendie 'placed a small dog about three years old upon a diet exclusively of pure refined sugar with distilled water for drink; he had both *ad libitum.*' By the third week the animal, already weakened, lost its appetite, and developed small ulcers in the centre of each cornea. The ulcers spread, and then the corneas liquefied. Shortly afterwards, the dog died.
>
> Magendie tried other nutritious foods. 'Everyone knows that dogs can live very well on bread alone,' he confidently asserted—but when he put this to the test, he found that 'a dog does not live above fifty days.' The most calorific foods in Magendie's pantry—wheat gluten, starches, sugar, olive oil—were not enough for life. This was totally unexpected. There was something missing—something available only as part of a varied diet—but what?"[415]

Turns out that it was vitamin A, isolated a hundred years later by two American teams, that was needed to keep the eyes from liquefying, though not enough to save the life. The addition of whole milk to the diet saved the life; no, not of the dog, but of children, soldiers, waifs and strays suffering from xerophthalmia in the years preceding the isolation of vitamin A. Of course, even then, experiments—on dogs, children, waifs, or strays—were not performed in the reverse to prove that you don't need the sugar. Carbohydrates have been considered essential since the dawn of agriculture.

"That transition from hunting and gathering to agriculture is generally considered a decisive step in our progress, when we at last acquired the stable food supply and leisure time prerequisite to the great accomplishments of modern civilization. In fact, careful examination of that transition suggests another conclusion: for most people the transition brought infectious diseases, malnutrition, and a shorter life span. For human society in general it worsened the relative lot of women and introduced class-based inequality. More than any other milestone along the path from chimpanzeehood to humanity, agriculture inextricably combines causes of our rise and our fall."[416]

Back to organ systems. As I was saying, we know how sugar by itself negatively affects many organs and organ systems, but little is known about how any specific diet permutation affects the (7b) integumentary (skin, hair and nails), (9) respiratory, (10) lymphatic, (11) immune,[417] or (12) reproductive system. Now, it surely can be inferred that, if we forgo the bolus insulin and carbohydrates, and eat just fat and protein, with type 1s only adding basal insulin, and we live a long, happy, healthy life, then all other organ systems must be doing just fine. But such circumstantial evidence doesn't necessarily *prove* that they're healthy in the court of public opinion, let alone in science. Unlike in evolution versus creationism, where, thankfully, evolution has been upheld,[418] no action has been brought against any carbohydrate-espousing proponent, by any low-carbohydrate proponent, in any jurisdiction. Thus, we have no precedent, no ruling, no adjudication, based upon any evidence, for or against any diet, from any court of law. Not that the vegans haven't tried.[419]

We live today in an environment similar to that initially championed by John Washington Butler,[420] except, instead of its realization deriving from a law forbidding public school teachers from denying the Biblical account of man's origin, we now navigate through an environment emotionally charged by a low-fat dogma; those that pray to it and live by its code do so influenced by the trinity of politics—playing into the public perceptions that they themselves or their forebearers created—faith and commerce, not science, serving it best by ensuring its promulgation into clinical practice guidelines, research, education, news and fixed media. This dogma, however, unlike the Butler Act, is enforced not just in public schools, but across nearly all demographics. Maybe by the time the 18th edition of this book is published, a precedent will be set upholding low-carbohydrate diets in a court of law, the above organ systems will be covered in more detail, and I will be able to provide a robust summary.

There is some information about how diet affects the (12) reproductive system, but most sources highlight the role of calories, not how any specific combination of macronutrients affects the reproductive system. At first glance, learning that a low-carbohydrate, ketogenic diet led to significant improvement in weight, percent free testosterone, and fasting insulin in women with obesity and Polycystic Ovary Syndrome (PCOS) over a 24 week period, it sounds like we can put one in the win column for a low-carbohydrate diet best supporting the reproductive system. Alas, PCOS is considered an endocrine disorder.[421]

Which really leaves only one organ system that I didn't cover. Well, half of one.

The (6b) Skeletal (bone) system, beyond studies about the correlation between osteoporosis and calcium, is supported by a low-carbohydrate diet in "The Effect of a Low-Carbohydrate Diet on Bone Turnover," by J. D. Carter, F. B. Vasey, and J. Valeriano. Here, the authors set out to determine whether or not a low-carbohydrate diet would lead to increased bone turnover. Thirty patients (15 study subjects and 15 controls) were recruited for this 3-month study. The 15 patients on the diet were instructed to consume less than 20 g of carbohydrates per day for the 1st month and then less than 40 g per day for months 2 and 3. Control subjects had no restrictions on their diet. And the conclusion? "Although the patients on the low-carbohydrate diet did lose significantly more weight than the controls did, the diet did not increase bone turnover markers compared with controls at any time point. Further, there was no significant change in the bone turnover ratio compared with controls."[422]

In what could be classified as the only compendium devoted to the relationship between the skeletal system and diet, *Nutrition and Bone Health* (2004) doesn't *advocate* any particular diet, although it does include an article—the book is a collection of independently written articles— describing both the plate model of the UK and the pyramid model of the US.[423] The authors used these models as an assumption of diet; that, and a reference to fat leading to heart disease, without quoting any specific, credible evidence in defense of either. As you read more and more health, diet, medical, reference books and articles, you'll find support of those two concepts without evidence common faults.[424] Mark Twain understated it best when he said "Be careful about reading health books. You could die of a misprint."

However, if I could choose one quote from the book to best embody its entirety, it is that "bone health is not a mononutrient issue."[425] Some specific examples include:

- "An inadequate intake of calcium and an inadequate level of vitamin D, alone and in combination, influence calcium-regulating hormone levels. Deficiency of either nutrient results in reduced calcium absorption and a lower circulating ionized concentration. The latter stimulates the secretion of parathyroid hormone (PTH), a potent bone-resorbing agent. Over time, a small increase in the circulating level of PTH leads to measurable and significant bone loss and increased risk of fracture."[426]

- "Vitamin A deficiency is characterized by xerophthalmia, night blindness, cessation of growth, and increased susceptibility to infections. On the other side, very vitamin A intake might affect, among others, bone and bone metabolism, as it has long been known. High vitamin A intake seems to accelerate bone loss."[427]

- "Fluorine is an indispensable trace element and plays a role in normal development and maintenance of the skeleton and teeth. As is true for other essential trace elements, deficiency or excess has clinical consequences: intakes below the recommended daily dose result in growth and development retardation, whereas long-term high intake leads to hyperostosis or even severe skeletal sclerosis."[428]

Low-fat endorsing as it may be perceived, one article clearly supports the use of fat in promoting bone health: "Dairy products are complex, containing many essential nutrients, and thus their effects on bone health are likely more that can be accounted for by any single constituent and the totality of their effects may be more than the sum of parts."[429]

But more interesting is the book's discussion on fruits and vegetables:

- "The approach of using food groups to examine the relationship between diet and disease is an appropriate and logical approach to examining the relationship between diet and osteoporosis. There is somewhat remarkable agreement among countries as to the proportions with which we should be eating food groups. The data suggest that milk and milk products (as providers of more than 50% of total dietary calcium) and fruit and vegetables are beneficial to bone health across the age ranges, although clearly more work on fracture reduction is required."[430]

- "Only two large population-based studies have examined the specific impact of dietary "quality"/food groups directly on indices of bone health, namely, the Aberdeen Prospective Osteoporosis Screening Study (APOSS) and the Framingham Offspring Study. Cluster analysis on 904 women (mean age 54 yr.), pre-, peri-, and postmenopausal, showed that a number of food groups, including fried foods, cakes, processed meats, and puddings, were associated with worsening hip bone loss…"[431]

- "These data support the findings of both the original APOSS baseline study and the older Framingham cohort and indicate that a high fruit and vegetable intake is protective to the skeleton, whereas high candy consumption is associated with lower bone mass, regardless of gender. These data also suggest that a high intake of fatty, sugary foods is detrimental to bone health around the time of menopause."[432]

This last quote conflicts with one of the most interesting cohort studies I've seen on the subject. In "Food Choices and Coronary Heart Disease: A Population Based Cohort Study of Rural Swedish Men with 12 Years of Follow-up," by Sara Holmberg, Anders Thelin, and Eva-Lena, the authors concluded: "Daily intake of fruit and vegetables was associated with a lower risk of coronary heart disease when combined with a high dairy fat consumption, but not when combined with a low dairy fat consumption. Choosing wholemeal bread or eating fish at least twice a week showed no association with the outcome."[433]

As with other nutritional controversies, we find the unifying answer to whether or not it's fruits and vegetables *per se* or in combination with other foods that reduces heart or bone disease risk from Gary Taubes, and here he delivers the last words: "As a matter of logic, though, it doesn't necessarily imply that the lack of vitamins are caused by the lack of fresh fruits and vegetables…It's possible that eating easily digestible carbohydrates and sugars increases our need for vitamins that we would otherwise derive from animal products in sufficient quantities."[434] "There is an increased need for these vitamins when more carbohydrate in the diet is consumed."[435]

APPENDIX A: BOOKS ON DIABETES

Title: *8 Weeks to Maximizing Diabetes Control: How to Improve Your Blood Glucose and Stay Healthy with Type 2 Diabetes*
Author: Laura Hieronymus, MSED, APRN, BC-ADM, CDE, and Christine Tobin, RN, MBA, CDE
Publisher: American Diabetes Association, Inc.
Year Published: 2008
Number of Pages: 161
Diet Advocated: Low-Fat Diet
Specific Page Reference(s): Page 25: "Nutrition experts recommend that about half the calories you eat come from carbohydrates."

Title: *The Diabetes Answer Book: Practical Answers to More than 300 Top Questions*
Author: David K. McCulloch, MD
Publisher: Sourcebooks, Inc.
Year Published: 2008
Number of Pages: 333
Diet advocated: Low-Fat Diet
Specific Page Reference(s): Page 173: "In the past few decades, nutritional research has shown quite consistent results. The kind of diet that will help reduce your risk of getting heart disease, high cholesterol, high blood pressure, or cancer is the same diet that helps prevent you from getting overweight. You should eat less fat (especially saturated fat), less protein (especially animal protein), and more unrefined carbohydrate (especially carbohydrate that is high in soluble such as lentils and beans), grains, and fresh vegetables."

Title: *Type 1 Diabetes For Dummies*
Author: Alan L. Rubin, MD
Publisher: Wiley Publishing, Inc.
Year Published: 2008
Number of Pages: 360
Diet Advocated: Low-Fat Diet
Specific Page Reference(s): Page 129: "Experts recommend that 40 to 50 percent of a person's daily calorie intake should be from carbohydrates (1 gram of carbohydrate contains 4 kilocalories). And yes, people with diabetes can eat real carbohydrates rather than artificial sweeteners so long as they don't eat too many total calories." Page 135: "Even though carbohydrates are the most important source of energy for everyone (especially folks with T1DM), you can't forget about protein and fat."

Title: *What To Expect When You Have Diabetes: 170 Tips for Living Well with Diabetes*
Author: American Diabetes Association, Inc.
Publisher: Good Books / American Diabetes Association, Inc.
Year Published: 2008
Number of Pages: 216
Diet Advocated: Low-Fat Diet
Specific Page Reference(s): Page 104: "A heart-healthy eating plan is low in saturated and dietary cholesterol, with total fat around 30% of total calories. This helps reduce blood cholesterol...The following suggestions can help you eat low-fat meals: Select lean meats and cook with little or no fat. Choose low-fat or fat-free milk products. Eat less meat, cheese, and bacon. Eat low-fat breads and starchy foods, such as potatoes, rice, and beans."

Title: *10 Steps to Better Living*
Author: Ginger Kanzer-Lewis, RN, BC, EdM, CDE
Publisher: American Diabetes Association, Inc.
Year Published: 2007
Number of Pages: 260
Diet Advocated: Low-Fat Diet
Specific Page Reference(s): Page 67: "Recommendations for a Healthy Meal Plan: Eat a variety of foods as recommended in the Food Pyramid to get a balanced intake of the nutrients your body needs: carbohydrates, proteins, fats, vitamins, and minerals. Reduce the amount of fat you eat by choosing fewer high-fat foods and cooking with less fat. Eat more whole grains." Page 75: "You can eat foods that contain sugar."

Title: *Diabetes on Your Own Terms*
Author: Janis Roszler, RD, CDE, LD/N
Publisher: Marlowe & Company
Year Published: 2007
Number of Pages: 196
Diet Advocated: Low-Fat Diet
Specific Page Reference(s): Page 112: "Limit your fats — Reduce the amount of fat in a recipe as much as possible without compromising the quality of the dish. Use low-fat or reduced-fat versions of regular cheese, deli meats, and salad dressings."

Title: *Dr. Bernstein's Diabetes Solution: The Complete Guide to Achieving Normal Blood Sugars*
Author: Richard K. Bernstein, MD
Publisher: Little, Brown and Company. Hachette Book Group USA
Year Published: 2007
Number of Pages: 519
Diet Advocated: Low-Carbohydrate Diet
Specific Page Reference(s): Page xi: "Finally, much of what I will cover in this book is in direct opposition to the recommendation of the American Diabetes Association (ADA) and

other national diabetes associations. Why? Because if I had followed those guidelines, they would have killed me long ago. Such conflicts include the Low-Carbohydrate diet I recommend; the avoidance of oral agents (such as sulfonylureas) that burn our surviving insulin-producing beta cells in type 2 diabetics; my utilization of certain nutrients to lower insulin resistance; my preference for certain insulins over others, which I avoid; my desire to preserve remaining beta cells (an alien concept to traditional practice); and my insistence that diabetics are entitled to the same, normal blood sugars that non-diabetics enjoy, rather than the ADA's current insistence upon higher levels. Most important, unlike the ADA guidelines, ours work."

Title: *Dr. Neal Barnard's Program for Reversing Diabetes: The Scientifically Proven System for Reversing Diabetes Without Drugs*
Author: Neal D. Barnard, MD
Publisher: Rodale, Inc.
Year Published: 2007
Number of Pages: 272
Diet Advocated: Low-Fat Diet (Vegan)
Specific Page Reference(s): Page 29: "These practices eliminate cholesterol and animal fat, keep fats in general very low, and guide you away from sugar and refined carbohydrates and toward healthy complex carbohydrates. As you will see, there is a special advantage to a vegetarian diet, or I should say vegan diet—meaning a menu that includes no animal products at all. Dietary cholesterol is found only in animal products." Page 46: "Nutrition Guidelines. Overall principals: Choose foods from plant sources. Avoid all animal products and keep vegetable oils to a bare minimum. Favor foods with a low glycemic index (GI). Focus on the New Four Food Groups. Whole grains (8 servings per day), Legumes (3 servings per day), Vegetables (4 or more servings per day), Fruits (3 servings or more per day)."

Title: *Guide to Insulin & Type 2 Diabetes*
Author: Marie McCarren
Publisher: American Diabetes Association, Inc.
Year Published: 2007
Number of Pages: 232
Diet Advocated: Low-Fat Diet
Specific Page Reference(s): Page 111: "Carbohydrate raises your blood glucose level. Insulin lowers your blood glucose level. When you balance insulin and carbohydrate, you'll have better glucose control. This is called carbohydrate (carb) counting."

Title: *Sex and Diabetes: For Him and For Her*
Author: Janis Roszler, RD, CDE, LDN & Donna Rice, MBA, BSN, RN, CDE
Publisher: American Diabetes Association, Inc.
Year Published: 2007

Number of Pages: 209

Diet Advocated: Low-Fat Diet

Specific Page Reference(s): Page 43: "Excessively low-carbohydrate diets are popular, but can be unhealthy. Your body uses carbohydrate-containing foods for energy. When these aren't available, it turns to fat and protein, which don't burn efficiently. When fat is metabolized, it releases undesirable by-products called ketones. They can make you feel light-headed and even nauseous. Extremely high levels of ketones in the body can be life threatening. The American Diabetes Association suggests that you consume at least 130 grams of carbohydrates each day. This is the amount needed to meet the needs of your brain and central nervous system. Less than that is not recommended."

Title: *Stop Prediabetes Now: The Ultimate Plan to Lose Weight and Prevent Diabetes*
Author: Jack Challem and Ron Hunninghake, M.D.
Publisher: John Wiley & Sons, Inc.
Year Published: 2007
Number of Pages: 294
Diet Advocated: Low-Carbohydrate Diet
Specific Page Reference(s): Page 62: "People with prediabetes often have difficulty losing weight on low-fat, high-carb diets. Instead, they are more likely to lose weight on low-carb, high-protein diets. The reason is that people with prediabetes are extremely sensitive to sugar and carbohydrate calories. They do better with protein, which does not trigger a strong glucose response."

Title: *American Medical Association Guide to Living With Diabetes: Preventing and Treating Type 2 Diabetes – Essential Information You and Your Family need to Know*
Author: Boyd E. Metzger, MD
Publisher: John Wiley & Sons, Inc.
Year Published: 2006
Number of Pages: 278
Diet Advocated: Low-Fat Diet
Specific Page Reference(s): Page 15: "A healthy diet (see chapter 4) is an essential part of preventing type 2 diabetes. You will need to make changes in your eating habits to improve both the quality and quantity of food you eat. Your doctor or dietician can help you develop a dietary plan that supplies all your nutritional needs and fits your lifestyle. Generally, a healthy diet is low in fat and calories; provides carbohydrates, proteins, and fats in percentages recommended by your doctor or dietician; and is rich in fiber. It includes plenty of fruits, vegetables, whole grains, and legumes, along with fish (at least two or three times a week), which provides heart-healthy omega-3 fatty acids." Page 37: "A diabetes-fighting diet is heart-healthy, calorie conscious, high in fiber and other important nutrients, and low in harmful fats and sweets. Specifically, it is rich in whole grains, vegetables, legumes, and fruits, and replaces unhealthy fats (such as those in fatty meats and snack foods) with healthy plant-based fats (such as olive oil) and omega-3 fatty acids (from fish)." Page 46:

Appendix A

"Carbohydrates—composed of simple and complex sugars—are the body's most important source of fuel. Because of their importance, carbohydrates should comprise 50 to 60 percent of your daily intake of calories."

Title: *Cheating Destiny: Living with Diabetes, America's biggest Epidemic*
Author: James S. Hirsch
Publisher: Houghton Mifflin Company
Year Published: 2006
Number of Pages: 307
Diet Advocated: Low-Carbohydrate Diet
Specific Page Reference(s): Pages 126-134: "Dr. Bernstein's Solution."

Title: *Diabetes Survival Guide: Understanding The Facts About Diagnosis, Treatment, And Prevention* (Originally published as *Controlling Diabetes The Easy Way*)
Author: Stanley Mirsky, M.D., and Joan Rattner Heilman
Publisher: Ballantine Books
Year Published: 2006
Number of Pages: 326
Diet Advocated: Low-Fat Diet
Specific Page Reference(s): Page 33: "This diet is not concerned with calories (unless, of course, you want to lose weight). It is only concerned with carbohydrates. You must eat no more than a certain number of grams of carbohydrates (though not refined sugar) at every meal. That is the only rule. Aside from that, you can eat anything you like if your weight is where you want it to be." Page 35: "To follow this diet, there is just one rule: avoid simple carbohydrates such as sugar, honey, and syrups and eat 40 to 45 grams of complex carbohydrates at every meal. (Exception: if you are engaging in strenuous exercise, you may need more.) Forty to 45 grams of carbohydrate amount to 50 to 60 percent of your daily food, approximating the typical American diet."

Title: *Diabetes; Sugar-Coated Crisis: Who Gets It, Who Profits And How To Stop It*
Author: David Spero, RN
Publisher: New Society Publishers
Year Published: 2006
Number of Pages: 223
Diet Advocated: Low-Carbohydrate Diet
Specific Page Reference(s): Page 69: "The diabetes establishment advocates eating 45-65% of calories from carbohydrates, a number significantly higher than the typical American diet (40-45%). Some ADA publications advocate "making starches the star" in diet plans and give advice for increasing starch intake. On the face of it, this seems strange advice." Page 166: "I'm going to suggest a general meal plan, based on Richard Bernstein and others."

Title: *Mayo Clinic on Managing Diabetes: How To Prevent, Control and Live Well With Diabetes*
Author: Maria Collazo-Clavell, M.D., Medical Editor in Chief
Publisher: Mayo Clinic
Year Published: 2006
Number of Pages: 229
Diet Advocated: Low-Fat Diet
Specific Page Reference(s): Page 57: "There is no diabetes diet. Contrary to popular myth, having diabetes doesn't mean that you have to start eating special foods or follow a complicated diet plan. For most people, having diabetes simply translates into eating a variety of foods in moderate amounts and sticking to regular mealtimes. This means choosing a diet that emphasizes vegetables, fruits and whole grains—and smaller servings of lean or low-fat animal foods, such as lean cuts of meat and low-fat dairy products." Page 58: "Carbohydrates: 45% to 65% of daily calories."

Title: *Type 2 Diabetes: Your Questions Answered: A Comprehensive Guide to Living Well*
Author: Rosemary Walker & Jill Rodgers
Publisher: American Diabetes Association, Inc.
Year Published: 2006
Number of Pages: 208
Diet Advocated: Low-Fat Diet
Specific Page Reference(s): Page 48: "Aim for complex carbohydrates (starches) and fiber (such as bread, pasta, and whole grains) to make up about a third of what you eat, with fruit and vegetables forming another third. Making up the rest of your food intake from protein foods and dairy products (2-3 servings daily from each group) will give you a healthy balance. Choosing lower fat alternatives where you can will help reduce your risk of heart disease."

Title: *Conquering Diabetes: A Cutting-Edge, Comprehensive Program for Prevention and Treatment*
Author: Anne Peters, MD
Publisher: Hudson Street Press
Year Published: 2005
Number of Pages: 349
Diet Advocated: Low-Fat Diet
Specific Page Reference(s): Page 121: "The goal is to have the carbohydrate intake between 40 and 45 percent of total calories, protein between 15 and 20 percent of total calories, and fat between 30 and 35 percent of total calories."

Title: *Guide to Healthy Restaurant Eating: Third Edition*
Author: Hope S. Warshaw, MMSc, RD, CDE, BC-ADM
Publisher: American Diabetes Association, Inc.
Year Published: 2005
Number of Pages: 734

Appendix A

Diet Advocated: Low-Fat Diet

Specific Page Reference(s): Page 2: "Eat more (six or more servings) grains, beans, and starchy vegetables each day. Make three of the servings whole grains."

Title: *The Diabetes Carbohydrate & Fat Gram Guide: Quick, Easy Meal Planning Using carbohydrate & Fat Gram Counts*

Author: Lea Ann Holzmeister, RD, CDE

Publisher: American Diabetes Association, Inc.

Year Published: 2005

Number of Pages: 603

Diet Advocated: Low-Fat Diet

Specific Page Reference(s): Page xx: "Carbohydrates raise your blood glucose level. A recommended range of carbohydrate intake is 45-65% of total calories. Carbohydrate and monounsaturated fat together should provide 60-70% of your total calorie intake."

Title: *The Diabetes Diet: Dr. Bernstein's Low-Carbohydrate Solution*

Author: Richard K. Bernstein, MD

Publisher: Little, Brown and Company. Time Warner Book Group

Year Published: 2005

Number of Pages: 291

Diet Advocated: Low Carbohydrate Diet

Specific Page Reference(s): From Chapter 1, "Why a Low-Carb Diet is the Only Answer for Diabetics and a Very Good Answer for Everyone Else," Page 20: "There is simply no question that a truly low carbohydrate diet—namely the one presented in these pages—is the solution for diabetics. Indeed, it's the solution to the obesity that plagues increasingly sedentary populations around the world." Page 21: "In general, a low-carbohydrate diet provides the nutrients that people need without the excess carbohydrate that causes high blood sugars and requires high levels of insulin. In addition, protein, fat, and slow-acting carbohydrate, such as leafy and whole-plant vegetables and some kinds of root vegetables, tend to be broken down more slowly and continuously, so people who follow this diet tend to feel satisfied much longer after eating. It has also been shown that people on low-carbohydrate diets can consume more calories while losing the same amount of weight as those on simple restricted-calorie diets."

Title: *The Joslin guide to Diabetes: A Program for Managing Your Treatment*

Author: Richard S. Beaser, M.D., with Amy P. Campbell. R.D., M.S., C.D.E.

Publisher: Simon & Schuster (A Fireside Book)

Year Published: 2005

Number of Pages: 431

Diet Advocated: Low-Fat Diet

Specific Page Reference(s): Page 37: "Carbohydrate provides energy to the cells in the body. There is now a Recommended Dietary Allowance for carbohydrate of 130 grams a day for adults and children. This amount is based on the average minimum amount of glucose that is used by the brain."

Title: *The Type 2 Diabetes Sourcebook For Women*
Author: M. Sarah Rosenthal, Ph.D.
Publisher: McGraw-Hill
Year Published: 2005
Number of Pages: 258
Diet Advocated: Low-Fat Diet
Specific Page Reference(s): Page 93: "Lowering Fat and Healthy Eating. Studies show that reducing dietary fat may also prevent cancers, such as colorectal and estrogen-dependent cancers (like breast cancer). Dietary guidelines from nutrition experts, government nutrition advisories and panels, and registered dieticians have not changed in fifty years. A good diet is a balanced diet representing all food groups, based largely on plant-based foods—carbohydrates—such as fruits, vegetables, legumes, and grains, with a balance of calories from animal-based foods—protein and fat—such as meats (red meat, poultry), fish, and dairy products."

Title: *Atkins Diabetes Revolution: The Groundbreaking Approach to Preventing and Controlling Type 2 Diabetes*
Author: Robert C. Atkins, M.D., with Mary C. Vernon, M.D., C.M.D., and Jacqueline A Eberstein, R.N.
Publisher: William Morrow, An Imprint of HarperCollins Publishers
Year Published: 2004
Number of Pages: 538
Diet Advocated: Low-Carbohydrate Diet
Specific Page Reference(s): Page 128: "To kick-start weight loss, limit your carbohydrate intake to 20 grams of Net Carbs a day."

Title: *1001 Tips For Living Well With Diabetes*
Author: American Diabetes Association, Inc.
Publisher: American Diabetes Association, Inc.
Year Published: 2004
Number of Pages: 1184
Diet Advocated: Low-Fat Diet
Specific Page Reference(s): Page 498: "I've heard that a low-carbohydrate, high-protein, high-fat diet will help me lose weight without cutting calories. Should I change from the high-carbohydrate, low-fat diet I've always followed? Probably not. A low-carbohydrate diet is very difficult to follow for a long period of time." Page 498: "Until there's more evidence, it's probably best to continue with a balanced carbohydrate meal plan."

Appendix A

Title: *A Field Guide to Type 2 Diabetes: The Essential Resource from the Diabetes Experts*
Author: American Diabetes Association, Inc
Publisher: American Diabetes Association, Inc.
Year Published: 2004
Number of Pages: 287
Diet Advocated: Low-Fat Diet
Specific Page Reference(s): Page 75: "In terms of overall health, some sections are better than others. Whole grains, beans, and starchy vegetables provide vitamins, minerals, and fiber. Notice that their section is the biggest, meaning a healthy diet has more servings from this section than from the other sections."

Title: *Complete guide to Carb Counting: How to take the mystery out of carb counting and unlock the secrets to blood sugar control: 2nd edition*
Author: Hope S. Warshaw, MMSc, RD, CDE, BC-ADM, and Karmeen Kulkarni, MS, RD, CDE, BC-ADM
Publisher: American Diabetes Association, Inc.
Year Published: 2004
Number of Pages: 251
Diet Advocated: Low-Fat Diet
Specific Page Reference(s): Page 8: "If carbs raise blood glucose, should you follow a low-carb diet? Once you realize that carbohydrates raise blood glucose, you might jump to the conclusion that, if you have diabetes, it's best to steer clear of them. And that certainly might be your conclusion if you read up on one of the low-carb diet regimens. These diets sound like they are made-to-order for people with type 2 diabetes. The reality is that at this point, the science to support the long-term use of low-carb diets (less than 40% of calories as carbohydrate) for long-term weight loss and maintenance simply doesn't exist."

Title: *Dr. Peter J. D'Adamo's Eat Right 4 Your type Health Library. Diabetes: Fight It With the Blood Type Diet. The Individualized Plan for Preventing and Treating Diabetes (Type I, Type II) and Pre-Diabetes*
Author: Dr. Peter J. D'Adamo
Publisher: G.P. Putnam's Sons, a member of Penguin Group (USA) Inc.
Year Published: 2004
Number of Pages: 188
Diet Advocated: Low-Carbohydrate Diet
Specific Page Reference(s): Page 51: "Grains and starches are the Achilles' heel of Blood Type O. You tend to do poorly on corn, wheat, sorghum, barley, and many of their by-products (sweeteners, etc.). These common grains have a very pronounced effect on increasing body fat and promoting insulin resistance in Blood Type O, and other grains are by no means necessary in your diet."

Title: *How To Prevent, Control & Cure Diabetes*
Author: Seymour L. Alterman, M.D., F.A.C.P. & Donals A. Kullman, M.D.
Publisher: Frederick Fell Publishers, Inc.
Year Published: 2004
Number of Pages: 305
Diet Advocated: Low-Fat Diet
Specific Page Reference(s): Page 46: "Carbohydrate 40-60% of calories, Protein 10-20% of calories, Fat less than 30% of calories."   Page 47: "Eat more starches and foods high in fiber. Page 190-193: The Pritikin Program, Diabetes And Atherosclerosis."

Title: *Prediabetes: What You Need to Know to Keep Diabetes Away*
Author: Gretchen Becker
Publisher: Marlowe & Company
Year Published: 2004
Number of Pages: 200
Diet Advocated: Low-Carbohydrate Diet
Specific Page Reference(s): Page 7-8: "Furthermore, more and more controlled studies have been done that show that low-carb diets do work without causing deleterious effects on lipid levels. In fact, the lipid levels usually improve."   Page 32: "Learn what processed, or refined, carbohydrates are—and avoid them."

Title: *The Complete Diabetes Prevention Plan: A Guide To understanding the Emerging Epidemic of Prediabetes and Halting Its Progression to Diabetes*
Author: Sandra Woodruff, M.S., R.D., LD/N, and Christopher Saudek, M.D.
Publisher: Avery, A Member of Penguin Group (USA) Inc.
Year Published: 2004
Number of Pages: 280
Diet Advocated: Low-Fat Diet
Specific Page Reference(s): Page 21: "Eat a healthy diet that is low in calories, fat, and saturated fat. Limit fat intake to 30 percent of calories and saturated fat to no more than 10% of calories. None of the studies tested specifically whether reducing fat or carbohydrates or both were most effective, but all emphasized limiting fat and total calories. Choose more vegetables, fruits, whole grains, lean meats, low-fat dairy products, and unsaturated fats."

Title: *The Diabetes Sourcebook*
Author: Diana W. Guthrie, Ph.D., A.R.N.P., C.D.E., and Richard A Guthrie, M.D., C.D.E.
Publisher: McGraw-Hill
Year Published: 2004
Number of Pages: 290
Diet Advocated: Low-Fat Diet
Specific Page Reference(s): Page 39: "The recommended proportions are 30 percent or less fat, 12 to 20 percent protein, and the rest in carbohydrates called simple sugars and complex

carbohydrates, such as cereal, fruits, and vegetables." From the chart on Page 41: "6-11 servings per day from bread, cereal, rice, and pasta group."

Title: *The Everything Diabetes book: From Diagnosis and Die to Insulin and Exercise, All You Need to Live a Healthy, Active Life*
Author: Paula Ford-Martin with Ian Blummer, MD
Publisher: Adams Media, an F+W Publications Company
Year Published: 2004
Number of Pages: 303
Diet Advocated: Low-Fat Diet
Specific Page Reference(s): Page 120: "To avoid all carbohydrate-containing foods is both impossible and un-advisable—your body needs the important micronutrients and phytochemicals contained in these foods. In fact, the World Health Organization (WHO) recommends that carbohydrates from a variety of foods account for 55 percent of the total calories in your daily diet."

Title: *The Johns Hopkins White Papers: Diabetes*
Author: Christopher D. Saudek, M.D. and Simeon Margolis, M.D., Ph.D.
Publisher: Johns Hopkins Medicine
Year Published: 2004
Number of Pages: 59
Diet Advocated: Low-Fat Diet
Specific Page Reference(s): Page 26: "Most experts recommend that people with diabetes eat a diet high in carbohydrates and low in fat. According to this school of thought, 50% to 60% of calories should come from carbohydrates and 30% or fewer from fat."

Title: The pH Miracle For Diabetics: The Revolutionary Diet Plan for Type 1 and Type 2 Diabetics
Author: Robert O. Young, Ph.D., and Shelley Redford Young
Publisher: Warner Books
Year Published: 2004
Number of Pages: 333
Diet Advocated: Low-Carbohydrate Diet
Specific Page Reference(s): Page 73: "There's nothing complicated about eating to stabilize your blood sugar. Eat plenty of less acidic food, and skip the very acidic foods. You need to eat lots of green vegetables, (good) water, and (good) fats. You need to not eat sugars and starches. you need to eat frequently, and you need to stop eating when you are satisfied." Page 78: "Your body promptly turns even complex carbohydrates into sugars, so stick with low-carbohydrate foods. Your focus should be mainly on green vegetables, largely forsaking grains such as wheat, rice, barley, oats, and especially corn, as well as the cereals, pastas, pastries, and myriad other foods made with them. Yes, I know this flies in the face of that famous USDA food pyramid, with its wide base of bread, cereal, rice, and pasta. All I can say

is, I believe that pyramid is a recipe for disaster for anyone, and especially diabetics. It's a setup for bombarding your body with sugars, in the fast lane to overacidity."

Title: *Think Like A Pancreas: A Practical Guide to Managing Diabetes With Insulin*
Author: Gary Scheiner, MS, CDE
Publisher: Marlowe & Company
Year Published: 2004
Number of Pages: 241
Diet Advocated: Low-Fat Diet
Specific Page Reference(s): Page 44: "A major part of "thinking like a pancreas" involves matching insulin to carbohydrate intake."

Title: *Understanding Diabetes*
Author: Marie Clark
Publisher: John Wiley & Sons, Inc.
Year Published: 2004
Number of Pages: 122
Diet Advocated: Low-Fat Diet
Specific Page Reference(s): Page 72: "Base your meals on starchy foods—fill up on these. This means such foods as bread, potatoes, rice, pasta, noodles, oats, crackers, breakfast cereals. These all provide starch, fiber, vitamins (Especially B) and minerals." Page 73: "Reduce your intake of fats and fatty and sugary foods. Fats in the diet is the main problem as far as heart disease, high blood cholesterol and weight gain are concerned."

Title: *American Dietetic Association Guide to Eating Right When You Have Diabetes: The Comprehensive Approach To Managing your Diabetes by Eating Well*
Author: Magie Powers, MS, RD, CDE
Publisher: John Wiley & Sons, Inc.
Year Published: 2003
Number of Pages: 275
Diet Advocated: Low-Fat Diet
Specific Page Reference(s): Page 39: "Build a healthy base: Let the Food Guide Pyramid guide your food choices. Eat a variety of grains daily, especially whole grains. Eat a variety of fruits and vegetables daily. Choose a diet that is low in saturated fat and cholesterol and moderate in total fat."

Title: *Diabetes A to Z: What You Need to Know About Diabetes – Simply Put*
Author: American Diabetes Association, Inc.
Publisher: American Diabetes Association, Inc.
Year Published: 2003
Number of Pages: 204
Diet Advocated: Low-Fat Diet

214

Specific Page Reference(s): Page 126: "Eat larger amounts and more servings from food groups that take up more space on the pyramid. The three food groups that take up more space are 1) grains, beans, and starchy vegetables; 2) vegetables; and 3) fruits."

Title: *Help! My Underwear is Shrinking! One woman's story of how to eat right, lose weight, and win the battle against diabetes*
Author: Jo Ann Hattner, MPH, RD, Ann Coulston, MS, RD, and E. Michael Goodkind, BA
Publisher: American Diabetes Association, Inc.
Year Published: 2003
Number of Pages: 137
Diet Advocated: Low-Fat Diet
Specific Page Reference(s): Page 121-131: "Appendix B. Sample Menus contain 165 grams of carbohydrate per day for a 5-foot tall person to 245 grams of carbohydrate per day for a 5-foot-10-inch tall person."

Title: *Insulin Pump Therapy Demystified: An Essential Guide for Everyone Pumping Insulin*
Author: Gabrielle Kaplan-Mayer
Publisher: Marlowe & Company
Year Published: 2003
Number of Pages: 192
Diet Advocated: Low-Fat Diet
Specific Page Reference(s): Page 103: "By counting the carbohydrates in the food you're eating, you'll be able to determine exactly how much insulin to take." Page 103: "Don't despair: It takes some time and practice to get a sense of just how much insulin to bolus to cover the carbohydrates in the food you eat."

Title: *The Diabetic's Total Health And Happiness Book*
Author: June Biermann and Barbara Toohey
Publisher: Jeremy P. Tarcher/Penguin, a member of Penguin Group (USA) Inc.
Year Published: 2003
Number of Pages: 354
Diet Advocated: Informational (but leans toward Low- Fat)
Specific Page Reference(s): Although this book gives equal information about Low-Fat and Low-Carbohydrate diets, even including quotes from Dr. Bernstein (See pages 51-56), the authors offer a recipe for "Mashed Potatoes with Green Onions" on Page 297: "For total comfort the only thing to serve with meat loaf is mashed potatoes. In fact, mashed potatoes are the ultimate comfort dish. This healthy version, flavor-heightened with scallions, is so fast and easy that you now have no excuse to ever again use instant mashed potatoes, which are a whopping 80 on the Glycemic index. Carbohydrate: 28 gm."

Title: *What Makes My Blood Glucose Go Up...And Down? And 101 Other Frequently Asked Questions about Your Blood Glucose Levels*
Author: Jennie Brand-Miller, Ph.D., Kaye Foster-Powell, M. Nutr. & Diet., & Rick Mendosa
Publisher: Marlowe & Company
Year Published: 2003
Number of Pages: 196
Diet Advocated: Low-Fat Diet
Specific Page Reference(s): Page 27: "How much carbohydrate should a person eat at one sitting? It depends on your overall calorie intake. If you are an average-weight man or woman who is moderately active, then your carbohydrate intake at one sitting should be about 60 grams per meal and 30 grams per snack. This amounts to half of your calories as carbohydrate, a level that is considered healthy."

Title: *A Field Guide to Type 1 Diabetes: The Essential Resource from the Diabetes Expert*
Author: American Diabetes Association, Inc.
Publisher: American Diabetes Association, Inc.
Year Published: 2002
Number of Pages: 210
Diet Advocated: Low-Fat Diet
Specific Page Reference(s): Page 80: "In terms of overall health, some sections are better than others. Whole grains, beans, and starchy vegetables provide vitamins, minerals, and fiber. Notice that their section is the biggest, meaning a healthy diet has more servings from this section than from the other sections."

Title: *Carol Guber's Type 2 Diabetes Life plan: Take Charge, Take Care, and Feel Better than Ever*
Author: Carol Guber with Betsy Thorpe
Publisher: Broadway Books
Year Published: 2002
Number of Pages: 234
Diet Advocated: Low-Fat Diet
Specific Page Reference(s): Page 60: "For most adults, 45 to 75 grams of carbohydrate per meal is sufficient depending on age, weight, and physical activity. This translates into three to five servings each meal every day. For good health, your carbohydrates should be spread out between whole grains, fruits and vegetables, and dairy products."

Title: *Eat Away Diabetes: Beat Type 2 Diabetes by Winning the Blood Sugar Battle*
Author: Kristine Napier, M.P.H., R.D., L.D.
Publisher: Prentice Hall Press
Year Published: 2002
Number of Pages: 366
Diet Advocated: Low-Fat Diet

Appendix A

Specific Page Reference(s): Page 30: "Goal #3: Eat less fat and especially less saturated fat." Page 31: "Goal #5 Eat plenty of fruits, vegetables, legumes, and whole grains, which are high in vitamins, minerals, fiber, and phytochemicals." Page 39: "When you consume 50 to 60 percent of your daily calories as carbohydrate calories (from specific foods), you can better control Type 2 diabetes and reduce the risk of associated heart disease."

Title: *Start Pumping For People with Diabetes: A Practical Approach to Mastering the Insulin Pump*
Author: Howard Wolpert, MD, Editor
Publisher: American Diabetes Association, Inc.
Year Published: 2002
Number of Pages: 181
Diet Advocated: Low-Fat Diet
Specific Page Reference(s): Page 125: "By now you know that of the nutrients you eat, carbohydrate has the biggest impact on your blood glucose and that matching your insulin boluses with the carbohydrates you eat is the cornerstone of your diabetes therapy." Page 131: "It's recommended that you get no more than 30% of our calories from fat, with less than 10% of that coming from saturated fats."

Title: *Tell Me What to Eat If I Have Type II Diabetes*
Author: Elaine Magee, M.P.H., R.D.
Publisher: Rosen Publishing
Year Published: 2002
Number of Pages: 232
Diet Advocated: Low-Fat Diet
Specific Page Reference(s): Page 48: "I don't blame you for being confused. Most of us health professionals are trying to figure it out too. Yes, having a moderate-fat diet (30 to 35 percent calories from fat) seems to add up to better blood sugars for some people with type II diabetes compared to a very low-fat diet (10 to 20 percent calories from fat). The fat helps slow down digestion in general, and "paces" the introduction of glucose. For a variety of reasons, fat also helps some people feel more satisfied after a meal or snack. The tricky part is knowing how much is enough for the diabetic benefits but not too much that it increases your risk of other chronic diseases as well as weight gain. I would try to stick to around 30 to 35 percent calories from fat and see what effect it has on your personal blood sugars, weight, and blood lipid levels. This way you could still have about 15 to 20 percent calories from protein, leaving around 45 to 55 percent calories from carbohydrates (hopefully mostly from whole grains, beans, fruits and vegetables)."

Title: *The Everyday Meal Planner for Type 2 Diabetics: Simple Tips for Healthy Dining at Home or on the Town*
Author: Kristen L. Carson, B.S., M.A., and Aaron Henry
Publisher: Contemporary Books, a Division of the McGraw-Hill Companies
Year Published: 2002

Number of Pages: 178

Diet Advocated: Low-Fat Diet

Specific Page Reference(s): Page 7: "...we do not advocate a high fat content in your diet because of its link to heart disease and other medical problems."

Title: *The Uncomplicated Guide to Diabetes Complications: What every person with diabetes should know about prevention, treatment, and self-care for complications of the Heart, Nerves, Feet, Eyes, Skin, Kidneys, More*

Author: Edited by Marvin E. Levin, MD, and Michael A Pfeifer, MD, MS, CDE, FACE

Publisher: American Diabetes Association, Inc.

Year Published: 2002

Number of Pages: 295

Diet Advocated: Low-Fat Diet

Specific Page Reference(s): Page 275: "A healthy diet is the same for everyone, including people with diabetes. The Food Guide Pyramid illustrates this kind of healthy eating pyramid. The ADA has developed a similar pyramid for people with diabetes."

Title: *What to Do When You Have type 2 Diabetes*

Author: American Diabetes Association, Inc.

Publisher: American Diabetes Association, Inc.

Year Published: 2002

Number of Pages: 59

Diet Advocated: Low-Fat Diet

Specific Page Reference(s): Page 6: "The pyramid scheme. No, it's not really a scheme. It's a way to picture what foods you should eat and how much of them to eat. Food is divided into 6 groups and put into the sections of a pyramid, called the Food Guide Pyramid. The American Diabetes Association developed the one on page 8 just for you. You eat more of the foods in the wide base and fewer servings of the foods in the smaller sections at the top." Page 7: "The healthy base of the pyramid is grains, beans, and starchy vegetables. Eat 6 or more servings of these each day."

Title: *Complete Guide to Convenience Food Counts*

Author: Lea Ann Holzmeister, RD, CDE

Publisher: American Diabetes Association, Inc.

Year Published: 2001

Number of Pages: 430

Diet Advocated: Low-Fat Diet

Specific Page Reference(s): Page 15: "Use the Pyramid as a guide. Write your menus and your list with the Food Pyramid in mind. Load up with grains, vegetables, and fruit. Choose smaller amounts of low-fat dairy, meats, fish, poultry, and legumes. Think carefully about fats, oils, and sweets."

Appendix A

Title: *Diabetic Cooking For Seniors: Delicious New Ways To Eat Well, Eat Right*
Author: Kathleen Stanley, CDE, CN, RD, LD, MSED
Publisher: American Diabetes Association, Inc.
Year Published: 2001
Number of Pages: 181
Diet Advocated: Low-Fat Diet
Specific Page Reference(s): Page 6: "Find out how much fat is allowed in your meal plan—a healthy diet will still contain some fat." Page 6: "Learn to cook without adding extra fat." Page 6: "When eating out, ask if dishes can be prepared without fat."

Title: *The Diabetes Food & Nutrition Bible: A Complete Guide to Planning, Shopping, Cooking, and Eating*
Author: Hope S. Warshaw, MMSc, RD, CDE, and Robyn Webb, MS
Publisher: American Diabetes Association, Inc.
Year Published: 2001
Number of Pages: 324
Diet Advocated: Low-Fat Diet
Specific Page Reference(s): Page 2: "Carbohydrate is your body's main and preferred energy source, whether it's energy to keep your heart beating or energy to walk around the block. Typically, carbohydrate makes up 40% to 60% of calorie intake."

Title: *The Diabetic Athlete: Prescriptions for Exercise and Sports*
Author: Sheri Colberg, PhD
Publisher: Human Kinetics
Year Published: 2001
Number of Pages: 260
Diet Advocated: High-Carbohydrate Diet in relation to Athleticism
Specific Page Reference(s): Page 24: "In general, carbohydrate is recommended during exercise due to its rapid metabolism and absorption compared to fat and protein."

Title: *The First Year: Type 2 Diabetes. An Essential Guide for the Newly Diagnosed*
Author: Gretchen Becker
Publisher: Marlowe & Company
Year Published: 2001
Number of Pages: 312
Diet Advocated: Informational
Specific Page Reference(s): Pages 36-42 discuss all diets and conclude with "There is no single "diabetic diet," and you need to find what works for you."

Title: *Alternative and Complimentary Diabetes Care: How to Combine Natural and Traditional Therapies*

Author: Diana W. Guthrie, Ph.D., F.A.A.N., C.D.E., and Richard A Guthrie, M.D., F.A.C.E., C.D.E.

Publisher: John Wiley & Sons, Inc.

Year Published: 2000

Number of Pages: 244

Diet Advocated: Low-Fat Diet

Specific Page Reference(s): Although this book gives a good overview of the different types of diets available, including Pritikin (page 83), Ornish (page 84), Atkins (page 85), Bernstein (page 86), Eades (page 87), Schwartzbein (page 88), Steward (page 89), and Sears (page 90), the authors conclude on page 99 that: "For individual meal plans it (carbohydrate) would consume 55 to 65 percent."

Title: *American College of Physicians Home Medical Guide to Diabetes*

Author: David R. Goldmann, MD, Medical Editor; David A. Horowitz, MD, Associate Medical Editor

Publisher: Dorling Kindersley Publishing, Inc.

Year Published: 2000

Number of Pages: 96

Diet Advocated: Low-Fat Diet

Specific Page Reference(s): Page 23: "Two-fifths of your meal should be composed of starchy, high-fiber food. Two-fifths of your meal should be composed of vegetables, salad, or fruit. The remaining one-fifth of your meal should be a protein source, such as meat, fish, eggs, legumes, or cheese." Page 24: "It is fine to use a small amount of ordinary sugar for baking cakes, but you should eat them as desserts and do not forget the calorie content." Page 24: "Starches: Bread, potatoes, rice, pasta cereals, and fruit and good examples. They tend to be absorbed more slowly and release their sugar into the blood more gradually. They are good sources of energy. Eat them regularly and include some with each meal."

Title: *Diabetes & Pregnancy: What to Expect: Your guide to A Healthy Pregnancy and a Happy, Healthy Baby*

Author: American Diabetes Association, Inc.

Publisher: American Diabetes Association, Inc.

Year Published: 2000

Number of Pages: 77

Diet Advocated: Low-Fat Diet

Specific Page Reference(s): Page 20: "In recent years, some changes have been made in nutrition guidelines for people with diabetes. You are now encouraged to eat more complex carbohydrates, such as vegetables, breads, and pasta; more fiber; and less fat. You may be able to eat small amounts of simple sugars (such as a small piece of unfrosted cake, a cookie, or a small scoop of ice cream) on special occasions — but first check with your RD and doctor to learn how to fit it into your meal plan, and, if necessary, to adjust your insulin dose."

Title: *Natural Treatments for Diabetes*
Author: Kathi Head, N.D.
Publisher: Prima Health, a Division of Prima Publishing
Year Published: 2000
Number of Pages: 157
Diet Advocated: Low-Fat Diet
Specific Page Reference(s): Page 23: "Most clinicians tend to recommend diets in the middle of the carbohydrate spectrum for the majority of their patients with diabetes — generally about 40 to 50% carbohydrate."

Title: *Syndrome X: The Complete Nutritional Program To Prevent and Reverse insulin Resistance*
Author: Jack Challem, Burton Berkson, M.D., and Melissa Diane Smith
Publisher: John Wiley & Sons, Inc.
Year Published: 2000
Number of Pages: 272
Diet Advocated: Low-Carbohydrate Diet
Specific Page Reference(s): Page 21: "So, are low-fat diets an alternative? No. In recent years, large numbers of people have adopted low-fat diets and regularly eat low-fat or zero-fat foods, in the belief that such diets are healthy and can help them to reduce weight and lower their risk of heart disease. However, low-fat diets are just one more fad in a seemingly endless succession of fad diets."

Title: *The Diabetes Travel Guide: How to Travel with Diabetes — Anywhere in the World*
Author: David F. Kruger, MSN, RN, CS, CDE
Publisher: American Diabetes Association, Inc.
Year Published: 2000
Number of Pages: 172
Diet Advocated: Low-Fat Diet
Specific Page Reference(s): Page 76: "Also, the meals and snacks should contain about the same amount of carbohydrate as the meals at home." Page 103: "To balance the blood glucose effect of the delicious (we hope) meals that you will be having, travel also offers an abundance of opportunities to get much more exercise than you usually do."

Title: *The Family & Friends Guide to Diabetes: Everything You Need to Know*
Author: Eve Gehling, M.Ed., R.D., C.D.E.
Publisher: John Wiley & Sons, Inc.
Year Published: 2000
Number of Pages: 282
Diet Advocated: Low-Fat Diet

Specific Page Reference(s): Page 76-77: "Instead of trying to control diabetes by restricting or adjusting the food eaten, diabetes can be controlled through eating a consistent amount of healthy food each day and adjusting, instead, the medication dose someone takes. Today, the diet for diabetes is one that allows a person to eat a variety of foods and promotes healthy eating habits for life." From the chart on Page 77: "Calories from fat: less than 30%; Calories from protein: 10-20%; Calories from carbohydrate: 50-60%)."

Title: *What you Can Do To Prevent Diabetes: Simple Changes to Improve your Life*
Author: Annette Maggi, M.S., R.D., and Jackie Boucher, M.S., R.D., C.D.E.
Publisher: John Wiley & Sons, Inc.
Year Published: 2000
Number of Pages: 146
Diet Advocated: Low-Fat Diet
Specific Page Reference(s): Page 50: "The goal for each of us is to get less than 30 percent of each day's calories from fat (65 grams of fat or less, for the average person), but most of us are still getting more than that."

Title: *Women & Diabetes: Staying Healthy in Body, Mind, and Spirit*
Author: Laurinda M. Poirier, MPH, RN, CDE, and Katharine M. Coburn, MPH
Publisher: American Diabetes Association, Inc.
Year Published: 2000
Number of Pages: 230
Diet Advocated: Low-Fat Diet
Specific Page Reference(s): Page 76: "My friend Alice always chose the restaurant we went to after bingo on Fridays. Her favorite was Lou's Diner. This was a real problem because we always had so few low-fat options." Page 203: "Eat a low-fat (healthy fats) meal plan."

Title: *101 Tips For improving your blood Sugar*
Author: University of New Mexico Diabetes Care Team
Publisher: American Diabetes Association, Inc.
Year Published: 1999
Number of Pages: 129
Diet Advocated: Low-Fat Diet
Specific Page Reference(s): Page 90: "Can I eat candy bars now that the ADA is including table sugar in meal plans? Sometimes. It is true that the most recent dietary guidelines for people with diabetes include simple sugars, including table sugar. Several studies have shown that table sugar eaten as part of a meal plan does not have any worse effect on blood glucose than rice or potatoes. This does not mean, however, that people with diabetes can eat sweets freely. Sugars must be included as part of your meal plan. And the reason you still want to limit the number of candy bars you eat is that most of the calories in candy bars come from fat. Fat should be limited in everybody's diet!"

Appendix A

Title: *16 Myths of a "Diabetic Diet"*
Author: Karen Hanson Chalmers, MS, RD, CDE and Amy E. Peterson, MS, RD, CDE
Publisher: American Diabetes Association
Year Published: 1999
Number of Pages: 238
Diet Advocated: Low-Fat Diet
Specific Page Reference(s): Page 4: "The Food Guide Pyramid and the Dietary Guidelines for Americans, Published by the US Departments of Agriculture and Health and human Services, provide nutritional guidelines for all healthy Americans and a precise approach to reshape the way Americans eat. They also serve as excellent guides for people with diabetes and their family members." Page 5: "Choose foods low in total fat, saturated fat, and cholesterol." Page 14: "The idea that it's necessary to avoid sugar is one of the biggest misconceptions in diabetes management today." Page 36: "7. Use low fat, low-calorie toppings on starchy foods instead of the high-fat toppings that add too many calories (for example, try using salsa on your baked potato instead of sour cream)."

Title: *My Doctor Says I Have A Little Diabetes: A Guide To Understanding And Controlling Type 2 Non-Insulin-Dependent Diabetes*
Author: Martha hope McCool, RN, CDE, and Sandra Woodruff, RD
Publisher: Avery Publishing Group
Year Published: 1999
Number of Pages: 138
Diet Advocated: Low-Fat Diet
Specific Page Reference(s): Page 31: "There is no doubt that a low-fat, balanced diet rich in vegetables, fruits, whole grains, and other wholesome foods is necessary for good health."

Title: *The Diabetes Problem Solver: Quick Answers to Your Questions About Treatment & Self-Care*
Author: Nancy Touchette, PhD
Publisher: American Diabetes Association, Inc.
Year Published: 1999
Number of Pages: 511
Diet Advocated: Low-Fat Diet
Specific Page Reference(s): Page 359: "Just remember that the foods you eat are not different than what people without diabetes eat. You don't have to eat special diabetic foods." Page 390: "Bread. Look for low-fat varieties that list whole grain as the first ingredient on the label." Page 390: "Good examples of low-fat snacks are pretzels or plain popcorn that has been air-popped with no added cheese or butter and that contain 2 grams of fat or less per serving." Page 390: "Try to avoid pastas or noodles that contain eggs and fat."

Title: *When A Child Has Diabetes*
Author: Dennis Daneman, MB, BCh, FRCPC, Marcia Frank, RN, MHSc, CDE, and Kusiel Perlman, MD, FRCPC

223

Publisher: Firefly Books
Year Published: 1999
Number of Pages: 217
Diet Advocated: Low-Fat Diet
Specific Page Reference(s): Page 55: "In fact, people with diabetes can and do eat sugar."
Page 56: "People with diabetes can eat sugar and foods containing added sugar, such as candy and chocolate, in moderation—up to 10% of their total calorie intake."

Title: *Diabetes Type 2 & What To Do*
Author: Virginia Valentine, R.N., M.S., C.D.E., June Bierman & Barbara Toohey
Publisher: Lowell House, a Division of NTC/Contemporary Publishing Group, Inc.
Year Published: 1998
Number of Pages: 210
Diet Advocated: Low-Fat Diet
Specific Page Reference(s): Page 99: "June And Barbara: Many experts agree that fat, not carbohydrate, is the real enemy. Avoiding fat is the cornerstone of the successful Pritikin weight-loss (and health gain!) diet and of the Martin Katahn T-Factor diet. It's also basic in Dr. James Anderson's high-carbohydrate, high-fiber, low-fat diet (HCF diet), which allows only 9 percent calories as fat..."

Title: *Healthy Living with Diabetes*
Author: Margot Joan Fromer
Publisher: New Harbinger Publications
Year Published: 1998
Number of Pages: 251
Diet Advocated: Low-Fat Diet
Specific Page Reference(s): Page 31-32: "What you really have to watch out for is fat—but everyone should be doing that. The damage that saturated fat does to the body has been so widely publicized that eating a low-fat diet has become the "in" thing to do for many people. You should now be one of them."

Title: *The Diabetic Male's Essential Guide to Living Well*
Author: Joseph Juliano, M.D.
Publisher: Henry Holt and Company
Year Published: 1998
Number of Pages: 204
Diet Advocated: Low-Fat Diet
Specific Page Reference(s): Page 112: "If dietary protein contributes 10-21 percent of the total caloric content of the diet, then 80-90 percent of the calories remain to be distributed between dietary fat and carbohydrates. Less than 10 percent of these calories should be from saturated fats and up to 10 percent calories from polyunsaturated fats, leaving 60-70 percent of the total calories derived from monounsaturated fats and carbohydrates. Individuals with

normal lipid levels and reasonable weight can follow the USDA Dietary Guidelines for Americans recommendations: less than 30 percent of the calories should be from total fat."

Title: *Diabetes is Not A Piece of Cake*
Author: Janet Meirelles, R.N., C.D.E.
Publisher: Lincoln Publishing Incorporated
Year Published: 1997
Number of Pages: 282
Diet Advocated: Low-Fat Diet
Specific Page Reference(s): Page 118: "50% to 60% carbohydrate; 12% to 18% protein; 25% to 30% fat."

Title: *Type 2 Diabetes: Your Healthy Living Guide: Tips, Techniques, and Practical Advice For Living Well With Diabetes*
Author: American Diabetes Association, Inc.
Publisher: American Diabetes Association, Inc.
Year Published: 1997
Number of Pages: 180
Diet Advocated: Low-Fat Diet
Specific Page Reference(s): Page 37: "The healthiest eating plan is low in saturated fat and cholesterol, moderate in protein, high in starches and fiber, and moderate in sodium, sugars, and sugar substitutes."

APPENDIX B: REFERENCE BOOKS

Title: *Lange 2009 Current Medical Diagnosis & Treatment*
Author: Edited by Stephen J. McPhee, MD, Maxine A. Papadakis, MD, and Lawrence M. Tierney, Jr., MD, Senior Editor
Publisher: McGraw-Hill Medical
Year Published: 2009
Number of Pages: 1708
Diet Advocated: Low-Fat Diet
Specific Page Reference(s): Page 1061: "A well-balanced, nutritious diet remains a fundamental element of therapy. The American Diabetes Association (ADA) recommends about 45-65% of total daily calories in the form of carbohydrates; 25-35% in the form of fat (of which less than 7% are from saturated fat), and 10-35% in the form of protein. In patients with type 2 diabetes, limiting the carbohydrate intake and substituting some of the calories with monounsaturated fats, such as olive oil, rapeseed (canola) oil, or the oils in nuts and avocados, can lower triglycerides and increase HDL cholesterol."

Title: *The Gale Encyclopedia of Alternative Medicine Third Edition: Volume 2*
Author: Laurie J. Fundukian, Editor
Publisher: Gale, Cengage Learning
Year Published: 2009
Number of Pages: 2688
Diet Advocated: Low-Fat Diet
Specific Page Reference(s): Page 688: "Both conventional and alternative medicine practitioners agree that diet and moderate exercise are the first treatments to be implemented in diabetes. For overweight and obese type 2 diabetics, weight loss is an important goal to help them to control their blood glucose levels. A well-balanced, nutritious diet provides approximately 50 to 60% of calories from carbohydrates, approximately 10 to 20% of calories from protein, and less than 30% of calories from fat."

Title: *Harrison's Principles of Internal Medicine, 17th Edition*
Author: Editors: Anthony S. Fauci, MD, Eugene Braunwald, MD, Dennis Kasper, MD, Stephen L. Hauser, MD, Dan Longo, MD, J. Larry Jameson, MD, PhD, and Joseph Loscalzo, MD, PhD.
Publisher: McGraw-Hill Medical
Year Published: 2008
Number of Pages: 2754
Diet Advocated: Low-Fat Diet

Specific Page Reference(s): Page 2294: "As for the general population, a diet that includes fruits, vegetables, fiber-containing foods, and low-fat milk is advised." Page 2295: Table 338-9: "Nutritional Recommendations for Adults with Diabetes: Fat: 20-35% of total caloric intake; Carbohydrate: 45-65% of total caloric intake (low-carbohydrate diets are not recommended); Protein: 10-35% of total caloric intake (high-protein diets are not recommended)."

Title: *Lange 2008 Current Medical Diagnosis & Treatment*
Author: Edited by Stephen J. McPhee, MD, Maxine A. Papadakis, MD, and Lawrence M. Tierney, Jr., MD, Senior Editor
Publisher: McGraw-Hill Medical
Year Published: 2008
Number of Pages: 1671
Diet Advocated: Low-Fat Diet
Specific Page Reference(s): Page 1041: "A well-balanced, nutritious diet remains a fundamental element of therapy. The American Diabetes Association (ADA) recommends about 45-65% of total daily calories in the form of carbohydrates; 25-35% in the form of fat (of which less than 7% are from saturated fat), and 10-35% in the form of protein. In patients with type 2 diabetes, limiting the carbohydrate intake and substituting some of the calories with monounsaturated fats, such as olive oil, rapeseed (canola) oil, or the oils in nuts and avocados, can lower triglycerides and increase HDL cholesterol."

Title: *Columbia University Children's Medical Guide: The Illustrated Quick-Reference Guide to Children's Symptoms and Their Treatment*
Author: Dr. Steve Caddle, Dr. Mary McCord, and Dr. Bernard Valman
Publisher: DK Publishing, Inc.
Year Published: 2008
Number of Pages: 216
Diet Advocated: Low-Fat Diet
Specific Page Reference(s): Page 191: "For a child over 5 years of age, just over a third of the diet should be made up of fats, about 15 percent should consist of protein, and the remainder should be carbohydrates."

Title: *The Gale Encyclopedia of Medicine Third Edition: Volume 2*
Author: Jacqueline L. Longe, Editor
Publisher: Thomson Gale, A Part of The Thomson Corporation
Year Published: 2006
Number of Pages: 4475
Diet Advocated: Low-Fat Diet
Specific Page Reference(s): Page 1158: "Diet and moderate exercise are the first treatments implemented in diabetes. For many Type II diabetics, weight loss may be an important goal in helping them to control their diabetes. A well-balanced, nutritious diet provides

approximately 50-60% of calories from carbohydrates, approximately 10-20% of calories from protein, and less than 30% of calories from fat."

Title: *The Encyclopedia of Children's Health and Wellness*
Author: Carol Turkington and Albert TZEEL, M.D., F.A.A.P.
Publisher: Facts On File, Inc.
Year Published: 2004
Number of Pages: 682
Diet Advocated: Low-Fat Diet
Specific Page Reference(s): Page 146: "Children with type 1 diabetes are treated with a healthful diet, physical activity, and insulin via injection or an insulin pump. The amount of insulin must be balanced with food intake and daily activities."

Title: *Cecil Textbook of Medicine 22nd Edition*
Author: Edited by Lee Goldman, MD, and Dennis Ausiello, MD
Publisher: Saunders, An Imprint of Elsevier
Year Published: 2004
Number of Pages: 2506
Diet Advocated: Low-Fat Diet
Specific Page Reference(s): Page 1435: "If properly managed and sufficiently motivated, diabetic patients should be able to consume the foods they enjoy and should be able to fully participate in exercise and sports." Page 1435: "The introduction of intensive insulin regimens has increased meal flexibility by allowing more latitude in varying the size, content, and timing of meals." Page 1435: "Restriction of saturated fat to <10% of total calories, to be replaced in the diet by carbohydrates and monounsaturated fats."

Title: *Griffith's 5-Minute Clinical Consult*
Author: Editor: Mark R. Dambro
Publisher: Lippincott Williams & Wilkins, A Wolters Kluwer Company
Year Published: 2004
Number of Pages: 1342
Diet Advocated: Low-Fat Diet
Specific Page Reference(s): Page 319: "Diet: Appropriate diabetes exchange (ADA) diet for age (carbohydrate-50%, protein-20%, fat-30%)."

Title: Johns Hopkins Symptoms and Remedies
Author: Medical Editor: Simeon Margolis, M.D., Ph.D.
Publisher: Rebus, Inc
Year Published: 2003
Number of Pages: 736
Diet Advocated: Low-Fat Diet

Specific Page Reference(s): Page 416: "A strict diet and schedule of meals are necessary to control blood glucose levels. Your doctor may recommend a diet low in fat, salt, and cholesterol, and may advise you to see a nutritionist for dietary planning."

Title: *American College of Physicians Home Medical Guide: The Authoritative Medical Reference for Today's Family*
Author: Editor-in-Chief: David R. Goldmann, MD, FACP; Associate Editor::David A. Horowitz, MD
Publisher: DK Publishing, Inc.
Year Published: 2003
Number of Pages: 1104
Diet Advocated: Low-Fat Diet
Specific Page Reference(s): Page 689: "Follow general guidelines for a healthy diet and seek the guidance of a dietitian if necessary. Try to keep fat intake low, and obtain energy from complex carbohydrates (such as bread and rice) to minimize fluctuations in blood glucose level."

Title: *Rudolph's Pediatrics 21st Edition*
Author: Colin D. Rudolph, Abraham M. Rudolph, Margaret K. Hostetter, George Lister, Norman J. Siegel
Publisher: McGraw-Hill, Medical Publishing Division
Year Published: 2003
Number of Pages: 2688
Diet Advocated: Low-Fat Diet
Specific Page Reference(s): Page 2111: "Maintenance of the glucose concentration of blood in a nearly normal range can prevent or minimize long-term damage. Assuring optimal management of this disorder over the patient's lifetime places a tremendous amount of responsibility on the patient, family, and health care team." Page 2128: "The food types from which caloric intake is derived are the same for children with diabetes mellitus as they are for the general population. Carbohydrates should constitute 45 to 60% of the total daily calories. Because of long-term concerns about atherosclerosis, 30% or less of total calories should come from fat, less than 10% from saturated fat. Protein should constitute 10 to 20% of daily caloric intake."

Title: *The Merck Manual Of Medical Information Second Home Edition*
Author: Mark H. Beers, MD, Editor-in-Chief
Publisher: Merck Research Laboratories
Year Published: 2003
Number of Pages: 1907
Diet Advocated: Low-Fat Diet
Specific Page Reference(s): Page 965: "Treatment of diabetes involves diet, exercise, education, and, for most people, drugs. If a person with diabetes keeps blood sugar levels

tightly controlled, complications are less likely to develop. Page 965-966: Doctors recommend a healthy, balanced diet and efforts to maintain a healthy weight. Some people benefit from meeting with a dietitian to develop an optimal eating plan."

Title: *Williams Textbook of Endocrinology Tenth Edition*
Author: P. Reed Larsen, MD, FACP, FRCP, Henry M Kronenber, MD, Shlomo Melmed, MD, Kenneth S. Polonsky, MD
Publisher: Saunders, An Imprint of Elsevier
Year Published: 2003
Number of Pages: 1927
Diet Advocated: Low-Fat Diet
Specific Page Reference(s): Page 1496: "The overriding principle in the treatment of the majority of patients with type 1 diabetes is that a health care team that includes a physician, diabetes nurse educator, nutritionist, and other health care professionals as appropriate should work closely with the patient to achieve blood glucose concentrations as close to normal as possible because these are associated with a reduced risk of diabetic complications. Although studies in animal models and epidemiological studies suggested that tighter glucose control was associated with better long-term outcomes for the diabetic patient in terms of a reduced risk of complications, the most definitive study in this regard has been the Diabetes Control and Complications Trial (DCCT) that was completed in 1993." Page 1497: "It is recognized that in order to achieve glucose control at this level patients need to monitor glucose levels at least three or four times per day and receive nutritional counseling and training in self-management of the insulin doses and problem solving to allow them to deal with the problems that they encounter in their daily lives. Hospitalization may be necessary for the initiation of therapy."

Title: *Current Pediatric Diagnosis & Treatment*
Author: Edited by William W. Hay, Jr., MD, Anthony R. Hayward, MD, PhD, Myron J. Levin, MD, and Judith M. Sondheimer, MD
Publisher: Lange Medical Books/McGraw-Hill
Year Published: 2003
Number of Pages: 1415
Diet Advocated: Low-Fat Diet
Specific Page Reference(s): Page 981: "The mainstays of dietary treatment are discussed in detail in understanding insulin Dependent Diabetes, the entire text of which is also to be found at http://www.uchsc.edu." Page 981: "The American Diabetes Association (ADA) no longer recommends any one diabetic diet or ADA diet. Instead, nutrition therapy for diabetics should be individualized, with consideration given to the patient's customary cultural eating habits and other lifestyle matters. Some families and children (particularly those with weight problems) find exchange diets helpful initially while they are learning categories of foods. Most centers now just use exchanges of carbohydrates, referred to below as 'carbohydrate-counting.'"

Title: *Childhood Diseases and Disorders Sourcebook*
Author: Edited by Chad T. Kimball
Publisher: Omnigraphics
Year Published: 2003
Number of Pages: 661
Diet Advocated: Informational
Specific Page Reference(s): Page 433: "Follow a healthy meal plan: A child or teen needs to follow a meal plan developed by a physician, diabetes educator, or a registered dietician. A meal plan outlines proper nutrition for growth. A meal plan also helps keep blood glucose levels in the target range. Children or adolescents and their families can learn how different types of food—especially carbohydrates such as breads, pasta, and rice—can affect blood glucose levels. Portion size, the right amount of calories for the child's age, and ideas for healthy food choices at meal and snack time also should be discussed."

Title: *The Encyclopedia of Diabetes*
Author: William A. Petit, Jr., M.D., F.A.C.P., F.A.C.E., and Christine Adamec
Publisher: Facts On File, Inc.
Year Published: 2002
Number of Pages: 374
Diet Advocated: Low-Fat Diet
Specific Page Reference(s): Page 48: "There is no evidence that complete restriction of sucrose (sugar) is helpful for people with diabetes. However, this does not mean that it's acceptable or advisable for people with diabetes to eat large amounts of sugar-filled foods. Instead, sugar should be consumed in moderation." Page 62: "Dietary adjustments can lower LDL levels; for example, foods that are high in starch and fiber can help to lower the LDL level, as well as foods that are low in fat and cholesterol." Page 91: "Typical meal plans or diets for patients with diabetes contain less than 30 percent of their calories from fat, 50-60 percent from carbohydrates, and 10-20 percent of calories from protein."

Title: *The Complete Home Wellness Handbook: Home Remedies, Prevention, Self-Care*
Author: John Edward Swartzberg, M.D., F.A.C.P., Sheldon Margen, M.D., and the editors of the UC Berkeley Wellness Letter
Publisher: Rebus, Inc
Year Published: 2001
Number of Pages: 672
Diet Advocated: Low-Fat Diet
Specific Page Reference(s): Page 236: "Improve your diet. Try to maintain a semivegetarian diet that is low in fat and emphasizes complex carbohydrates over simple sugars. Such a diet is also known to lower the risk of heart disease and some cancers."

Appendix B

Title: *Family Medicine Principles & Practice Fifth Edition*
Author: Editor: Robert B. Taylor
Publisher: Springer-Verlag
Year Published: 1998
Number of Pages: 1191
Diet Advocated: Low-Fat Diet
Specific Page Reference(s): Pages 1068-1069: "Education should also focus on dietary principles. For individuals with diabetes, the current dietary recommendations are a diet containing at least 50% carbohydrate, less than 30% fat, and 20% or less protein."

APPENDIX C: LOW-CARBOHYDRATE ARTICLES

Many scientific articles referring to low-carbohydrate — ketogenic — diets you may be interested in reviewing have been provided in this appendix. The title of the article, author(s) (where available), journal, and PubMed ID number have been included to enable your search within the PubMed database, a service of the US National Library of Medicine and the National Institutes of Health.

Visit: http://www.ncbi.nlm.nih.gov/sites/entrez?db=pubmed. Please note that some of the articles have a free abstract available, some do not. Also, some of the articles are available to view online free of charge, but most require a fee.

Ketones suppress brain glucose consumption
LaManna JC, Salem N, Puchowicz M, Erokwu B, Koppaka S, Flask C, Lee Z
Adv Exp Med Biol. 2009;645:301-6.
PMID: 19227486

Dietary fat and carbohydrates differentially alter insulin sensitivity during caloric restriction
Kirk E, Reeds DN, Finck BN, Mayurranjan MS, Klein S
Gastroenterology. 2009 Jan 24.
PMID: 19208352

Clinical experience with a relatively low carbohydrate, calorie-restricted diet improves insulin sensitivity and associated metabolic abnormalities in overweight, insulin resistant South Asian Indian women
Backes AC, Abbasi F, Lamendola C, McLaughlin TL, Reaven G, Palaniappan LP
Asia Pac J Clin Nutr. 2008;17(4):669-71.
PMID: 19114407

Physiological, performance, and nutritional profile of the Brazilian Olympic Wushu (kung-fu) team
Artioli GG, Gualano B, Franchini E, Batista RN, Polacow VO, Lancha AH Jr.
J Strength Cond Res. 2009 Jan;23(1):20-5.
PMID: 19077742

Circadian rhythms, diet, and neuronal excitability
Allen CN
Epilepsia. 2008 Nov;49 Suppl 8:124-6. Review.

PMID: 19049609

Cultural challenges in using the ketogenic diet in Asian countries
Seo JH, Kim HD
Epilepsia. 2008 Nov;49 Suppl 8:50-2. Review.
PMID: 19049587

Low-carbohydrate (low & high-fat) versus high-carbohydrate low-fat diets in the treatment of obesity in adolescents
Demol S, Yackobovitch-Gavan M, Shalitin S, Nagelberg N, Gillon-Keren M, Phillip M
Acta Paediatr. 2009 Feb;98(2):346-51. Epub 2008 Sep 29.
PMID: 18826492

Low-carbohydrate weight-loss diets. Effects on cognition and mood
D'Anci KE, Watts KL, Kanarek RB, Taylor HA
Appetite. 2009 Feb;52(1):96-103. Epub 2008 Aug 29.
PMID: 18804129

Improved glucose regulation on a low carbohydrate diet in diabetic rats transplanted with macroencapsulated porcine islets
Vinerean HV, Gazda LS, Hall RD, Rubin AL, Smith BH
Cell Transplant. 2008;17(5):567-75.
PMID: 18714676

Systematic review of randomized controlled trials of low-carbohydrate vs. low-fat/low-calorie diets in the management of obesity and its comorbidities
Hession M, Rolland C, Kulkarni U, Wise A, Broom J
Obes Rev. 2009 Jan;10(1):36-50. Epub 2008 Aug 11.
PMID: 18700873

Acute effects of the very low carbohydrate diet on sleep indices
Afaghi A, O'Connor H, Chow CM
Nutr Neurosci. 2008 Aug;11(4):146-54.
PMID: 18681982

Comparison of the effects of four commercially available weight-loss programmes on lipid-based cardiovascular risk factors
Morgan L, Griffin B, Millward D, Delooy A, Fox K, Baic S, Bonham M, Wallace J, Macdonald I, Taylor M, Truby H
Public Health Nutr. 2008 Jul 23:1-9.
PMID: 18647427

Appendix C

Weight loss with a low-carbohydrate, Mediterranean, or low-fat diet
Shai I, Schwarzfuchs D, Henkin Y, Shahar DR, Witkow S, Greenberg I, Golan R, Fraser D, Bolotin A, Vardi H, Tangi-Rozental O, Zuk-Ramot R, Sarusi B, Brickner D, Schwartz Z, Sheiner E, Marko R, Katorza E, Thiery J, Fiedler GM, Blüher M, Stumvoll M, Stampfer MJ; Dietary Intervention Randomized Controlled Trial (DIRECT) Group.
N Engl J Med. 2008 Jul 17;359(3):229-41.
PMID: 18635428

Metabolic effects of the very-low-carbohydrate diets: misunderstood 'villains' of human metabolism
Manninen AH
J Int Soc Sports Nutr. 2004 Dec 31;1(2):7-11.
PMID: 18500949

Low-carbohydrate diet in type 2 diabetes: stable improvement of bodyweight and glycemic control during 44 months follow-up
Nielsen JV, Joensson EA
Nutr Metab (Lond). 2008 May 22;5:14.
PMID: 18495047

The ketogenic diet increases mitochondrial glutathione levels
Jarrett SG, Milder JB, Liang LP, Patel M
J Neurochem. 2008 Aug;106(3):1044-51. Epub 2008 May 5.
PMID: 18466343

Low-carbohydrate diet versus caloric restriction: effects on weight loss, hormones, and colon tumor growth in obese mice
Wheatley KE, Williams EA, Smith NC, Dillard A, Park EY, Nunez NP, Hursting SD, Lane MA
Nutr Cancer. 2008;60(1):61-8.
PMID: 18444137

Dietary carbohydrate restriction induces a unique metabolic state positively affecting atherogenic dyslipidemia, fatty acid partitioning, and metabolic syndrome
Volek JS, Fernandez ML, Feinman RD, Phinney SD
Prog Lipid Res. 2008 Sep;47(5):307-18. Epub 2008 Mar 15.
PMID: 18396172

Adipocytokine changes caused by low-carbohydrate compared to conventional diets in obesity
Seshadri P, Samaha FF, Stern L, Ahima RS, Daily D, Iqbal N
Metab Syndr Relat Disord. 2005;3(1):66-74.

PMID: 18370712

Effects of continuous low-carbohydrate diet after long-term exercise on GLUT-4 protein content in rat skeletal muscle
Kubota M, Koshinaka K, Kawata Y, Koike T, Oshida Y
Horm Metab Res. 2008 Jan;40(1):24-8.
PMID: 18335580

Effects of weight loss from a very-low-carbohydrate diet on endothelial function and markers of cardiovascular disease risk in subjects with abdominal obesity
Keogh JB, Brinkworth GD, Noakes M, Belobrajdic DP, Buckley JD, Clifton PM
Am J Clin Nutr. 2008 Mar;87(3):567-76.
PMID: 18326593

How the ideology of low fat conquered America
La Berge AF
J Hist Med Allied Sci. 2008 Apr;63(2):139-77. Epub 2008 Feb 23.
PMID: 18296750

South Beach Diet associated ketoacidosis: a case report
Chalasani S, Fischer J
J Med Case Reports. 2008 Feb 11;2:45.
PMID: 18267031

Low-carbohydrate-diet score and risk of type 2 diabetes in women
Halton TL, Liu S, Manson JE, Hu FB
Am J Clin Nutr. 2008 Feb;87(2):339-46.
PMID: 18258623

Physiogenomic comparison of human fat loss in response to diets restrictive of carbohydrate or fat
Seip RL, Volek JS, Windemuth A, Kocherla M, Fernandez ML, Kraemer WJ, Ruaño G
Nutr Metab (Lond). 2008 Feb 6;5:4.
PMID: 18254975

Diet-induced obesity alters protein synthesis: tissue-specific effects in fasted versus fed mice
Anderson SR, Gilge DA, Steiber AL, Previs SF
Metabolism. 2008 Mar;57(3):347-54.
PMID: 18249206

Suppression of myocardial 18F-FDG uptake by preparing patients with a high-fat, low-carbohydrate diet

Williams G, Kolodny GM
AJR Am J Roentgenol. 2008 Feb;190(2):W151-6.
PMID: 18212199

Benefit of low-fat over low-carbohydrate diet on endothelial health in obesity
Phillips SA, Jurva JW, Syed AQ, Syed AQ, Kulinski JP, Pleuss J, Hoffmann RG, Gutterman DD
Hypertension. 2008 Feb;51(2):376-82. Epub 2008 Jan 14.
PMID: 18195164

Metabolic effects of weight loss on a very-low-carbohydrate diet compared with an isocaloric high-carbohydrate diet in abdominally obese subjects
Tay J, Brinkworth GD, Noakes M, Keogh J, Clifton PM
J Am Coll Cardiol. 2008 Jan 1;51(1):59-67.
PMID: 18174038

A comparison of the effectiveness, tolerability and safety of high and low carbohydrate diets in women with gestational diabetes
Cypryk K, Kamińska P, Kosiński M, Pertyńska-Marczewska M, Lewiński A
Endokrynol Pol. 2007 Jul-Aug;58(4):314-9.
PMID: 18058723

Comparison of low fat and low carbohydrate diets on circulating fatty acid composition and markers of inflammation
Forsythe CE, Phinney SD, Fernandez ML, Quann EE, Wood RJ, Bibus DM, Kraemer WJ, Feinman RD, Volek JS
Lipids. 2008 Jan;43(1):65-77. Epub 2007 Nov 29.
PMID: 18046594

Comparison of a low carbohydrate and low fat diet for weight maintenance in overweight or obese adults enrolled in a clinical weight management program
Lecheminant JD, Gibson CA, Sullivan DK, Hall S, Washburn R, Vernon MC, Curry C, Stewart E, Westman EC, Donnelly JE
Nutr J. 2007 Nov 1;6:36.
PMID: 17976244

A low-carbohydrate diet is more effective in reducing body weight than healthy eating in both diabetic and non-diabetic subjects
Dyson PA, Beatty S, Matthews DR
Diabet Med. 2007 Dec;24(12):1430-5. Epub 2007 Oct 29.
PMID: 17971178

Low-fat or low-carbohydrate diet for cardiovascular health
Best D, Grainger P
Can J Cardiovasc Nurs. 2007;17(3):19-26. Review.
PMID: 17941565

Effects of calorie-restricted low-carbohydrate diet on glucose and lipid metabolism in Otsuka Long Evans Tokushima Fatty rats
Koide N, Oyama T, Miyashita Y, Shirai K
J Atheroscler Thromb. 2007 Oct;14(5):253-60. Epub 2007 Oct 12.
PMID: 17938540

Three-year weight change in successful weight losers who lost weight on a low-carbohydrate diet
Phelan S, Wyatt H, Nassery S, Dibello J, Fava JL, Hill JO, Wing RR
Obesity (Silver Spring). 2007 Oct;15(10):2470-7.
PMID: 17925473

Effects of moderate variations in the macronutrient content of the diet on cardiovascular disease risk factors in obese patients with the metabolic syndrome
Muzio F, Mondazzi L, Harris WS, Sommariva D, Branchi A
Am J Clin Nutr. 2007 Oct;86(4):946-51.
PMID: 17921369

Blood ketones are directly related to fatigue and perceived effort during exercise in overweight adults adhering to low-carbohydrate diets for weight loss: a pilot study
White AM, Johnston CS, Swan PD, Tjonn SL, Sears B
J Am Diet Assoc. 2007 Oct;107(10):1792-6.
PMID: 17904939

Clinical use of evidence-based medicine: studies used to assess harm
Fett N, Smalley R, Kiehn K, Feldstein DA
WMJ. 2007 Jul;106(4):181-2. Review.
PMID: 17844705

Is weight loss sustainable with a low-carbohydrate diet?
Standard-Goldson A
Am Fam Physician. 2007 Jul 1;76(1):32, 35; author reply 35. No abstract available.
PMID: 17672007

Ketogenic diet for the treatment of refractory epilepsy: a 10 year experience in children
Freitas A, Paz JA, Casella EB, Marques-Dias MJ
Arq Neuropsiquiatr. 2007 Jun;65(2B):381-4.

PMID: 17665000

Increasing the fat-to-carbohydrate ratio in a high-fat diet prevents the development of obesity but not a prediabetic state in rats
Sinitskaya N, Gourmelen S, Schuster-Klein C, Guardiola-Lemaitre B, Pévet P, Challet E
Clin Sci (Lond). 2007 Nov;113(10):417-25.
PMID: 17608620

Carbohydrate versus energy restriction: effects on weight loss, body composition and metabolism
Williams EA, Perkins SN, Smith NC, Hursting SD, Lane MA
Ann Nutr Metab. 2007;51(3):232-43. Epub 2007 Jun 18.
PMID: 17587795

Energy balance and hypothalamic effects of a high-protein/low-carbohydrate diet
Kinzig KP, Hargrave SL, Hyun J, Moran TH
Physiol Behav. 2007 Oct 22;92(3):454-60. Epub 2007 Apr 22.
PMID: 17512959

Psychological benefits of a high-protein, low-carbohydrate diet in obese women with polycystic ovary syndrome — a pilot study
Galletly C, Moran L, Noakes M, Clifton P, Tomlinson L, Norman R
Appetite. 2007 Nov;49(3):590-3. Epub 2007 Apr 4.
PMID: 17509728

Nutrition strategies for the marathon: fuel for training and racing
Burke LM
Sports Med. 2007;37(4-5):344-7.
PMID: 17465604

Beneficial effects of ketogenic diet in obese diabetic subjects
Dashti HM, Mathew TC, Khadada M, Al-Mousawi M, Talib H, Asfar SK, Behbahani AI, Al-Zaid NS
Mol Cell Biochem. 2007 Aug;302(1-2):249-56. Epub 2007 Apr 20.
PMID: 17447017

The ketogenic diet: one decade later
Freeman JM, Kossoff EH, Hartman AL
Pediatrics. 2007 Mar;119(3):535-43. Review.
PMID: 17332207

Low-carbohydrate diet and coronary heart disease in women

Hrdy DB
N Engl J Med. 2007 Feb 15;356(7):750; author reply 750-2. No abstract available.
PMID: 17310524

Effects of low-carbohydrate diet on vascular health: more than just weight loss
Phillips SA
Am J Physiol Heart Circ Physiol. 2007 May;292(5):H2037-9. Epub 2007 Feb 16. No abstract available.
PMID: 17308015

Low-carbohydrate diet and coronary heart disease in women
Esposito K, Ciotola M, Giugliano D
N Engl J Med. 2007 Feb 15;356(7):750; author reply 750-2. No abstract available.
PMID: 17301311

Effects of a low-fat versus a low-carbohydrate diet on adipocytokines in obese adults
de Luis DA, Aller R, Izaola O, Gonzalez Sagrado M, Bellioo D, Conde R
Horm Res. 2007;67(6):296-300. Epub 2007 Feb 6.
PMID: 17284923

Restoration of coronary endothelial function in obese Zucker rats by a low-carbohydrate diet
Focardi M, Dick GM, Picchi A, Zhang C, Chilian WM
Am J Physiol Heart Circ Physiol. 2007 May;292(5):H2093-9. Epub 2007 Jan 12.
PMID: 17220180

Low-carbohydrate-diet score and the risk of coronary heart disease in women
Halton TL, Willett WC, Liu S, Manson JE, Albert CM, Rexrode K, Hu FB
N Engl J Med. 2006 Nov 9;355(19):1991-2002.
PMID: 17093250

High-fat/low-carbohydrate diets regulate glucose metabolism via a long-term transcriptional loop
Sparks LM, Xie H, Koza RA, Mynatt R, Bray GA, Smith SR
Metabolism. 2006 Nov;55(11):1457-63.
PMID: 17046547

Low-carb diets, fasting and euphoria: Is there a link between ketosis and gamma-hydroxybutyrate (GHB)?
Brown AJ
Med Hypotheses. 2007;68(2):268-71. Epub 2006 Oct 2.
PMID: 17011713

Appendix C

Low-carbohydrate diet and oxidative stress in diabetic and nondiabetic rats
Kamuren ZT, Sanders R, Watkins JB 3rd
J Biochem Mol Toxicol. 2006;20(5):259-69.
PMID: 17009256

Low carbohydrate diets for weight loss: historical & environmental perspective
Seshadri P, Iqbal N
Indian J Med Res. 2006 Jun;123(6):739-47. Review.
PMID: 16885595

The effects of a low-carbohydrate versus low-fat diet on adipocytokines in severely obese
adults: three-year follow-up of a randomized trial
Cardillo S, Seshadri P, Iqbal N
Eur Rev Med Pharmacol Sci. 2006 May-Jun;10(3):99-106.
PMID: 16875041

A low-carbohydrate diet rapidly and dramatically reduces intrahepatic triglyceride content
Browning JD, Davis J, Saboorian MH, Burgess SC
Hepatology. 2006 Aug;44(2):487-8. No abstract available.
PMID: 16871586

A very low-carbohydrate diet improves gastroesophageal reflux and its symptoms
Austin GL, Thiny MT, Westman EC, Yancy WS Jr, Shaheen NJ
Dig Dis Sci. 2006 Aug;51(8):1307-12. Epub 2006 Jul 27.
PMID: 16871438

Pancreatic exocrine response to long-term high-fat diets in rats
Lee KY, Ahn HC, Kim C, Kim SH, Kim DK, Park HS
JOP. 2006 Jul 10;7(4):397-404.
PMID: 16832137

The skinny on low-carbohydrate diets: should they be recommended to patients with the
metabolic syndrome?
Stevens Ohlson M
J Cardiovasc Nurs. 2006 Jul-Aug;21(4):314-21.
PMID: 16823286

A low-carbohydrate diet may prevent end-stage renal failure in type 2 diabetes. A case report
Nielsen JV, Westerlund P, Bygren P
Nutr Metab (Lond). 2006 Jun 14;3:23.
PMID: 16774676

Low-carbohydrate diet in type 2 diabetes. Stable improvement of bodyweight and glycemic control during 22 months follow-up
Nielsen JV, Joensson E
Nutr Metab (Lond). 2006 Jun 14;3:22.
PMID: 16774674

The reduced energy intake of rats fed a high-protein low-carbohydrate diet explains the lower fat deposition, but macronutrient substitution accounts for the improved glycemic control
Blouet C, Mariotti F, Azzout-Marniche D, Bos C, Mathé V, Tomé D, Huneau JF
J Nutr. 2006 Jul;136(7):1849-54.
PMID: 16772448

Information from your family doctor. Is a low-carbohydrate diet right for me?
American Academy of Family Physicians
Am Fam Physician. 2006 Jun 1;73(11):1951. No abstract available.
PMID: 16770924

The ketogenic diet causes a reversible decrease in activity level in Long-Evans rats
Murphy P, Burnham WM
Exp Neurol. 2006 Sep;201(1):84-9. Epub 2006 Jun 5.
PMID: 16750194

Are the eating and exercise habits of successful weight losers changing?
Phelan S, Wyatt HR, Hill JO, Wing RR
Obesity (Silver Spring). 2006 Apr;14(4):710-6.
PMID: 16741274

The effect of a low-carbohydrate diet on bone turnover
Carter JD, Vasey FB, Valeriano J
Osteoporos Int. 2006;17(9):1398-403. Epub 2006 May 23.
PMID: 16718399

Effects of prior exercise and a low-carbohydrate diet on muscle sarcoplasmic reticulum function during cycling in women
Duhamel TA, Green HJ, Perco JG, Ouyang J
J Appl Physiol. 2006 Sep;101(3):695-706. Epub 2006 May 18.
PMID: 16709650

Comparative effects of a low-carbohydrate diet and exercise plus a low-carbohydrate diet on muscle sarcoplasmic reticulum responses in males
Duhamel TA, Green HJ, Perco JG, Ouyang J

Am J Physiol Cell Physiol. 2006 Oct;291(4):C607-17. Epub 2006 May 17.
PMID: 16707551

Long term effects of ketogenic diet in obese subjects with high cholesterol level
Dashti HM, Al-Zaid NS, Mathew TC, Al-Mousawi M, Talib H, Asfar SK, Behbahani AI
Mol Cell Biochem. 2006 Jun;286(1-2):1-9. Epub 2006 Apr 21.
PMID: 16652223

The effect of liposuction and diet on ghrelin, adiponectin, and leptin levels in obese Zucker rats
Schreiber JE, Singh NK, Shermak MA
Plast Reconstr Surg. 2006 May;117(6):1829-35.
PMID: 16651955

Use of glargine and lente insulins in cats with diabetes mellitus
Weaver KE, Rozanski EA, Mahony OM, Chan DL, Freeman LM
J Vet Intern Med. 2006 Mar-Apr;20(2):234-8.
PMID: 16594577

Dietary treatment of diabetes mellitus in the pre-insulin era (1914-1922)
Westman EC, Yancy WS Jr, Humphreys M
Perspect Biol Med. 2006 Winter;49(1):77-83.
PMID: 16489278

A low carbohydrate diet in type 1 diabetes: clinical experience — a brief report
Nielsen JV, Jönsson E, Ivarsson A
Ups J Med Sci. 2005;110(3):267-73.
PMID: 16454166

Low-carbohydrate diets: nutritional and physiological aspects
Adam-Perrot A, Clifton P, Brouns F
Obes Rev. 2006 Feb;7(1):49-58. Review.
PMID: 16436102

The metabolic response to a high-protein, low-carbohydrate diet in men with type 2 diabetes mellitus
Nuttall FQ, Gannon MC
Metabolism. 2006 Feb;55(2):243-51.
PMID: 16423633

Postprandial glycogen and lipid synthesis in prednisolone-treated rats maintained on high-protein diets with varied carbohydrate levels

Obeid OA, Boukarim LK, Al Awar RM, Hwalla N
Nutrition. 2006 Mar;22(3):288-94. Epub 2006 Jan 18.
PMID: 16412611

Ketoacidosis during a low-carbohydrate diet
Shah P, Isley WL
N Engl J Med. 2006 Jan 5;354(1):97-8. No abstract available.
PMID: 16394313

Low-fat dietary pattern and weight change over 7 years: the Women's Health Initiative
Dietary Modification Trial
Howard BV, Manson JE, Stefanick ML, Beresford SA, Frank G, Jones B, Rodabough RJ,
Snetselaar L, Thomson C, Tinker L, Vitolins M, Prentice R.
JAMA. 2006 Jan 4;295(1):39-49.
PMID: 16391215

The effect of low carbohydrate on energy metabolism
Erlanson-Albertsson C, Mei J
Int J Obes (Lond). 2005 Sep;29 Suppl 2:S26-30. Review.
PMID: 16385748

Metabolic and antioxidative changes in liver steatosis induced by high-fat, low-carbohydrate
diet in rabbits
Birkner E, Kasperczyk S, Kasperczyk A, Zalejska-Fiolka J, Zwirska-Korczala K, Stawiarska-
Pieta B, Grucka-Mamczar E
J Physiol Pharmacol. 2005 Dec;56 Suppl 6:45-58.
PMID: 16340038

Cost-effectiveness of a low-carbohydrate diet and a standard diet in severe obesity
Tsai AG, Glick HA, Shera D, Stern L, Samaha FF
Obes Res. 2005 Oct;13(10):1834-40.
PMID: 16286532

Altered hypothalamic signaling and responses to food deprivation in rats fed a low-
carbohydrate diet
Kinzig KP, Scott KA, Hyun J, Bi S, Moran TH
Obes Res. 2005 Oct;13(10):1672-82.
PMID: 16286514

A ketogenic diet reduces amyloid beta 40 and 42 in a mouse model of Alzheimer's disease.
Van der Auwera I, Wera S, Van Leuven F, Henderson ST
Nutr Metab (Lond). 2005 Oct 17;2:28.

Appendix C

PMID: 16229744

Efficacy of a low-carbohydrate diet for short-term weight loss
Hadi S, Jensen GL
Nutr Clin Pract. 2005 Feb;20(1):17-20. Review. No abstract available.
PMID: 16207643

The case for not restricting saturated fat on a low carbohydrate diet
Volek JS, Forsythe CE
Nutr Metab (Lond). 2005 Aug 31;2:21. No abstract available.
PMID: 16135250

Recovery of muscle glycogen concentrations in sled dogs during prolonged exercise
McKenzie E, Holbrook T, Williamson K, Royer C, Valberg S, Hinchcliff K, Jose-Cunilleras E,
Nelson S, Willard M, Davis M
Med Sci Sports Exerc. 2005 Aug;37(8):1307-12.
PMID: 16118576

Variability in exercise capacity and metabolic response during endurance exercise after a low
carbohydrate diet
Claassen A, Lambert EV, Bosch AN, Rodger M, St Clair Gibson A, Noakes TD
Int J Sport Nutr Exerc Metab. 2005 Apr;15(2):97-116.
PMID: 16089270

Lasting improvement of hyperglycaemia and bodyweight: low-carbohydrate diet in type 2
diabetes. A brief report.
Nielsen JV, Jönsson E, Nilsson AK
Ups J Med Sci. 2005;110(2):179-83.
PMID: 16075898

Safety of low-carbohydrate diets
Crowe TC
Obes Rev. 2005 Aug;6(3):235-45. Review.
PMID: 16045639

The case for low carbohydrate diets in diabetes management
Arora SK, McFarlane SI
Nutr Metab (Lond). 2005 Jul 14;2:16.
PMID: 16018812

Free fatty acids, insulin resistance, and corrected qt intervals in morbid obesity: effect of
weight loss during 6 months with differing dietary interventions

Seshadri P, Samaha FF, Stern L, Chicano KL, Daily DA, Iqbal N
Endocr Pract. 2005 Jul-Aug;11(4):234-9.
PMID: 16006297

Energetics of obesity and weight control: does diet composition matter?
Schoeller DA, Buchholz AC
J Am Diet Assoc. 2005 May;105(5 Suppl 1):S24-8. Review.
PMID: 15867892

Effect of a low-carbohydrate diet on appetite, blood glucose levels, and insulin resistance in obese patients with type 2 diabetes
Boden G, Sargrad K, Homko C, Mozzoli M, Stein TP
Ann Intern Med. 2005 Mar 15;142(6):403-11. Summary for patients in: Ann Intern Med. 2005 Mar 15;142(6):I44.
PMID: 15767618

Summaries for patients. Short-term effects of low-carbohydrate diet compared with usual diet in obese patients with type 2 diabetes.
[No authors listed]
Ann Intern Med. 2005 Mar 15;142(6):I44. No abstract available.
PMID: 15767614

Diet-induced weight loss is associated with decreases in plasma serum amyloid a and C-reactive protein independent of dietary macronutrient composition in obese subjects
O'Brien KD, Brehm BJ, Seeley RJ, Bean J, Wener MH, Daniels S, D'Alessio DA
J Clin Endocrinol Metab. 2005 Apr;90(4):2244-9. Epub 2005 Jan 25.
PMID: 15671108

Insulin resistance, low-fat diets, and low-carbohydrate diets: time to test new menus
Schwenke DC
Curr Opin Lipidol. 2005 Feb;16(1):55-60. Review.
PMID: 15650564

The role of energy expenditure in the differential weight loss in obese women on low-fat and low-carbohydrate diets
Brehm BJ, Spang SE, Lattin BL, Seeley RJ, Daniels SR, D'Alessio DA
J Clin Endocrinol Metab. 2005 Mar;90(3):1475-82. Epub 2004 Dec 14.
PMID: 15598683

Fad diets and obesity — Part III: a rapid review of some of the more popular low-carbohydrate diets
Moyad MA

Urol Nurs. 2004 Oct;24(5):442-5.
PMID: 15575116

A low-carbohydrate diet in overweight patients undergoing stable statin therapy raises high-density lipoprotein and lowers triglycerides substantially
Gann D
Clin Cardiol. 2004 Oct;27(10):563-4.
PMID: 15553308

Dietary recommendations in the prevention and treatment of coronary heart disease: do we have the ideal diet yet?
Chahoud G, Aude YW, Mehta JL
Am J Cardiol. 2004 Nov 15;94(10):1260-7. Review.
PMID: 15541241

Metabolic aspects of low carbohydrate diets and exercise
Peters SJ, Leblanc PJ
Nutr Metab (Lond). 2004 Sep 30;1(1):7.
PMID: 15507161

Ketogenic diets and physical performance
Phinney SD
Nutr Metab (Lond). 2004 Aug 17;1(1):2.
PMID: 15507148

Atkins and other low-carbohydrate diets: hoax or an effective tool for weight loss?
Astrup A, Meinert Larsen T, Harper A
Lancet. 2004 Sep 4-10;364(9437):897-9. Review.
PMID: 15351198

Effect of a high-protein, low-carbohydrate diet on blood glucose control in people with type 2 diabetes
Gannon MC, Nuttall FQ
Diabetes. 2004 Sep;53(9):2375-82.
PMID: 15331548

Beneficial effect of low carbohydrate in low calorie diets on visceral fat reduction in type 2 diabetic patients with obesity
Miyashita Y, Koide N, Ohtsuka M, Ozaki H, Itoh Y, Oyama T, Uetake T, Ariga K, Shirai K
Diabetes Res Clin Pract. 2004 Sep;65(3):235-41.
PMID: 15331203

High-unsaturated-fat, high-protein, and low-carbohydrate diet during pregnancy and lactation modulates hepatic lipid metabolism in female adult offspring
Zhang J, Wang C, Terroni PL, Cagampang FR, Hanson M, Byrne CD
Am J Physiol Regul Integr Comp Physiol. 2005 Jan;288(1):R112-8. Epub 2004 Aug 19.
PMID: 15319218

Enzymatic regulation of glucose disposal in human skeletal muscle after a high-fat, low-carbohydrate diet
Pehleman TL, Peters SJ, Heigenhauser GJ, Spriet LL
J Appl Physiol. 2005 Jan;98(1):100-7. Epub 2004 Aug 13.
PMID: 15310747

Does a low-carbohydrate diet affect biomarkers for CVD?
Onega T
JAAPA. 2004 Apr;17(4):44-6. Review. No abstract available.
PMID: 15305498

Weight loss leads to reductions in inflammatory biomarkers after a very-low-carbohydrate diet and a low-fat diet in overweight men
Sharman MJ, Volek JS
Clin Sci (Lond). 2004 Oct;107(4):365-9.
PMID: 15265001

More fat and fewer seizures: dietary therapies for epilepsy
Kossoff EH
Lancet Neurol. 2004 Jul;3(7):415-20. Review.
PMID: 15207798

Comparison of a low-fat diet to a low-carbohydrate diet on weight loss, body composition, and risk factors for diabetes and cardiovascular disease in free-living, overweight men and women
Meckling KA, O'Sullivan C, Saari D
J Clin Endocrinol Metab. 2004 Jun;89(6):2717-23.
PMID: 15181047

The effects of low-carbohydrate versus conventional weight loss diets in severely obese adults: one-year follow-up of a randomized trial
Stern L, Iqbal N, Seshadri P, Chicano KL, Daily DA, McGrory J, Williams M, Gracely EJ, Samaha FF
Ann Intern Med. 2004 May 18;140(10):778-85.
PMID: 15148064

Appendix C

A low-carbohydrate, ketogenic diet versus a low-fat diet to treat obesity and hyperlipidemia: a randomized, controlled trial
Yancy WS Jr, Olsen MK, Guyton JR, Bakst RP, Westman EC
Ann Intern Med. 2004 May 18;140(10):769-77.
PMID: 15148063

Short-term low-carbohydrate diet dissociates lactate and ammonia thresholds in men
Langfort J, Czarnowski D, Zendzian-Piotrowska M, Zarzeczny R, Górski J
J Strength Cond Res. 2004 May;18(2):260-5.
PMID: 15142017

Very low-carbohydrate and low-fat diets affect fasting lipids and postprandial lipemia differently in overweight men
Sharman MJ, Gómez AL, Kraemer WJ, Volek JS
J Nutr. 2004 Apr;134(4):880-5.
PMID: 15051841

Comparison of a very low-carbohydrate and low-fat diet on fasting lipids, LDL subclasses, insulin resistance, and postprandial lipemic responses in overweight women
Volek JS, Sharman MJ, Gómez AL, DiPasquale C, Roti M, Pumerantz A, Kraemer WJ
J Am Coll Nutr. 2004 Apr;23(2):177-84.
PMID: 15047685

Effects of a low-carbohydrate diet
McDougall J
Mayo Clin Proc. 2004 Mar;79(3):431; author reply 431-2. No abstract available.
PMID: 15008619

Effects of a low-carbohydrate diet
Brower RE
Mayo Clin Proc. 2004 Mar;79(3):431; author reply 431-2. No abstract available.
PMID: 15008618

Long-term effects of a high-protein, low-carbohydrate diet on weight control and cardiovascular risk markers in obese hyperinsulinemic subjects
Brinkworth GD, Noakes M, Keogh JB, Luscombe ND, Wittert GA, Clifton PM
Int J Obes Relat Metab Disord. 2004 May;28(5):661-70. Erratum in: Int J Obes Relat Metab Disord. 2004 Sep;28(9):1187.
PMID: 15007396

Effects of the ketogenic diet in the glucose transporter 1 deficiency syndrome
Klepper J, Diefenbach S, Kohlschütter A, Voit T

Prostaglandins Leukot Essent Fatty Acids. 2004 Mar;70(3):321-7.
PMID: 14769490

Low-carbohydrate diets: what are the potential short- and long-term health implications?
Bilsborough SA, Crowe TC
Asia Pac J Clin Nutr. 2003;12(4):396-404.
PMID: 14672862

The development of diabetes mellitus in Wistar rats kept on a high-fat/low-carbohydrate diet
for long periods
Wang Y, Wang PY, Qin LQ, Davaasambuu G, Kaneko T, Xu J, Murata S, Katoh R, Sato A
Endocrine. 2003 Nov;22(2):85-92.
PMID: 14665711

Is carb-cutting a safe way to diet? New research suggests that a high-protein, low-
carbohydrate diet is less risky than many experts had thought. Does that mean it's a healthy
way to eat?
[No authors listed]
Harv Womens Health Watch. 2003 Nov;11(3):1-2. No abstract available.
PMID: 14633476

Low carbohydrate diet. Its effects on selected body parameters of obese patients
Alnasir FA, Fateha BE
Saudi Med J. 2003 Sep;24(9):949-52.
PMID: 12973475

An isoenergetic very low carbohydrate diet improves serum HDL cholesterol and
triacylglycerol concentrations, the total cholesterol to HDL cholesterol ratio and postprandial
pipemic responses compared with a low fat diet in normal weight, normolipidemic women
Volek JS, Sharman MJ, Gómez AL, Scheett TP, Kraemer WJ
J Nutr. 2003 Sep;133(9):2756-61.
PMID: 12949361

Maternal consumption of a high-meat, low-carbohydrate diet in late pregnancy: relation to
adult cortisol concentrations in the offspring
Herrick K, Phillips DI, Haselden S, Shiell AW, Campbell-Brown M, Godfrey KM
J Clin Endocrinol Metab. 2003 Aug;88(8):3554-60.
PMID: 12915635

Plasma leptin is influenced by diet composition and exercise
Koutsari C, Karpe F, Humphreys SM, Frayn KN, Hardman AE
Int J Obes Relat Metab Disord. 2003 Aug;27(8):901-6.

Appendix C

PMID: 12861230

Low-carbohydrate diet effective for adults
Carter DF
J Fam Pract. 2003 Jul;52(7):515-6. No abstract available.
PMID: 12841960

Influence of diet on the modeling of adipose tissue triglycerides during growth
Brunengraber DZ, McCabe BJ, Kasumov T, Alexander JC, Chandramouli V, Previs S
Am J Physiol Endocrinol Metab. 2003 Oct;285(4):E917-25. Epub 2003 Jun 10.
PMID: 12799315

Is the Atkins diet on to something? No, it's not a healthy way to eat. But the high-protein, low-carbohydrate diet may hold a few important lessons about weight loss and healthy eating.
[No authors listed]
Harv Health Lett. 2003 May;28(7):1-2. No abstract available.
PMID: 12770829

A randomized trial of a low-carbohydrate diet for obesity
Foster GD, Wyatt HR, Hill JO, McGuckin BG, Brill C, Mohammed BS, Szapary PO, Rader DJ, Edman JS, Klein S
N Engl J Med. 2003 May 22;348(21):2082-90.
PMID: 12761365

A low-carbohydrate as compared with a low-fat diet in severe obesity
Samaha FF, Iqbal N, Seshadri P, Chicano KL, Daily DA, McGrory J, Williams T, Williams M, Gracely EJ, Stern L
N Engl J Med. 2003 May 22;348(21):2074-81.
PMID: 12761364

Efficacy and safety of low-carbohydrate diets: a systematic review
Bravata DM, Sanders L, Huang J, Krumholz HM, Olkin I, Gardner CD, Bravata DM
JAMA. 2003 Apr 9;289(14):1837-50. Review.
PMID: 12684364

A randomized trial comparing a very low carbohydrate diet and a calorie-restricted low fat diet on body weight and cardiovascular risk factors in healthy women
Brehm BJ, Seeley RJ, Daniels SR, D'Alessio DA
J Clin Endocrinol Metab. 2003 Apr;88(4):1617-23.
PMID: 12679447

Effects of a low-carbohydrate diet on weight loss and cardiovascular risk factor in overweight adolescents
Sondike SB, Copperman N, Jacobson MS
J Pediatr. 2003 Mar;142(3):253-8.
PMID: 12640371

Whole-body fat oxidation rate and plasma triacylglycerol concentrations in men consuming an ad libitum high-carbohydrate or low-carbohydrate diet
Landry N, Bergeron N, Archer R, Samson P, Corneau L, Bergeron J, Dériaz O
Am J Clin Nutr. 2003 Mar;77(3):580-6.
PMID: 12600846

Hepatic de novo lipogenesis in normoinsulinemic and hyperinsulinemic subjects consuming high-fat, low-carbohydrate and low-fat, high-carbohydrate isoenergetic diets
Schwarz JM, Linfoot P, Dare D, Aghajanian K
Am J Clin Nutr. 2003 Jan;77(1):43-50.
PMID: 12499321

Effects of a hypocaloric, low-carbohydrate diet on weight loss, blood lipids, blood pressure, glucose tolerance, and body composition in free-living overweight women
Meckling KA, Gauthier M, Grubb R, Sanford J
Can J Physiol Pharmacol. 2002 Nov;80(11):1095-105.
PMID: 12489929

Effects of a low carbohydrate diet and graded exercise during the follicular and luteal phases on the blood antioxidant status in healthy women
Kłapcińska B, Sadowska-Krepa E, Manowska B, Pilis W, Sobczak A, Danch A
Eur J Appl Physiol. 2002 Aug;87(4-5):373-80. Epub 2002 Jun 28.
PMID: 12172876

Glucose intolerance induced by a high-fat/low-carbohydrate diet in rats effects of nonesterified fatty acids
Wang Y, Miura Y, Kaneko T, Li J, Qin LQ, Wang PY, Matsui H, Sato A
Endocrine. 2002 Apr;17(3):185-91.
PMID: 12108518

Effect of 6-month adherence to a very low carbohydrate diet program
Westman EC, Yancy WS, Edman JS, Tomlin KF, Perkins CE
Am J Med. 2002 Jul;113(1):30-6.
PMID: 12106620

Weight loss in obese dogs: evaluation of a high-protein, low-carbohydrate diet

Diez M, Nguyen P, Jeusette I, Devois C, Istasse L, Biourge V
J Nutr. 2002 Jun;132(6 Suppl 2):1685S-7S. No abstract available.
PMID: 12042493

Muscle glycogen content and glucose uptake during exercise in humans: influence of prior exercise and dietary manipulation
Steensberg A, van Hall G, Keller C, Osada T, Schjerling P, Pedersen BK, Saltin B, Febbraio MA
J Physiol. 2002 May 15;541(Pt 1):273-81.
PMID: 12015435

Exercise with low muscle glycogen augments TCA cycle anaplerosis but impairs oxidative energy provision in humans
Gibala MJ, Peirce N, Constantin-Teodosiu D, Greenhaff PL
J Physiol. 2002 May 1;540(Pt 3):1079-86.
PMID: 11986392

The 'carnivore connection' — evolutionary aspects of insulin resistance
Colagiuri S, Brand Miller J
Eur J Clin Nutr. 2002 Mar;56 Suppl 1:S30-5. Review.
PMID: 11965520

High-meat, low-carbohydrate diet in pregnancy: relation to adult blood pressure in the offspring
Shiell AW, Campbell-Brown M, Haselden S, Robinson S, Godfrey KM, Barker DJ
Hypertension. 2001 Dec 1;38(6):1282-8.
PMID: 11751704

Improvement of gastroesophageal reflux disease after initiation of a low-carbohydrate diet: five brief case reports
Yancy WS Jr, Provenzale D, Westman EC
Altern Ther Health Med. 2001 Nov-Dec;7(6):120, 116-9.
PMID: 11712463

Human skeletal muscle PDH kinase activity and isoform expression during a 3-day high-fat/low-carbohydrate diet
Peters SJ, Harris RA, Wu P, Pehleman TL, Heigenhauser GJ, Spriet LL
Am J Physiol Endocrinol Metab. 2001 Dec;281(6):E1151-8.
PMID: 11701428

Exercise prevents the accumulation of triglyceride-rich lipoproteins and their remnants seen when changing to a high-carbohydrate diet

Koutsari C, Karpe F, Humphreys SM, Frayn KN, Hardman AE
Arterioscler Thromb Vasc Biol. 2001 Sep;21(9):1520-5.
PMID: 11557682

The effect of low-carbohydrate diet on the pattern of hormonal changes during incremental, graded exercise in young men
Langfort JL, Zarzeczny R, Nazar K, Kaciuba-Uscilko H
Int J Sport Nutr Exerc Metab. 2001 Jun;11(2):248-57.
PMID: 11402256

Effects of isoenergetic high-carbohydrate compared with high-fat diets on human cholesterol synthesis and expression of key regulatory genes of cholesterol metabolism
Vidon C, Boucher P, Cachefo A, Peroni O, Diraison F, Beylot M
Am J Clin Nutr. 2001 May;73(5):878-84.
PMID: 11333840

Popular diets: correlation to health, nutrition, and obesity
Kennedy ET, Bowman SA, Spence JT, Freedman M, King J
J Am Diet Assoc. 2001 Apr;101(4):411-20. Review.
PMID: 11320946

Type 2 diabetes in an aviator, protein diet vs. traditional diet: case report
Hilton AD, Hursh TA
Aviat Space Environ Med. 2001 Mar;72(3):219-20.
PMID: 11277288

The low-carbohydrate diet in primary care OB/GYN
Bachman JM
Prim Care Update Ob Gyns. 2001 Jan;8(1):12-17.
PMID: 11164346

Fasting lipoprotein and postprandial triacylglycerol responses to a low-carbohydrate diet supplemented with n-3 fatty acids
Volek JS, Gómez AL, Kraemer WJ
J Am Coll Nutr. 2000 Jun;19(3):383-91.
PMID: 10872901

The effects of carbohydrate variation in isocaloric diets on glycogenolysis and gluconeogenesis in healthy men
Bisschop PH, Pereira Arias AM, Ackermans MT, Endert E, Pijl H, Kuipers F, Meijer AJ, Sauerwein HP, Romijn JA
J Clin Endocrinol Metab. 2000 May;85(5):1963-7.

Appendix C

PMID: 10843182

Diet high in monounsaturated fat does not have a different effect on arterial elasticity than a low-fat, high-carbohydrate diet
Ashton EL, Pomeroy S, Foster JE, Kaye RS, Nestel PJ, Ball M
J Am Diet Assoc. 2000 May;100(5):537-42.
PMID: 10812378

Fat and carbohydrate balances during adaptation to a high-fat.
Smith SR, de Jonge L, Zachwieja JJ, Roy H, Nguyen T, Rood JC, Windhauser MM, Bray GA
Am J Clin Nutr. 2000 Feb;71(2):450-7.
PMID: 10648257

The effect of fat and carbohydrate content of the diet on voluntary ethanol intake in golden hamsters
DiBattista D, Joachim D
Alcohol. 1999 Jun-Jul;18(2-3):153-7.
PMID: 10456566

The zone diet and athletic performance
Cheuvront SN
Sports Med. 1999 Apr;27(4):213-28. Review.
PMID: 10367332

Carbohydrate intake and multiple sprint sports: with special reference to football (soccer)
Balsom PD, Wood K, Olsson P, Ekblom B
Int J Sports Med. 1999 Jan;20(1):48-52.
PMID: 10090462

Utility of a short-term 25% carbohydrate diet on improving glycemic control in type 2 diabetes mellitus
Gutierrez M, Akhavan M, Jovanovic L, Peterson CM
J Am Coll Nutr. 1998 Dec;17(6):595-600.
PMID: 9853539

Dietary carbohydrate intake plays an important role in preventing alcoholic fatty liver in the rat
Tsukada H, Wang PY, Kaneko T, Wang Y, Nakano M, Sato A
J Hepatol. 1998 Nov;29(5):715-24.
PMID: 9833908

The efficacy of the ketogenic diet-1998: a prospective evaluation of intervention in 150 children
Freeman JM, Vining EP, Pillas DJ, Pyzik PL, Casey JC, Kelly L
Pediatrics. 1998 Dec;102(6):1358-63.
PMID: 9832569

Control of dental caries by a low carbohydrate diet
PANKEY LD
J Fla State Dent Soc. 1948 Oct;19(10):5-7.
PMID: 18889992

APPENDIX D: DCCT BIBLIOGRAPHY

1. The Diabetes Control and Complications Trial Research Group. The effect of intensive diabetes therapy on measures of autonomic nervous system function in the Diabetes Control and Complications Trial (DCCT). *Diabetologia*, 41:416-423, 1998. Available on SpringerLink online at http://www.springerlink.com/content/100410/?sortorder=asc. Retrieved on 4/12/09.

2. The Diabetes Control and Complications Trial Research Group. Effect of intensive therapy on residual Beta-cell function in patients with type 1 diabetes in the Diabetes Control and Complications Trial: A randomized, controlled trial. *Annals of Internal Medicine*, 128:517-523, 1998. Available online at http://www.annals.org/cgi/content/full/128/7/517#group. Retrieved on 4/12/09.

3. The Diabetes Control and Complications Trial Research Group. Early worsening of diabetic retinopathy in the Diabetes Control and Complications Trial. *Archives of Ophthalmology*, 116:874-886, 1998.

4. Purnell JQ, Hokanson JE, Marcovina SM, Steffes MW, Cleary PA and Brunzell JD. Effect of excessive weight gain with intensive therapy of type 1 diabetes on lipid levels and blood pressure: Results from the DCCT. *Journal of the American Medical Association*, 280:140-146, 1998.

5. The Diabetes Control and Complications Trial Research Group. Clustering of long-term complications in families with diabetes in the Diabetes Control and Complications Trial. *Diabetes*, 46:1829-1839, 1997.

6. The Diabetes Control and Complications Trial Research Group. Hypoglycemia in the Diabetes Control and Complications Trail. *Diabetes*, 46:271-286, 1997.

7. The Diabetes Control and Complications Trial Research Group. The absence of a glycemic threshold for the development of long-term complications: The perspective of the Diabetes Control and Complications Trial. *Diabetes*, 45:1289-1298, 1996.

8. The Diabetes Control and Complications Trial Research Group. Lifetime benefits and costs of intensive therapy as practiced in the Diabetes Control and Complications Trial. *Journal of the American Medical Association*, 276:1409-1415, 1996.

9. The Diabetes Control and Complications Trial Research Group. Pregnancy outcomes in the Diabetes Control and Complications Trial. *American Journal of Obstetrics and Gynecology*, 174:1343-1353, 1996.

10. The Diabetes Control and Complications Trial Research Group. Influence of intensive diabetes treatment on quality-of-life outcomes in the Diabetes Control and Complications Trial. *Diabetes Care*, 19:195-203, 1996.

11. The Diabetes Control and Complications Trial Research Group. Effects of intensive diabetes therapy on neuropsychological function in adults in the Diabetes Control and Complications Trial. *Annals of Internal Medicine*, 124:379-388, 1996. Available online at http://www.annals.org/cgi/content/full/124/4/379. Retrieved on 4/12/09.

12. Leiter L, and the Diabetes Control and Complications Trial Research Group. Use of bioelectrical impedance analysis measurements in patients with diabetes. *American Journal of Clinical Nutrition*, 64 (suppl.): 515S-518S, 1996.

13. The Diabetes Control and Complications Trial Research Group. Effect of intensive diabetes treatment on nerve conduction in the Diabetes Control and Complications Trial. *Annals of Neurology*, 38:869-880, 1995.

14. The Diabetes Control and Complications Trial Research Group. Adverse events and their association with treatment regimens in the Diabetes Control and Complications Trial. *Diabetes Care*, 18:1415-1427, 1995.

15. The Diabetes Control and Complications Trial Research Group. Resource utilization and costs of care in the Diabetes Control and Complications Trial. *Diabetes Care*, 18:1468-1478, 1995.

16. Purnell JQ, Marcovina SM, Hokanson JE, Kennedy H, Cleary PA, Steffes MW, and Brunzell JD. Levels of lipoprotein (a), apolipoprotein B, and lipoprotein cholesterol distribution in IDDM. Results from follow-up in the Diabetes Control and Complications Trial. *Diabetes*, 44:1218-1226, 1995.

17. The Diabetes Control and Complications Trial Research Group. The relationship of glycemic exposure (HbA$_{1c}$) to the risk of development and progression of retinopathy in the Diabetes Control and Complications Trial. *Diabetes*, 44:968-983, 1995.

18. The Diabetes Control and Complications Trial Research Group. Effect of intensive diabetes management on macrovascular events and risk factors in the Diabetes Control and Complications Trial. *The American Journal of Cardiology*, 75:894-903, 1995.

Appendix D

19. The Diabetes Control and Complications (DCCT) Research Group. Effect of intensive therapy on the development and progression of diabetic nephropathy in the Diabetes Control and Complications Trial. *Kidney International*, 47:1703-1720, 1995.

20. The Diabetes Control and Complications Trial Research Group. The effect of intensive diabetes therapy on the development and progression of neuropathy. *Annals of Internal Medicine*, 122:561-568, 1995.

21. The Diabetes Control and Complications Trial Research Group; and Klein R, Moss S. A comparison of the study populations in the Diabetes Control and Complications Trial and the Wisconsin Epidemiologic Study of Diabetic Retinopathy. *Archives of Internal Medicine*, 155:745-754, 1995.

22. The Diabetes Control and Complications Trial Research Group. Progression of retinopathy with intensive versus conventional treatment in the Diabetes Control and Complications Trial. *Ophthalmology*, 102:647-661, 1995.

23. The Diabetes Control and Complications Trial Research Group. The effect of intensive diabetes treatment on the progression of diabetic retinopathy in insulin-dependent diabetes mellitus: The Diabetes Control and Complications Trial. *Archives of Ophthalmology*, 113:36-51, 1995.

24. Diabetes Control and Complications Trial Research Group. Implementation of treatment protocols in the Diabetes Control and Complications Trial. *Diabetes Care*, 18:361-376, 1995.

25. The Diabetes Control and Complications Trial Research Group. Psychological aspects of the DCCT. In *The Technology of Diabetes Care: Converging Medical and Psychosocial Perspectives*, 122-139, 1994.

26. Leiter LA, Lukaski HC, Kenny DJ, Barnie A, Camelon K, Ferguson RS, MacLean S, Simkins S, Zinman B and Cleary PA for the DCCT Research Group. The use of Bioelectrical Impedance Analysis (BIA) to estimate body composition in the Diabetes Control and Complications Trial (DCCT). *International Journal of Obesity*, 18:829-835, 1994.

27. Schmidt LE, Cox MS, Buzzard IM, and Cleary PA, for the DCCT Research Group. Reproducibility of a comprehensive diet history in the Diabetes Control and Complications Trial. *Journal of the American Dietetic Association*, 94:1392-1397, 1994.

28. Diabetes Control and Complications Trial Research Group. Effect of intensive diabetes treatment on the development and progression of long-term complications in

adolescents with insulin-dependent diabetes mellitus: Diabetes Control and Complications Trial. *The Journal of Pediatrics*, 125:177-188, 1994.

29. The DCCT Research Group. A screening algorithm to identify clinically significant changes in neuropsychological functions in the Diabetes Control and Complications Trial. *Journal of Clinical and Experimental Neuropsychology*, 16:303-316, 1994.

30. Siebert C and Clark CM. Operational and policy considerations of data monitoring in clinical trials: the Diabetes Control and Complications Trial experience. *Controlled Clinical Trials*, 14(1): 30-44, 1993.

31. The DCCT Research Group. The impact of the trial coordinator in the Diabetes Control and Complications Trial. *Diabetes Educator*, 19:509-512, 1993.

32. Levey AS, Greene T, Schluchter MD, Cleary PA, Teschan PE, Lorenz RA, Molitch ME, Mitch WE, Siebert C, Hall PM, and Steffes MW, for the Modification of Diet in Renal Disease Study Group and the Diabetes Control and Complications Trial Research Group. Glomerular filtration rate measurements in clinical trials. *Journal of the American Society of Nephrology*, 4:1159-1171, 1993.

33. The Diabetes Control and Complications Trial Research Group. Nutrition interventions for intensive therapy in the Diabetes Control and Complications Trial. *The Journal of the American Dietetic Association*, 93:768-772, 1993.

34. The DCCT Research Group. Expanded role of the dietitian in the Diabetes Control and Complications Trial: Implications for clinical practice. *The Journal of the American Dietetic Association*, 93:758-767, 1993.

35. The Diabetes Control and Complications Trial Research Group. The effect of intensive treatment of diabetes on the development and progression of long-term complications in insulin-dependent diabetes mellitus. *The New England Journal of Medicine*, 329:977-986, 1993.

36. The Diabetes Control and Complications Trial Research Group. Baseline analysis of renal function in the Diabetes Control and Complications Trial. *Kidney International*, 43:668-674, 1993.

37. The DCCT Research Group. Lipid and lipoprotein levels in patients with IDDM: Diabetes Control and Complications Trial Experience. *Diabetes Care*, 15:886-894, 1992.

38. Ryan CM, Adams KA, Heaton RK, Grant I, Jacobson AM and the DCCT Research Group. Neurobehavioral assessment of medical patients in clinical trials: The DCCT

Appendix D

Experience. In *Handbook of Clinical Trials; The Neurobehavioral Approach*. Erich Mohr and Pim Brouwers, Eds. Amsterdam/Lisse: Swets and Zeitlinger, 215-241, 1991.

39. The DCCT Research Group. Epidemiology of severe hypoglycemia in the Diabetes Control and Complications Trial. *The American Journal of Medicine*, 90:450-59, 1991.

40. The DCCT Research Group. The Diabetes Control and Complications Trial (DCCT): Update. *Diabetes Care*, 13:427-433, 1990.

41. The DCCT Research Group. The Diabetes Control and Complications Trial (DCCT): The trial coordinator perspective. *Diabetes Educator*, 15:236-241, 1989.

42. The DCCT Research Group. The DCCT: Will it answer the questions? *Diabetes 1988*, R. Larkins, P. Zimmet, D. Chisolm, editors, Elsevier Science Publishers B.V. (Biomedical Division), 847-855, 1989.

43. The DCCT Research Group. The Diabetes Control and Complications Trial (DCCT): Results of the feasibility study and design of the full-scale clinical trial. *Pediatric and Adolescent Endocrinology*, Laron Z, Karp M (eds) Basel, Karger, 18:15-21, 1989.

44. The DCCT Research Group. Implementation of a multicomponent process to obtain informed consent in the Diabetes Control and Complications Trial. *Controlled Clinical Trials*, 10:83-96, 1989.

45. The DCCT Research Group. Update. *Diabetes Spectrum*, 1:187-190, 1988.

46. The DCCT Research Group. Reliability and validity of diabetes quality-of-life measure for the Diabetes Control and Complications Trial (DCCT). *Diabetes Care*, 11:725-732, 1988.

47. The DCCT Research Group. Weight gain associated with intensive therapy in the Diabetes Control and Complications Trial. *Diabetes Care*, 11:567-573, 1988.

48. Schumer M, Burton G, Burton C, Crum D, Pfeifer MA, the DCCT Study Group. Diabetic autonomic neuropathy-Part I: Autonomic nervous system data analysis by a computerized central unit in a multicenter trial. *The American Journal of Medicine*, 85 (suppl. 5A):137-143, 1988.

49. Hanssen KF, The DCCT Research Group, and Brunetti P. Is there a need for a continuation of the DCCT in 1988? *Diabetes Nutrition and Metabolism*, 1:151-159, 1988.

50. The DCCT Research Group. Factors in development of diabetic neuropathy: Baseline analysis of neuropathy in feasibility phase of the Diabetes Control and Complications Trial (DCCT). *Diabetes*, 37:476-481, 1988.

51. The DCCT Research Group. Are continuing studies of metabolic control and microvascular complications in insulin-dependent diabetes mellitus justified? The Diabetes Control and Complications Trial. *The New England Journal of Medicine*, 318:246-250, 1988.

52. The Diabetes Control and Complications Trial Research Group. Color photography vs. fluorescein angiography in the detection of diabetic retinopathy in the Diabetes Control and Complications Trial. *Archives of Ophthalmology*, 105:1344-1351, 1987.

53. The DCCT Research Group. Diabetes Control and Complications Trial (DCCT): results of feasibility study. *Diabetes Care*, 10:1-19, 1987.

54. The DCCT Research Group. Feasibility of centralized measurements of glycated hemoglobin in the Diabetes Control and Complications Trial: A multicenter study. *Clinical Chemistry*, 33:2267-2271, 1987.

55. The DCCT Research Group. Effects of age, duration and treatment of insulin-dependent diabetes mellitus on residual Beta-cell function: Observations during eligibility testing for the Diabetes Control and Complications Trial (DCCT). *Journal of Clinical Endocrinology and Metabolism*, 65:30-36, 1987.

56. The DCCT Research Group. Treatment regimen design in the Diabetes Control and Complications Trial (DCCT). *Transplantation Proceedings*, XVIII(6):1678-1680, 1986.

57. The DCCT Research Group. The Diabetes Control and Complications Trial (DCCT): Design and methodologic considerations for the feasibility phase. *Diabetes*, 35:530-545, 1986.

Notes

PREFACE TO THE SECOND EDITION

[1] "The QWERTY arrangement on a keyboard has no rational explanation, only a historic one. It was introduced in response to a problem in the early days of the typewriter. The keys used to jam. The idea was to minimize the collision problem by separating those keys that followed one another frequently...Once adopted, it resulted in many millions of typewriters and...the social cost of change...mounted with the vested interest created by the fact that so many fingers now knew how to follow the QWERTY keyboard. QWERTY has stayed on despite the existence of other, more "rational" systems." See Papert, Seymour. *Mindstorms: Children, Computers and Powerful Ideas*. New York: Basic Books, 1980, p. 33. *Op cit.* Dennett, Daniel C. *Darwin's Dangerous Idea: Evolution and the Meanings of Life*. New York: Simon & Schuster Paperbacks, 1995, p. 122-123.

PREFACE

[2] Walter Wellesley "Red" Smith (September 25, 1905 in Green Bay, Wisconsin – January 15, 1982 in Stamford, Connecticut) was an American sportswriter who rose to become one of America's most widely read sports columnists. After graduating from Green Bay East High School, site of Packers home games until 1957, Smith moved on to the University of Notre Dame. After graduation, he worked for the *Milwaukee Sentinel*, *St. Louis Journal*, and *Philadelphia Record*. After 18 years, Smith joined the *New York Herald Tribune*. He cemented his reputation with the *Herald-Trib*, as his column was widely read and often syndicated. When the paper folded in 1966, he became a freelance writer. He joined the *New York Times* in 1971 as a contract writer. By this time, his reputation was secured as one of the foremost sportswriters in America. During his time with the *Times*, Smith garnered many awards. In 1976, he was the first sportswriter to win the Pulitzer Prize for Commentary. He also received the J. G. Taylor Spink Award from the Baseball Hall of Fame in 1976. Furthermore, the Associated Press awarded him the first Red Smith Award for "outstanding contributions to sports journalism." Smith died at the age 76 of heart failure. Red Smith Middle School in Green Bay is named in his honor. Also named in his honor is the Red Smith Handicap, a race for Thoroughbred horses run at Belmont Park on Long Island, New York. "There's nothing to writing. All you do is sit down at a typewriter and open a vein." [p. 7, *No More Rejections: 50 Secrets to Writing A Manuscript That Sells*, by Alice Orr, Writer's Digest, Cincinnati, 2004]. Biography courtesy of Wikipedia. See http://en.wikipedia.org/wiki/Red_Smith_%28sportswriter%29. Retrieved on 11/22/08.

[3] What follows is abridged from the Wikipedia article entitled "Inspector Morse," available online at http://en.wikipedia.org/wiki/Inspector_Morse. Retrieved on 7/26/09.

[4] What follows is abridged from the Wikipedia article entitled "Claus von Bülow," available online at http://en.wikipedia.org/wiki/Claus_von_B%C3%BClow. Retrieved on 7/26/09.

[5] Taubes, Gary. *Good Calories, Bad Calories*. First Anchor Books Edition. New York: Anchor Books, 2008, page xvii.

[6] *Ibid*, pages 293-294.

[7] *Ibid*, page 297.

[8] *Ibid*, page 124.

[9] *Ibid*, pages 132-133.

[10] *Ibid*, page 153.

[11] *Ibid*, page 168.

AT THE LIBRARY

[12] A national library is a library specifically established by the government of a nation to serve as the preeminent repository of information for that country. Unlike public libraries, these rarely allow citizens to borrow books. Often, they include numerous rare, valuable, or significant works; such as the Library of Congress' Gutenberg Bible. National libraries are usually notable for their size, compared to that of other libraries in the same country. Some national libraries may be thematic or specialized in some specific domains, beside or in replacement of the 'main' national library. For a comprehensive list of national libraries and further resources, see the Wikipedia article "List of National Libraries," online at http://en.wikipedia.org/wiki/List_of_national_libraries. Retrieved on 4/5/09.

[13] In "We knew the web was big..." posted by Jesse Alpert & Nissan Hajaj, Software Engineers, Web Search Infrastructure Team, GOOGLE (July 25, 2008), on the blog http://googleblog.blogspot.com/2008/07/we-knew-web-was-big.html, the authors were surprised to find that content hit a milestone: 1 trillion (as in 1,000,000,000,000) unique URLs on the web at once. Retrieved on 3/31/09.

[14] See Abelson, Hal, Ledeen, Ken, and Lewis, Harry. *Blown to Bits: Your Life, Liberty, and Happiness After the Digital Explosion.* Upper Saddle River, NJ: Addison-Wesley, 2008, page 112.

[15] A library classification is a system of coding and organizing library materials (books, serials, audiovisual materials, computer files, maps, manuscripts, realia) according to their subject and allocating a call number to that information resource. Similar to classification systems used in biology, bibliographic classification systems group entities that are similar together typically arranged in a hierarchical tree structure. A different kind of classification system, called a faceted classification system, is also widely used which allows the assignment of multiple classifications to an object, enabling the classifications to be ordered in multiple ways.

Library classification of a piece of work consists of two steps. Firstly the 'aboutness' of the material is ascertained. Next, a call number, (essentially a book's address), based on the classification system in use at the particular library will be assigned to the work using the notation of the system.

It is important to note that unlike subject heading or Thesauri where multiple terms can be assigned to the same work, in library classification systems, each work can only be placed in one class. This is due to shelving purposes: a book can have only one physical place. However, in classified catalogs one may have main entries as well as added entries. Most classification systems like DDC and Library of Congress classification, also add a cutter number to each work which adds a code for the author of the work.

Classification systems in libraries generally play two roles. Firstly they facilitate subject access by allowing the user to find out what works or documents the library has on a certain subject. Secondly, they provide a known location for the information source to be located (e.g., where it is shelved).

Until the 20th century, most libraries had closed stacks, so the library classification only served to organize the subject catalog. In the 20th century, libraries opened their stacks to the public and started to shelve the library material itself according to some library classification to simplify subject browsing.

Some classification systems are more suitable for aiding subject access, rather than for shelf location. For example, UDC which uses a complicated notation including plus, colons are more difficult to use for the purpose of shelf arrangement but are more expressive compared to DDC in terms of showing relationships between subjects. Similarly faceted classification schemes are more difficult to use for shelf arrangement, unless the user has knowledge of the citation order.

Depending on the size of the library collection, some libraries might use classification systems solely for one purpose or the other. In extreme cases a public library with a small collection might just use a classification system for location of resources but might not use a complicated subject classification system. Instead all resources might just be put into a couple of wide classes (Travel, Crime, Magazines etc). This is known as a "mark and park" classification method, more formally called reader interest classification.

There are many standard system of library classification in use, and many more have been proposed over the years. However in general, classification systems can be divided into three types depending on how they are used: (1) Universal schemes covering all subjects. Examples include Dewey Decimal Classification, Universal Decimal Classification and Library of Congress Classification. (2) Specific classification schemes. Examples include Iconclass, British classification of Music, and Dickinson classification. (3) National schemes specially created for certain countries. An example is the Swedish library classification system, SAB (Sveriges Allmänna Biblioteksförening).

In terms of functionality, classification systems are often described as (1) enumerative: produce an alphabetical list of subject headings, assign numbers to each heading in alphabetical order, (2) hierarchical: divides subjects hierarchically, from most general to most specific, (3) faceted or analytico-synthetic: divides subjects into mutually exclusive orthogonal facets.

There are few completely enumerative systems or faceted systems, most systems are a blend but favoring one type or the other. The most common classification systems, LCC and DDC, are essentially enumerative, though with some hierarchical and faceted elements (more so for DDC), especially at the broadest and most general level. The first true faceted system was the Colon classification of S. R. Ranganathan.

Universal classification systems used in English-speaking world: Bliss bibliographic classification (BC), Dewey Decimal Classification (DDC), Library of Congress Classification (LCC), EnglishHarvard-Yenching Classification - An English classification system for Chinese language materials.

Universal classification systems in other languages: A System of Book Classification for Chinese Libraries (Liu's Classification), Nippon Decimal Classification (NDC), Chinese Library Classification (CLC), Korean Decimal Classification (KDC), Library-Bibliographic Classification (BBK) from Russia.

Universal classification systems that rely on synthesis (faceted systems): Bliss bibliographic classification, Colon classification, Cutter Expansive Classification, Universal Decimal Classification, Brinkler classification.

Newer classification systems tend to use the principle of synthesis (combining codes from different lists to represent the different attributes of a work) heavily, which is comparatively lacking in LC or DDC. Abridged from the Wikipedia article "Library Classification," online at http://en.wikipedia.org/wiki/Library_classification. Retrieved on 4/5/09.

[16] Abridged from the Wikipedia article "Library of Congress," online at http://en.wikipedia.org/wiki/Library_of_congress. Retrieved on 3/31/09.

[17] See the Library of Congress web page "About the Library" online at http://www.loc.gov/about/. Retrieved on 3/31/09.

[18] For information about Thomas Jefferson's library, see the article "Thomas Jefferson's Library" posted by Douglas Galbi, February, 2008, on the Purple Motes web site at http://purplemotes.net/2008/02/03/thomas-jeffersons-library/. Retrieved on 3/31/09. See also the Library of Congress web page "Preservation" online at http://www.loc.gov/preserv/history/growing.html. Retrieved on 3/31/09.

[19] See the online article "Jefferson's Legacy: A Brief History of the Library of Congress" published by the Library of Congress, at http://www.loc.gov/loc/legacy/loc.html. Retrieved on 4/5/09.

[20] *Ibid.*

[21] *Ibid.*

[22] See Thomas Jefferson's personal library at Library Thing, based on scholarship, online at http://www.librarything.com/catalog.php?view=ThomasJefferson. Retrieved on 4/5/09. See also "Library Thing Profile Page for Thomas Jefferson's library," summarizing contents and indicating sources online at http://www.librarything.com/profile/ThomasJefferson. Retrieved on 4/5/09.

[23] See the online article "Jefferson's Legacy: A Brief History of the Library of Congress" published by the Library of Congress, at http://www.loc.gov/loc/legacy/loc.html. Retrieved on 4/5/09.

[24] See Gutenberg's Bibles—Where to Find Them online at http://www.approvedarticles.com/Article/Gutenberg-s-Bibles--Where-to-Find-Them/1088. Retrieved on 4/5/09. See also http://www.octavo.com/editions/gtnbbl/index.html. Retrieved on 4/5/09. See also http://www.loc.gov/rr/rarebook/guide/europe.html. Retrieved on 4/5/09.

[25] See the article "About the Serial and Government Publications Division," published by The Library of Congress online at http://www.loc.gov/rr/news/brochure.html. Retrieved on 4/5/09.

[26] See the article "Mandatory Deposit," online at http://www.copyright.gov/help/faq/mandatory_deposit.html. Retrieved on 4/5/09.

[27] See the article "Fascinating Facts," published by the Library of Congress online at http://www.loc.gov/about/facts.html. Retrieved on 4/5/09.

[28] See the article "Did You Know?" published by the British Library online at http://www.bl.uk/about/didyou.html. Retrieved on 4/5/09.

[29] See the Library of Congress web page "About the Library" online at http://www.loc.gov/about/. Retrieved on 3/31/09. See also the article "Did You Know?" published by the British Library online at http://www.bl.uk/about/didyou.html. Retrieved on 4/5/09.

[30] See the article "Library of Congress General Information," published by the Library of Congress online at http://www.loc.gov/about/generalinfo.html. Retrieved on 4/5/09.

[31] See the article "Entire Library of Congress," online at http://outgoing.typepad.com/outgoing/2005/06/entire_library_.html. Retrieved on 4/5/09.

[32] See the article "Library of Congress General Information," published by the Library of Congress online at http://www.loc.gov/about/generalinfo.html. Retrieved on 4/5/09.

[33] The Thomas Jefferson Building is located between Independence Avenue and East Capitol Street on First Street SE. It first opened in 1897 as the main building of the Library and is the oldest of the three buildings. Known originally as the Library of Congress Building or Main Building, it took its present name on June 13, 1980. The John Adams Building is located between Independence Avenue and East Capitol Street on 2nd Street SE. It opened in 1938 as an annex to the main building. Between April 13, 1976 and June 13, 1980, the John Adams Building was known as the Thomas Jefferson Building. The James Madison Memorial Building is located between First and Second Streets on Independence Avenue SE. It opened in 1981 as the new headquarters of the Library. The James Madison Memorial Building also serves as the official memorial to James Madison. It houses, among other materials, the Law Library of Congress. See the Wikipedia article "Library of Congress" online at http://en.wikipedia.org/wiki/Library_of_congress. Retrieved on 4/4/09.

Notes

[34] See the article "Interlibrary Loan (Collections Access, Management and Loan Division, Library of Congress," published on the Library of Congress website online at http://www.loc.gov/rr/loan/. Retrieved on 4/5/09.

[35] Abridged from the Wikipedia article "Library of Congress Classification," online at http://en.wikipedia.org/wiki/Library_of_Congress_Classification. Retrieved on 4/5/09.

[36] Not listed in the Library of Congress search database, Matthew Dobson (1731-1784) wrote *Experiments and Observations on the Urine in Diabetes (Medical Observations and Inquiries)*, published in London, in 1776. Matthew Dobson from Yorkshire graduated MD at Edinburgh in 1756. By evaporating the urine of a diabetic patient, Dobson was the first to prove the presence of sugar in urine. He also made the crucial observation of the excess of sugar in blood, and demonstrated that diabetes is a systemic disorder rather than, as had been previously thought, a primary disease of the kidneys. See the Royal College of Physicians of Edinburgh webpage online at http://www.rcpe.ac.uk/library/exhibitions/diabetes/diabetes.php. Retrieved on 4/30/09.

[37] For a picture of the book cover, and others from the same time period, see the Royal College of Physicians of Edinburgh webpage online at http://www.rcpe.ac.uk/library/exhibitions/diabetes/diabetes.php. Retrieved on 4/30/09.

[38] See "The Google Book Search Project: Is Online Indexing a Fair Use Under Copyright Law?" by Robin Jeweler, Legislative Attorney, American Law Division, December 28, 2005. Available online at http://assets.opencrs.com/rpts/RS22356_20051228.pdf. Retrieved on 4/30/09.

[39] Participating libraries include those at the University of Michigan, Harvard University, Stanford University, Oxford, and the New York Public Library. For details, see http://books.google.com/googlebooks/partners.html. Retrieved on 4/30/09.

[40] See http://books.google.com/googlebooks/library.html. Retrieved on 4/30/09. For more background on the program, see GOOGLE's website at http://books.google.com/googlebooks/about.html. Retrieved on 4/30/09.

[41] McGraw-Hill Companies, Inc. v. GOOGLE, No. 05 CV 8881 (S.D.N.Y., filed Oct. 19, 2005); The Author's Guild v. GOOGLE, No. 05 CV 8136 (S.D.N.Y., filed Sept. 20, 2005).

[42] 17 U.S.C. § 106.

[43] 336 F.3d 811 (9th Cir. 2003). For more background on Kelly v. Arriba Soft Corp., see CRS Report RS21206, *Fair Use on the Internet: Copyright's Reproduction and Public Display Rights,* by Robin Jeweler.

[44] Adapted from "Scanning Project Digitizes 25,000 US Library of Congress Books," by Art Chimes, Washington, DC, January 23, 2009. Available online at http://www.voanews.com/english/archive/2009-01/2009-01-23-voa29.cfm?moddate=2009-01-23. Retrieved on 5/1/09.

[45] Portable Document Format (PDF) is a file format created by Adobe Systems in 1993, for document exchange. PDF is used for representing two-dimensional documents in a manner independent of the application software, hardware, and operating system.

[46] Purdy, Charles Wesley. *Diabetes: Its Causes, Symptoms, and Treatment.* Philadelphia and London: F.A. Davis Publisher, 1890, pages 80-87. Entire book available online at http://www.archive.org/stream/diabetesitscause00purduoft/diabetesitscause00purduoft_djvu.txt. Retrieved on 5/1/09.

[47] Williamson, M.D., M.R.C.P., R.T. *Diabetes Mellitus and Its Treatment.* Edinburgh & London: Young J. Pentland; New York: The Macmillan Company, 1898, pages 322-323. Available through GOOGLE Book Search online at

http://books.google.com/books?id=QrsnAAAAYAAJ&pg=PR3&lpg=PR3&dq=Williamson,+M.D.,+M.R.
C.P.,+R.T.++Diabetes+Mellitus+and+Its+Treatment.&source=bl&ots=0Gr_k5umq7&sig=IN_EaRtR9e0eQC
cuLTfqI_fecDc&hl=en&ei=q438SeiiCKP4tAOMg7HoAQ&sa=X&oi=book_result&ct=result&resnum=1.
Retrieved on 5/2/09.

[48] *Ibid*, page 325.

[49] *Ibid*, page 330.

[50] *Ibid*, pages 330-331.

[51] *Ibid*, page 337.

[52] *Ibid*, page 343.

[53] "The diabetic dietaries recommended by most authors agree generally with that just given, but the following are minor points of difference: Sir William Roberts adds "torrified" bread and celery to the articles sanctioned.

Pavy sanctions also turnips, French beans, cauliflower, asparagus, and vegetable marrow, but only in moderate quantity, and when boiled in a large amount of water; also radishes and celery.

Seegen allows the following in moderate quantities: Cauliflower, carrots, turnips, white cabbage, green peas, berries (such as strawberries, raspberries, currants); also oranges and almonds. But he forbids other fruits, such as grapes, cherries, peaches, apricots, plums, and all kinds of dried fruits.

In addition to the articles mentioned, v. Noorden sanctions mussels, oysters, lobster, cauliflower, spinach, onions, leeks, asparagus, sorrel, French beans. He also allows the following (amongst other articles), but only in very limited quantities: Celery, green peas, beans, carrots, mushrooms, radishes, two medium-sized tomatoes, a thin slice of cocoanut, a thin slice of melon, one small acid apple, one or one and a half peach, one tablespoon of wild raspberries or strawberries, four spoonfuls of currants, six greengages[53], twelve cherries, half a medium-sized pear.

Cantini prescribes a very rigid diet of nitrogenous and fatty foods only. He allows: Bouillon of various kinds. Beef, tongue, veal, mutton (but liver is forbidden), duck, goose, chicken, pigeon, and game of all kinds. Fish, crustacea, lobster, crabs.

In the cooking and preparation of the above he forbids the use of flour, sugar, wine, butter, vinegar, and lemon juice; but he sanctions the use of olive oil and fats, and recommends dilute acetic acid in place of inegar [sic.], and citric acid in place of lemon juice.

Cantini allows 500 to 600 grms. of nitrogenous food daily. In order to improve the digestion, and to increase the strength of emaciated patients, he recommends 60 to 200 grms. of pancreatic fat. The fresh pancreas of a cow, calf, or lamb is cut into small pieces, and mixed with pig's suet. After three hours it is lightly roasted." See *Ibid*, Appendix, pages 406-408.

[54] Dickson, Paul. *The Library in America, A Celebration in Words and Pictures.* New York: Facts on File Publications, 1986, page 1.

[55] *Fundamentals of Collection Development & Management.* Peggy Johnson. American Library Association. Chicago, 2004, page 4.

[56] *Ibid*, pages 6-7.

[57] This number is significantly lower than the total of 116,393 libraries as stated by *The Whole Library Handbook 4*, because it doesn't include "school library media centers" which in 2004 totaled 93,861. See *The Whole Library Handbook 4*, edited by George M. Eberhart, American Library Association, 2006, page 3.

Notes

58 *American Library Directory, 61st Edition*. Medford, New Jersey: Information Today, Inc., 2008, page xiii.

59 *Ibid*, page 260.

60 Nationwide public library statistics are collected and disseminated annually through the Federal-State Cooperative System for public library data (FSCS). Statistics are collected from nearly 9,000 public libraries. The FSCS web site is at: http://nces.ed.gov/pubsearch/getpubcats.asp?sid=041#052. The HAPLR Index includes 15 factors. The focus is on circulation, staffing, materials, reference service, and funding levels. The Index does not include data on audio and video collections, or interlibrary loan, among other items that could have been calculated from the FSCS data. Perhaps most prominently absent from the data are any measures of electronic use or Internet service. While such measures would have been desirable, the FSCS data simply are simply not sufficient for such comparisons at this time. Internet, electronic services and audiovisual services are excluded because there is simply not enough data reported by enough libraries to make comparisons meaningful. What remains is fairly traditional data for print services, book checkouts, reference service, funding and staffing. It is likely that in the future, additional measures can be added to the FSCS data to begin to evaluate such other library services as internet use, electronic services, and non-print services. The FSCS data have only been collected on a consistent national basis since 1981. Since then the data have been refined to be more consistent and to include more information. That trend is likely to accelerate, making the additional comparisons possible soon. See Hennen's American Public Library Ratings, available online at http://www.haplr-index.com/index.html. Retrieved on 1/24/09.

61 Abridged Dewey Decimal Classification, Edition 12. Devised by Melvil Dewey. Edited by John P. Camaromi. New York: Forest Press, a Division of OCLC Online Computer Library Center, Inc., 1990, page 6. Originally published in 1894.

62 *Ibid*, page 7.

63 *Ibid*.

64 *Ibid*, page 8.

65 *Fundamentals of Collection Development & Management*. Peggy Johnson. American Library Association. Chicago, 2004, pages 3-4.

66 *Circulating Collection Management Manual*. Ann Lockett, Collection Management Coordinator. Santa Clara City Library, January, 1999, page 52.

67 When starting a collection, libraries frequently consult the *Public Library Catalog*, a list of recommended reference and nonfiction books for adults, classified by subject. There are seven books on diabetes within the 616.4 classification listed for inclusion in any collection, of which three were on the shelf. The seven books listed are: (1) *American Diabetes Association Complete Guide to Diabetes; The Ultimate Home Reference from the Diabetes Experts*. 3rd edition, completely rev. American Diabetes Assn., 2002, 517 pages, (2) *The Joslin Guide to Diabetes; A Program for Managing Your Treatment*; [by] Richard S. Beaser, with Joan C.V. Hill and the Joslin Education Committee. Simon & Schuster, 1995, 351 pages, (3) *Diabetes Sourcebook*; edited by Dawn D. Matthews. 3rd edition. Omnigraphics, 2003, 621 pages, (4) *The Thyroid Guide*; [by] Beth Ann Ditkoff and Paul loGerfo. HarperPerennial, 2000, 171 pages, (5) *Mayo Clinic on Managing Diabetes*; Maria Collazo-Clavell, editor in chief. Mayo Clinic; [distributed by] Mason Crest, 2002, 194 pages, (6) *Women & Diabetes: Staying healthy in Body, Mind, and Spirit*; by Laurinda M. Poirier and Katharine M. Coburn. 2nd edition. American diabetes Assn., 2000, 230 pages, and (7) *The John Hopkins Guide to Diabetes: for Today and Tomorrow*; [by] Christopher D. Saudek, Richard R. Rubin, and Cynthia S. Shump. John Hopkins Univ. Press. 1997, 422 pages. See *Public Library Catalog 12th Edition: Guide to Reference Books and Adult Nonfiction*. Edited by Juliette Yaakov. The H.W. Wison Company. 2004.

SUPERMASSIVE BLACK HOLES & THE DCCT

[68] See http://chandra.harvard.edu/xray_sources/blackholes_stellar.html. Retrieved on 1/19/09.

[69] See *Ibid.*

[70] See *Ibid.*

[71] See *Ibid.*

[72] See *Ibid.*

[73] See *Ibid.*

[74] See *Ibid.*

[75] See *Ibid.*

[76] See *Ibid.*

[77] See *Ibid.*

[78] Ferguson, Kitty. *Prisons of light: Black Holes.* NY: Cambridge University Press, 1996, page 15.

[79] See http://chandra.harvard.edu/xray_sources/blackholes_sm.html. Retrieved on 1/19/09.

[80] See *Ibid.*

[81] See *Ibid.*

[82] For a good, authorized biography of Stephen Hawking, see *Stephen Hawking: Quest for a Theory of the Universe,* by Kitty Ferguson (New York: Franklin Watts, 1991). Kitty Ferguson is a remarkable person, receiving both a bachelor's and master's from the Julliard School. For many years she was a successful professional musician, conducting and performing oratorio, early music and chamber music, before renewing her lifelong interest in physics and cosmology by auditing graduate lectures and seminars at the Department of Applied Mathematics and Theoretical Physics at Cambridge University.

[83] See "General Treatment of Diabetes," D. A. Pyke, *Br Med J.* 1970 Aug 1;3(5717):269. Available online at http://www.ncbi.nlm.nih.gov/pubmed/5448803. Retrieved on 3/7/09.

[84] Singh, Inder. "Low-Fat Diet and Therapeutic Doses of Insulin in Diabetes Mellitus." *Lancet,* 1955, Feb 26; 268(6861): p. 422.

[85] *Ibid,* p. 423.

[86] Kinsell, L.W. "The Diabetic Diet." In: *Diabetes Mellitus: Diagnosis and Treatment,* edited by G.J. Hamwi and T.S. Danowski. New York, American Diabetic Association, 1967, vol. II, pp. 97-99. See also Pyke, D.A. General Treatment of Diabetes. *Brit. Med. J.* 3: 268, 1970.

[87] Bierman, E.L., M.J. Albrink, R.A. Arky, W.E. Conner, et al. "Special Report. Principles of Nutrition and Dietary Recommendations for Patients with Diabetes Mellitus." *Diabetes.* 20: 633, 1971.

[88] Singh, Inder. "Low-Fat Diet and Therapeutic Doses of Insulin in Diabetes Mellitus." *Lancet.* 1955, Feb 26; 268(6861): p. 422. Anderson, J.W. "Influence of High Carbohydrate Diets on Glucose Tolerance of Normal and Diabetic Men." *Proc. Int. Sugar Res.* Symposium. Washington, D.C., March, 1974. Kempner, W., R.L. Peschel and C. Schlayer. "Effect of Rice Diet on Diabetes Mellitus Associated with Vascular Disease." *Postgrad. Med.* 24: 359, 1958. Brunzell. J.D., R.L. Lerner, W.R. Hazzard, D. Porte, Jr., et al.

Notes

"Improved Glucose Tolerance with High Carbohydrate Feeding in Mild Diabetes." *N. Engl. J. Med.* 284: 521, 1971. Brunzell, J.D., R.L. Lerner, D. Porte, Jr., and E.L. Bierman. "Effect of a Fat Free, High Carbohydrate Diet on Diabetic Subjects with Fasting hyperglycemia. *Diabetes.* 23: 138, 1974.

[89] Tae G. Kiehm, M.D., James W. Anderson, M.D., and Kyleen Ward, R.D. "Beneficial Effects of a High Carbohydrate, High Fiber Diet on Hyperglycemic Diabetic Men," *Am. J. Clin. Nutr.* 29: 1976, p. 895.

[90] *Ibid.*

[91] See "High-carbohydrate diets and insulin-dependent diabetics," by R W Simpson, J I Mann, J Eaton, R D Carter, and T D Hockaday, *Br Med J.* 1979 September 1; 2(6189): 523–525. Available online at http://www.pubmedcentral.nih.gov/pagerender.fcgi?artid=1596170&pageindex=1#page. Retrieved on 5/3/09.

[92] In a randomised cross-over study 18 nondependent (NIDDM) and 9 insulin-dependent (IDDM) diabetics were put on to a high carbohydrate diet containing leguminous fibre (HL) for 6 weeks, and also a standard low carbohydrate diet (LC) for 6 weeks. During two identical 24 hour metabolic profiles mean preprandial and mean 2 hour postprandial blood glucoses were significantly lower on HL in both groups, as were also several overall measures of diabetic control, including the degree of glycosuria. Total cholesterol was reduced significantly on HL in both groups, and the HDL/LDL cholesterol ratio increased significantly on HL in the NIDDM group.

See "A high carbohydrate leguminous fibre diet improves all aspects of diabetic control," by Simpson HC, Simpson RW, Lousley S, Carter RD, Geekie M, Hockaday TD, and Mann JI. *Lancet.* 1981 Jan 3;1(8210):1-5. Available online at http://www.ncbi.nlm.nih.gov/pubmed/6109047. Retrieved on 5/3/09.

[93] This study investigated the possible beneficial effects of the digestible carbohydrate component. A diet rich in carbohydrate was compared with a traditional low carbohydrate diet in 10 Type 2 (non-insulin-dependent) diabetic patients, using a crossover design; both diets contained < 20 g dietary fibre/day. During 24-h metabolic profiles carried out after 4 weeks on each diet, the mean basal plasma glucose (mean of 03.00, 05.00 and 07.00 h values) was 5.3 mmol/l on the high carbohydrate diet and 5.9 mmol/l on the low carbohydrate diet (p < 0.05), despite the 2-h postprandial glucose (mean of three main meals) being higher on the high carbohydrate diet than on the low carbohydrate diet (8.7 versus 7.3 mmol/1, p < 0.01). Overall diabetic control was the same throughout the study, as judged by a mean 24-h plasma glucose of 6.7 mmol/1 on the high carbohydrate and 6.6 mmol/1 on the low carbohydrate diet, and haemoglobin Alc percentage of 8.3 on both diets. Mean cholesterol was 4.55 mmol/1 on both diets and fasting plasma triglyceride was 2.83 mmol/1 on the high carbohydrate and 2.55 mmol/1 on the low carbohydrate diet (p = NS).

See "Digestible Carbohydrate—an Independent Effect on Diabetic Control in Type 2 (Non-Insulin-Dependent) Diabetic Patients?" by H. C. R. Simpson, R. D. Carter, S. Lousley, and J. I. Mann. *Diabetologia* (1982) 23:235-239. Available online at http://www.springerlink.com/content/x272687026872634/fulltext.pdf. Retrieved on 5/3/09.

[94] "What carbohydrate foods should diabetics eat?" by J I Mann. *Br Med J* (Clin Res Ed). 1984 April 7; 288(6423): 1025. Available online at http://www.pubmedcentral.nih.gov/pagerender.fcgi?artid=1442616&pageindex=1#page. Retrieved on 5/3/09.

[95] *Ibid.*

[96] *Ibid.*

[97] See Ravnskov, Uffe. *Fat and Cholesterol are Good for You! What Really Causes Heart Disease,* Sweden: GB Publishing, 2009, page 76.

⁹⁸ Taubes, Gary. *Good Calories, Bad Calories*. First Anchor Books Edition. New York: Anchor Books, 2008, page 395.

⁹⁹ *Ibid*, pages 395-396.

¹⁰⁰ This tale is adapted from the Wikipedia article entitled "Thrifty Gene hypothesis," available online at http://en.wikipedia.org/wiki/Thrifty_gene_hypothesis. Retrieved on 3/8/09.

¹⁰¹ Neel JV (1962). "Diabetes mellitus: a "thrifty" genotype rendered detrimental by "progress"?" *Am. J. Hum. Genet.* 14: 360. PMID 13937884. Available online at http://www.ncbi.nlm.nih.gov/pubmed/13937884. Retrieved on 3/8/09.

¹⁰² *Ibid*, p.359

¹⁰³ *Ibid*, p.355

¹⁰⁴ *Ibid*, p.353

¹⁰⁵ Neel, J.V. 1982. "The Thrifty Genotype Revisited." In: *The Genetics of Diabetes Mellitus*, ed. J. Kobberling and R. Tattersall. New York: Academic Press, 293-93.

¹⁰⁶ Speilman, R.S., S.S. Fajans, J.V. Neel, S. Pek, J.C. Floyd, and W.J. Oliver. 1982. "Glucose Tolerance in Two Unacculturated Indian Tribes of Brazil." *Diabetologia*. Aug.;23(2):90-93.

¹⁰⁷ Neel, J.V. 1989. "Update to 'The Study of Natural Selection in Primitive and Civilized Human Populations.'" *Human Biology*. Oct.-Dec.;61(5-6):811-23.

¹⁰⁸ Neel, J.V. 1999. "The 'Thrifty Genotype' in 1998." *Nutrition Reviews* May; 57(5, pt.2):S2-9.

¹⁰⁹ Speakman JR (2007). "A nonadaptive scenario explaining the genetic predisposition to obesity: the "predation release" hypothesis." *Cell Metab.* 6 (1): 5–12; doi: 10.1016/j.cmet.2007.06.004. PMID 17618852. Available online at http://www.ncbi.nlm.nih.gov/pubmed/17618852. Retrieved on 3/8/09.

¹¹⁰ Baschetti R (1998). "Diabetes epidemic in newly westernized populations: is it due to thrifty genes or to genetically unknown foods?" *J R Soc Med*. 91 (12): 622–625. See also Lee, R.B. 1968. "What Hunters Do for a Living, or, How to Make Out on Scarce Resources." In: Lee and Devores, eds. 1968.

¹¹¹ Speakman JR (2007). "A nonadaptive scenario explaining the genetic predisposition to obesity: the "predation release" hypothesis." *Cell Metab.* 6 (1): 5–12; doi: 10.1016/j.cmet.2007.06.004. PMID 17618852. Available online at http://www.ncbi.nlm.nih.gov/pubmed/17618852. Retrieved on 3/8/09.

¹¹² Taubes, Gary. *Good Calories, Bad Calories*. First Anchor Books Edition. New York: Anchor Books, 2008, page 456.

¹¹³ Reprinted with permission from the National Academies Press, Copyright 2005, National Academy of Sciences, "Dietary Carbohydrates: Sugars and Starches," in *Dietary Reference Intakes for Energy, Carbohydrate, Fiber, Fat, Fatty Acids, Cholesterol, Protein, and Amino Acids (Macronutrients) (2005)*. Food and Nutrition Board, 2005, pages 275-279. License number 2241560984249. Available online at http://www.nap.edu/catalog.php?record_id=10490. Retrieved on 3/7/09. Established in 1970 under the charter of the National Academy of Sciences, the Institute of Medicine (http://www.iom.edu/) provides independent, objective, evidence-based advice to policymakers, health professionals, the private sector, and the public. The mission of the Institute of Medicine embraces the health of people everywhere.

¹¹⁴ Taubes, Gary. *Good Calories, Bad Calories*. First Anchor Books Edition. New York: Anchor Books, 2008, page 456.

Notes

[115] *Family Medicine Principles & Practice, Fifth Edition.* Editor: Robert B. Taylor. Springer-Verlag, 1998, page 1067.

[116] *Rudolph's Pediatrics 21st Edition.* Edited by Colin D. Rudolph, Abraham M. Rudolph, Margaret K. Hostetter, George Lister, Norman J. Siegel. McGraw-Hill, Medical Publishing Division, 2003, page 2123.

[117] *Cecil Textbook of Medicine 22nd Edition.* Edited by Lee Goldman, MD, and Dennis Ausiello, MD. Saunders, an imprint of Elsevier, 2004, pages 1432-1433.

[118] *Harrison's Principles of Internal Medicine, 17th Edition.* Edited by Anthony S. Fauci, MD, et al. McGraw-Hill Medical, 2008, page 2286.

[119] *Williams Textbook of Endocrinology, Tenth Edition.* P. Reed Larsen, MD, FACP, FRCP, Henry M. Kronenber, MD, Shlomo Melmed, MD, and Kenneth S. Polansky, MD. Saunders, an imprint of Elsevier, 2003, page 1496.

[120] *International Textbook of Diabetes Mellitus.* Editors-in-chief: R.A. Defronzo, E. Ferrannini, H. Keen, and P. Zimmet. John Wiley & Sons, Ltd., 2004, page 1067.

[121] *Joslin's Diabetes Mellitus.* Edited by C. Ronald Kahn, Gordon C. Weir, George L. King, Alan M. Jacobson, Alan C. Moses, Robert J. Smith. Lippincott Williams & Wilkin & The Joslin Diabetes Center. Page 2.

[122] *Lange 2009 Current Medical Diagnosis & Treatment.* Edited by Stephen J. McPhee, MD, Maxine A. Papadakis, MD, and Lawrence M. Tierney, Jr., MD, Senior Editor. McGraw-Hill Medical, 2009, pages 1059-1060.

[123] See the Biostatistics Center of the George Washington University website, available online at http://www.bsc.gwu.edu/bsc/studies/dcct.html. Retrieved on 1/19/09.

[124] See *Ibid.*

[125] The DCCT Research Group (1993). The effect of intensive treatment of diabetes on the development and progression of long-term complications in insulin-dependent diabetes mellitus. *The New England Journal of Medicine* 329: 977-986.

[126] The DCCT Research Group (1995). Adverse events and their association with treatment regimens in the Diabetes Control and Complications Trial. *Diabetes Care* 18: 1415-1427.

[127] The DCCT Research Group (1995). The relationship of glycemic exposure (HbA1c) to the risk of development and progression of retinopathy in the Diabetes Control and Complications Trial. *Diabetes* 44: 968-983. See also The DCCT Research Group (1996). The absence of a glycemic threshold for the development of long-term complication: the perspective of the Diabetes Control and Complications Trial. *Diabetes* 45: 1289-1298.

[128] The DCCT Research Group (1997). Hypoglycemia in the Diabetes Control and Complications Trial. *Diabetes* 45: 271-286.

[129] See the Biostatistics Center of the George Washington University website, available online at http://www.bsc.gwu.edu/bsc/studies/dcct.html. Retrieved on 1/19/09.

[130] See *Ibid.*

[131] Diabetes Control and Complications Trial (DCCT). *N Engl J Med* 1993;329:977-986.

[132] "The Diabetes Control and Complications Trial (DCCT) Design and Methodologic Considerations for the Feasibility Phase," *Diabetes* 1986; 35:534.

[133] *Ibid.*

[134] The DCCT was supported under cooperative agreements and a research contract with the Division of Diabetes, Endocrinology, and Metabolic Diseases of the National Institute of Diabetes and Digestive and Kidney Diseases and by the National Heart, Lung, and Blood Institute, the National Eye Institute, the National Center for Research Resources, and various corporate sponsors listed in *Diabetes Care* 1987;10:1-19). In addition, the Epidemiology of Diabetes Intervention and Complications (EDIC) ongoing funding was $58 million. See the National Institutes of Health Fact Sheet online at http://www.aimbe.org/assets/84_nihresearchintowhatworksb.pdf. Retrieved on 4/11/09.

[135] For a particularly enlightening article explaining how claimed research findings may often be simply accurate measures of the prevailing bias, see Ioannidis JPA (2005) Why Most Published Research Findings Are False. PLoS Med 2(8): e124; doi: 10.1371/journal.pmed.0020124. Available online at http://medicine.plosjournals.org/perlserv/?request=get-document&doi=10.1371/journal.pmed.0020124. Retrieved on 3/24/09.

[136] For a good discussion of all the different types of cognitive bias, see the Wikipedia article "List of Cognitive Biases" online at http://en.wikipedia.org/wiki/List_of_cognitive_biases. Retrieved on 3/22/09.

[137] McCullough DK, Mitchell RD, Ambler J, et al. A prospective comparison of "conventional" and high-carbohydrate/high-fibre/low-fat diets in adults with type 1 diabetes. *Diabetologia* 1985;28:208-212.

[138] Gutierrez M, Akhavan M, et al. Utility of a short-term 25% carbohydrate diet on improving glycemic control in type II diabetes mellitus. *J Am Coll Nutr* 1998;17:595-600.

[139] Hays JH, et al. Abstract presented at the 81st Annual Meeting of the Endocrine Society, 1999.

[140] O'Neill DF, Westman EC, Bernstein RK. The effects of a low-carbohydrate regimen on glycemic control and serum lipids in diabetes mellitus. *Metabolic Syndrome and Related Disorders*. Volume 1, number 4, 2003, p. 291-298.

[141] See Osler W, McCrae T. *The Principle and Practice of Medicine.* New York: D. Appleton and Company, 1923. *Op Cit.* O'Neill (2003).

[142] See "Dietary carbohydrate restriction in type 2 diabetes mellitus and metabolic syndrome: time for a critical appraisal," by Anthony Accurso, Richard K Bernstein, Annika Dahlqvist, Boris Draznin, Richard D Feinman, Eugene J Fine, Amy Gleed, David B Jacobs, Gabriel Larson, Robert H Lustig, Anssi H Manninen, Samy I McFarlane, Katharine Morrison, Jørgen Vesti Nielsen, Uffe Ravnskov, Karl S Roth, Ricardo Silvestre, James R Sowers, Ralf Sundberg,, Jeff S Volek, Eric C Westman, Richard J Wood, Jay Wortman, and Mary C Vernon. *Nutrition & Metabolism* 2008, 5:9; doi: 10.1186/1743-7075-5-9. Available online at http://www.nutritionandmetabolism.com/content/5/1/9#B29. Retrieved on 5/8/09.

For another good review of low-carbohydrate diets in the treatment of diabetes, as reprinted in my previous book *Thrive With Diabetes*, see Surender K Arora and Samy I McFarlane. "The Case for Low Carbohydrate Diets in Diabetes Management." *Nutr Metab* (Lond). 2005; 2: 16. Published online July 14, 2005; doi: 10.1186/1743-7075-2-16. Available online at http://www.pubmedcentral.nih.gov/articlerender.fcgi?tool=pmcentrez&artid=1188071. Retrieved on 3/14/08.

[143] See "Dietary carbohydrate restriction in type 2 diabetes mellitus and metabolic syndrome: time for a critical appraisal," by Anthony Accurso, Richard K Bernstein, Annika Dahlqvist, Boris Draznin, Richard D Feinman, Eugene J Fine, Amy Gleed, David B Jacobs, Gabriel Larson, Robert H Lustig, Anssi H Manninen, Samy I McFarlane, Katharine Morrison, Jørgen Vesti Nielsen, Uffe Ravnskov, Karl S Roth, Ricardo Silvestre, James R Sowers, Ralf Sundberg, Jeff S Volek, Eric C Westman, Richard J Wood, Jay Wortman, and Mary C Vernon. *Nutrition & Metabolism* 2008, 5:9; doi: 10.1186/1743-7075-5-9. Available online at http://www.nutritionandmetabolism.com/content/5/1/9#B29. Retrieved on 5/8/09.

[144] For a good, brief history detailing three other possible attributions of the word "meme" see "A Note on the Origin of 'Memes'/'Mnemes,'" by John Laurent, School of Science, Griffith University, available online at http://cfpm.org/jom-emit/1999/vol3/laurent_j.html. Retrieved on 4/9/09.

For a comprehensive list of Mimetics publications on the web including those of Susan Blackmore, Richard Dawkins, Daniel Dennett, Liane Gabora, Derek Gatherer, Francis Heylighen, Aaron Lynch, and Paul Marsden, et al., compiled by Dave Gross, see http://users.lycaeum.org/~sputnik/Memetics/. Retrieved on 4/9/09.

For a compelling short video replete with written transcript, see "Dan Dennett on Dangerous Memes," on TED.com, recorded February, 2002, in Monterey, CA, (video duration: 15:39), online at http://blog.ted.com/2007/07/dan_dennett_on_2.php. Retrieved on 4/9/09.

See also Dennett, Daniel C. *Darwin's Dangerous Idea: Evolution and the Meanings of Life*. New York: Simon & Schuster Paperbacks, 1995,

For further resources, see also the Wikipedia article "Meme" online at http://en.wikipedia.org/wiki/Meme. Retrieved on 4/9/09.

[145] Pinker, Steven. *How the Mind Works*. New York: W.W. Norton & Company, 1997, page 208.

[146] Dawkins, Richard. *The Selfish Gene*. New York: Oxford University Press, 30th Anniversary Edition, 2006, page 192.

[147] Pinker, Steven. *How the Mind Works*. New York: W.W. Norton & Company, 1997, page 208.

THE WAY THINGS OUGHT TO BE (PART I)

[148] Bronowski, J. *The Ascent of Man*. Boston, MA: Little, Brown and Company, 1973, pages 44-45.

[149] Tel (alternate spelling: tell) meaning "hill" or "mound," is a type of archaeological site in the form of an earthen mound that results from the accumulation and subsequent erosion of material deposited by long human occupation. A tell mostly consists of architectural building materials containing a high proportion of stone, mudbrick, or loam as well as, to a minor extent, domestic refuse. The distribution of this phenomenon spans from the Indus valley in the east to Central Europe in the west. There are about 50,000 visible tells in the Middle East, a testament to the long settlement of the area. Definition from the article "Tell" on Wikipedia online at http://en.wikipedia.org/wiki/Tell. Retrieved on 4/4/09.

[150] Bronowski, J. *The Ascent of Man*. Boston, MA: Little, Brown and Company, 1973, pages 64-68.

[151] *Ibid*, page 69.

[152] Jacob Bronowski (18 January 1908 – 22 August 1974) was a British mathematician and biologist of Polish-Jewish origin. He is best remembered as the presenter and writer of the 1973 BBC television documentary series, *The Ascent of Man*.

Jacob Bronowski was born in Łódź, Congress Poland, Russian Empire in 1908. His family moved to Germany during the First World War, and then to England in 1920. Although, according to Bronowski, he knew only two English words on arriving in Great Britain, he gained admission to the Central Foundation Boys' School in London and went on to study at the University of Cambridge.

As a mathematics student at Jesus College, Cambridge, Bronowski co-edited—with William Empson—the literary periodical *Experiment*, which first appeared in 1928. Bronowski would pursue this sort of dual activity, in both the mathematical and literary worlds, throughout his professional life. He was also a strong chess player, earning a half-blue while at Cambridge and composing numerous chess problems for the British Chess Magazine between 1926 and 1970. He received a Ph.D. in mathematics in 1935, writing a dissertation in algebraic geometry. From 1934 to 1942 he taught mathematics at the University College of Hull. For a time in the 1930s he lived near Laura Riding and Robert Graves in Majorca.

During the Second World War Bronowski worked in operations research, and afterward became Director of Research for the National Coal Board in the UK. Following his experiences as an official observer of the after-effects of the Nagasaki and Hiroshima bombings, he turned to biology, as did his friend Leo Szilard, to better understand the nature of violence. Bronowski was an associate director of the Salk Institute from 1964.

Jacob Bronowski married Rita Coblentz in 1941. The couple had four children, all daughters, the eldest being the British academic Lisa Jardine and another being the filmmaker Judith Bronowski.

In 1967 Bronowski delivered the six Silliman Foundation lectures at Yale University and chose as his subject the role of imagination and symbolic language in the progress of scientific knowledge. Transcripts of the lectures were published posthumously in 1978 as *The Origins of Knowledge* and *Imagination* and remain in print.

He first became familiar to the British public through appearances on the BBC television version of *The Brains Trust* in the late 1950s, but is better known for his thirteen part series *The Ascent of Man* (1973). This was an inspiration for Carl Sagan to make *Cosmos* in 1980. During the making of *The Ascent of Man*, Bronowski was interviewed by Michael Parkinson, and Bronowski's description of a visit to Auschwitz — he had lost many family members during the Nazi era — was described by Parkinson as one of his most memorable interviews.

Jacob Bronowski died in 1974 of a heart attack in East Hampton, New York a year after *The Ascent of Man* was completed, and was buried in the western side of London's Highgate Cemetery, near the entrance. The seventeen books he wrote are: *The Poet's Defence* (1939), *William Blake: A Man Without a Mask* (1943), *The Common Sense of Science* (1951), *The Face of Violence* (1954), *Science and Human Values* (1956), *William Blake: The Penguin Poets Series* (1958), *The Western Intellectual Tradition, From Leonardo to Hegel* (1960) - with Bruce Mazlish, *Biography of an Atom* (1963) - with Millicent Selsam, *Insight* (1964), *The Identity of Man* (1965), *Nature and Knowledge: The Philosophy of Contemporary Science* (1969), *William Blake and the Age of Revolution* (1972), *The Ascent of Man* (1974), *A Sense of the Future* (1977), *Magic Science & Civilization* (1978), *The Origins of Knowledge and Imagination* (1978), and *The Visionary Eye: Essays in the Arts, Literature and Science* (1979) - edited by Piero Ariotti and Rita Bronowski.

Biography courtesy of the article "Jacob Bronowski" from Wikipedia, available online at http://en.wikipedia.org/wiki/Jacob_Bronowski. Retrieved on 4/4/09.

[153] Chalem, Laurence D. *Thrive With Diabetes: Lead an Optimistic, Fun, Challenging, Fit, Tenacious, Enlightened, Innovative & Heroic Life*. South Carolina: BookSurge Publishing, 2008, p. 68.

[154] Barrow, John D. *New Theories of Everything: The Quest for Ultimate Explanation*. New York: Oxford University Press Inc., 2007, pages 10-13; 231-232; 243-244. Used by permission of Oxford University Press.

[155] *Ibid*, page 213.

[156] *Ibid*, page 231.

[157] See the page "Interactive Personalized Metabolic Management" on the Proactive Metabolics Co. website at http://www.mangesius.com/Technology/ipmm.html. Retrieved on 3/2/08. See also Horm Metab Res Suppl. 1990;24:10-9. A model-based system for the individual prediction of metabolic responses to improve therapy in type I diabetes. Salzsieder E, Fischer U, Stoewhas H, Thierbach U, Rutscher A, Menzel R, Albrecht G. Central Institute of Diabetes Gerhard Katsch, Karlsburg, German Democratic Republic. As stated, there are many, many mathematical models of the Glucose-Insulin system. For summaries of the literature and individual articles, the reader is referred to the following sources: A critical review of

mathematical models and data used in diabetology, A Boutayeb and A Chetouani, Department of Mathematics Faculty of Sciences, Oujda, Morocco. *BioMedical Engineering Online* 2006, 5:43; doi: 10.1186/1475-925X-5-43. Available online at: http://www.biomedical-engineering-online.com/content/5/1/43. Retrieved on 1/10/08. See also http://math.la.asu.edu/~kuang/paper/lkm.pdf. Retrieved on 1/10/08. See also Berger M, Rodbard D (1989): Computer Simulation of Plasma Insulin and Glucose Dynamics After Subcutaneous Insulin Injection. *Diabetes Care* 12(10), 725-736. See also Pacini G (1994): Mathematical Models of Insulin Secretion in Physiological and Clinical Investigations. *Computer Methods and Programs in Biomedicine* 41, 269-285. See also Rutscher A, Salszieder E, Fischer U, Freyse E-J (1994): KADIS: Model-Aided Education in Type I Diabetes. *Computer Methods and Programs in Biomedicine* 41, 205-215. See also Salszieder E, Albrecht G, Fischer U, Freyse E-J (1995): Kinetic Modeling of the Glucoregulatory System to Improve Insulin Therapy. *IEEE Transactions on Biomedical Engineering.* BME-32, 846-855. For a particularly good web-based mathematical model and free computer-based model of the body-wide glucose-insulin system, see A Web-Based Educational Simulation Package for Glucose-Insulin Levels in the Human Body, subtitled GlucoSim: Process Modeling, Monitoring, and Control Research, by the Illinois Institute of Technology, available online at http://216.47.139.196/glucosim/gsimul.html. Retrieved on 1/10/08.

[158] For a good discussion of insulin resistance, see Taubes, Gary. *Good Calories, Bad Calories.* First Anchor Books Edition. New York: Anchor Books, 2008, pages 180-183 and 395-397.

[159] Insulin glargine, marketed by Sanofi-Aventis under the name Lantus®, is a long-acting basal insulin analogue, given once daily to help control the blood sugar level of those with diabetes. Its advantage is that it has a duration of action of 24 hours, with no pronounced peak. Thus, it more closely resembles the basal insulin secretion of the normal pancreatic beta cells. See http://www.lantus.com/hcp/default.aspx. Retrieved on 6/23/09.

The same can be said for Insulin detemir, a long-acting human insulin analogue for maintaining the basal level of insulin. Novo Nordisk markets Insulin detemir under the trade name Levemir®. See http://www.levemir-us.com/. Retrieved on 6/30/09.

Lantus is produced by E. coli bacteria; Levemir is produced by baker's yeast. See "Lantus and Levemir: What's the Difference?" by Linda von Wartburg, Jul 17, 2007. Available online at http://www.diabeteshealth.com/read/2007/07/17/5316/lantus-and-levemir--whats-the-difference/. Retrieved on 6/30/09.

For a comparison of Levemir & Lantus, see the article entitled "Lantus vs. Levemir Summary November 2006," at the Iowa Medicaid Enterprise website online at http://www.iowamedicaidpdl.com/uploads/nm/eM/nmeM9o6uTen5x1JSJyV2wg/Insulin-glargine-vs-Insulin-Detemir_-Nov-2006.pdf. Retrieved on 6/30/09.

"In the two clinical trials comparing Lantus and Levemir, the majority of patients with either type 1 or type 2 diabetes required twice daily administration of Levemir to achieve comparable A1C reductions to once daily administration of Lantus.

To achieve glycemic control comparable to Lantus, the dose of Levemir required appears to be greater especially in patients with type 2 diabetes. Caution should be exercised when converting from 1 basal insulin to the other.

Levemir had a lower risk of nocturnal hypoglycemia in patients with type 1 diabetes compared to Lantus; however, in patients with type 2 diabetes both basal insulins had similar risk of nocturnal, minor, and major hypoglycemia. Weight gain was observed with both basal insulins however, in patients receiving Levemir twice daily the difference in weight between the Levemir and Lantus treatment arms was not significant."

See also D.R. Owens, G.B. Bolli. Diabetes Technology & Therapeutics. October 2008, 10(5): 333-349; doi: 10.1089/dia.2008.0023. Available online at http://www.liebertonline.com/doi/abs/10.1089/dia.2008.0023?cookieSet=1&journalCode=dia. Retrieved on 6/30/09.

"The new rDNA and DNA-derived "basal" insulin analogs, glargine and detemir, represent significant advancement in the treatment of diabetes compared with conventional NPH insulin. This review describes blood glucose homeostasis by insulin in people without diabetes and outlines the physiological application of exogenous insulin in patients with type 1 and type 2 diabetes."

In mid-2009, the European Association for the Study of Diabetes (EASD) made an urgent call for more research into a possible link between use of insulin glargine and increased risk of cancer, following evidence from studies in Germany, Sweden and Scotland. The studies are reported in *Diabetologia* (the journal of EASD). See http://www.diabetologia-journal.org/cancer.html#press. Retrieved on 6/30/09.

"The concerns about a possible link between use of Lantus insulin and increased cancer risk were raised by a German study of around 127,000 insulin-treated patients in an insurance database. The research identified a statistically significant link between patients who had used Lantus insulin and those who had been diagnosed with cancer. Compared with people using similar doses of human insulin, out of every 100 people who used Lantus insulin over an average of about one-and-a-half years, one additional person was diagnosed with cancer. Of particular note in this study was the finding that the increased risk of cancer was dose-dependent. Thus for patients given a dose of 10U, Lantus insulin alone increased the risk of cancer by 9% compared with human insulin; but for a dose of 50U, the increased risk was 31%. The study did not consider insulin detemir (Levemir), an insulin analogue whose action is prolonged by a different principle from Lantus.

Professor Edwin Gale, Editor of Diabetologia, and Professor Ulf Smith, President of EASD, realised the significance of these findings but wanted them replicated in other studies from other European countries before announcing them formally. Studies were thus carried out using databases from Sweden, Scotland, and the UK. The Swedish study found that compared with patients on insulins other than Lantus insulin, patients on lantus insulin alone had double the risk of breast cancer. The Scottish study found a non-significant increased risk for breast cancer specifically. The UK study found no link between insulin glargine and cancer.

Prof Gale and Prof Smith emphasize the limitations to the studies. The main one is that, although the data were adjusted for a number of variables, the characteristics of the groups of patients taking lantus insulin alone (generally older, higher blood pressure, more overweight) were different to those on other forms of insulin. Thus any difference in cancer risk could be attributed to the pre-treatment characteristics of the groups, rather than the treatment itself. Also, the numbers of cases of breast cancer in the Swedish and Scottish studies were very small, meaning the findings could have occurred due to chance. They state categorically that Lantus and other insulins do not cause cancer, but these studies expose the possibility that Lantus insulin could cause existing cancer cells to grow and divide more rapidly-which might explain why more cancers came to be diagnosed over 1-3 years of observation. They say: "We believe people are entitled to know that use of Lantus insulin might be associated with greater risk, but this must also be balanced against the possibility that we might be causing unnecessary alarm by raising these concerns."

[160] "Frequent light exercise" is the ideal, as deduced in my previous book. See Chalem, Laurence. *Thrive with Diabetes: Lead an Optimistic, Fun, Challenging, Fit, Tenacious, Enlightened, Innovative & Heroic Life*. South Carolina: BookSurge, 2008, Part III.

[161] In one sample, sleep duration and quality were significant predictors of HbA$_{1c}$. Combined with existing evidence linking sleep loss to increased diabetes risk, these data suggest that optimizing sleep duration and quality should be tested as an intervention to improve glucose control in patients with Type 2 diabetes. See *Arch Intern Med*. 2006;166:1768-1774. Available online at http://archinte.ama-assn.org/cgi/reprint/166/16/1768.pdf. Retrieved 3/1/08. The article references eleven other studies.

[162] According to the National Diabetes Information Clearinghouse (NDIC) normal fasting blood sugar range is 70-110 mg/dL, see http://diabetes.niddk.nih.gov/dm/pubs/hypoglycemia/. The American Diabetes Association states a normal fating blood sugar range for diabetics is 70-130 mg/dL, see

http://diabetes.org/type-1-diabetes/blood-glucose-checks.jsp; the Joslin Diabetes Center states that the normal blood sugar range for non-diabetics should be less than 110 mg/dL, and the goal for diabetics should be between 90-130 mg/dL, see http://www.joslin.org/Beginners_guide_523.asp; the National Diabetes Education Program states that blood sugar ranges before meals should be between 90-130 mg/dL, see http://www.ndep.nih.gov/diabetes/control/4Steps.htm#Step1; on page 13 of "Definition and Diagnosis of Diabetes Mellitus and Intermediate Hyperglycemia," a Report of a WHO/IDF Consultation, the World Health Organization stated "One approach to addressing the issue of defining categories of intermediate hyperglycemia is to define normal glucose tolerance. However, this seemingly simple question is difficult to answer. Each of the ADA publications on the diagnostic criteria for diabetics has defined normal plasma glucose levels. The 2003 ADA statement defined a normal fasting plasma glucose as less than 5.6 mmol/l (approx. less than 101 mg/dL). See http://www.who.int/diabetes/publications/Definition%20and%20diagnosis%20of%20diabetes_new.pdf. See also http://www.who.int/diabetes/en/index.html. Retrieved on 3/22/08.

163 There was much research done even before the late 1960s regarding fat, serum cholesterol, and diet as it related to atherosclerosis. In "Dietary Fat, Heart Attacks, and Strokes," the committee stated "...It should be borne in mind that moderate amounts of fat, particularly those containing an appreciable quantity of the poly-unsaturated type, are necessary for good health. Fat is an economical, and in limited amounts, a wholesome food. Food faddism of any sort should be avoided and significant changes in diet should not be undertaken without medical advice." The statement by the committee concluded with "More complete information must be obtained before final conclusions can be reached. See "Dietary Fat and Its Relation to Heart Attacks and Strokes," by The Central Committee for Medical and Community Program of the American Heart Association, Ad Hoc Committee on Dietary Fat and Atherosclerosis, Irvine H. Page, Edgar V. Allen, Francis L. Chamberlain, Ancel Keys, Jeremiah Stamler and Frederick J. Stare. *Circulation.* 1961;23;133-136. Available online at http://circ.ahajournals.org/cgi/reprint/23/1/133?maxtoshow=&HITS=10&hits=10&RESULTFORMAT= &fulltext=ancel+keyes&searchid=1&FIRSTINDEX=20&resourcetype=HWCIT. Retrieved on 3/2/08. All of the articles used as reference were from the 1950s.

164 See "The Soft Science of Dietary Fat" by Gary Taubes. Available online by the National Association of Science Writers at http://www.nasw.org/awards/2001/01Taubesarticle1.htm. Retrieved on 3/2/08. You are encouraged to see also *"What if It's All Been a Big Fat Lie,"* by Gary Taubes, published on July 8, 2002 in FrontPage Magazine. Available online at http://www.frontpagemag.com/Articles/Printable.aspx?GUID={367127E3-4395-4DB8-90E0-AC52B2D86AF4}. Retrieved on 3/18/08.

Gary Taubes (born April 30, 1956) is an American science writer. He is the author of *Nobel Dreams* (1987), *Bad Science: the Short Life and Weird Times of Cold Fusion* (1993), and *Good Calories, Bad Calories* (2007). He has won the *Science In Society Award* of the National Association of Science Writers three times and was awarded a MIT Knight Science Journalism Fellowship for 1996-97.

Born in Rochester, New York, Taubes studied applied physics at Harvard and aerospace engineering at Stanford (MS, 1978). After receiving a master's degree in journalism at Columbia University in 1981, Taubes joined Discover magazine as a staff reporter in 1982. Since then he has written numerous articles for Discover, Science and other magazines. Originally focusing on physics issues, his interests have more recently turned to medicine and nutrition. Taubes' books have all dealt with scientific controversies. *Nobel Dreams* takes a critical look at the politics and experimental techniques behind the Nobel Prize-winning work of physicist Carlo Rubbia. *Bad Science* is a chronicle of the short-lived media frenzy surrounding the Pons-Fleischmann cold fusion experiments of 1989. Taubes gained prominence in the low-carb diet debate following the publication of his 2002 New York Times Magazine piece, *What if It's All Been a Big Fat Lie?*

The article questioned the efficacy and health benefits of low-fat diets and was seen as defending the Atkins diet against the medical establishment. In 2007, he published his book *Good Calories, Bad Calories: Challenging the Conventional Wisdom on Diet, Weight Control, and Disease,* ISBN 978-1400040780, which aims at examining how a hypothesis got to become dogma and claims to show how the scientific method was circumvented so one man's hypothesis could be claimed as correct. The book uses data and studies compiled from dietary research from as early as the 1800's. Taubes includes information and studies which indicate that physical exercise increases appetite to a degree that makes it an inefficient tool in weight loss. He tracks the origins of commonly accepted dietary advice and aims to show that information that is filtered to the public often contradicts scientific evidence. On October 19, 2007, Taubes appeared on Larry King Live to discuss his book. Although Taubes has no formal training in nutrition or medicine, his book was praised as "raising interesting and valuable points" by Dr. Andrew Weil and Dr. Mehmet Oz who both appeared on the same program.

Biography courtesy of Wikipedia, available online at http://en.wikipedia.org/wiki/Gary_Taubes. Retrieved on 5/12/08.

[165] For background, see Dawber TR, Meadors GF, Moore FE Jr. Epidemiological approaches to heart disease: The Framingham Study. Am J Public Health 1951;41:279-81. Available online at http://www.ajph.org/cgi/reprint/41/3/279?ijkey=3a284c08840688facaf375b751546378d05dea63&keytyp e2=tf_ipsecsha. Retrieved on 3/10/08. See also http://www.nhlbi.nih.gov/about/framingham/design.htm. Retrieved on 3/10/08. For more information about the Framingham Heart Study, see their website at http://www.framinghamheartstudy.org/index.html. Retrieved on 3/10/08.

[166] See the Framingham Heart Study article, available online at http://www.framinghamheartstudy.org/about/history.html. Retrieved on 3/10/08.

[167] Castelli, William, *Archives of Internal Medicine*, Jul 1992, 152:7:1371-1372. Op Cit., Fallon, Sally, and Enig, Mary. *Nourishing Traditions: The Cookbook that Challenges Politically Correct Nutrition and the Diet Dictocrats*. Washington, DC; NewTrends Publishing, Inc., 2001, page 5.

[168] See Hubert H., et al, *Circulation*, 1983, 67:968; Smith, R and ER Pinckney, *Diet, Blood Cholesterol, and Coronary Heart Disease: A Critical Review of the Literature*, Vol 2, 1991, Vector Enterprises, Sherman Oaks, CA. Op cit. Fallon, Sally, and Enig, Mary. *Nourishing Traditions: The Cookbook that Challenges Politically Correct Nutrition and the Diet Dictocrats*. Washington, DC: NewTrends Publishing, Inc., 2001, page 5.

[169] Fallon, Sally, and Enig, Mary. *Nourishing Traditions: The Cookbook that Challenges Politically Correct Nutrition and the Diet Dictocrats*. Washington, DC: NewTrends Publishing, Inc., 2001, page 5.

[170] Rose G, et al, *The Lancet*, 1983, 1:1062-1065. Op cit. Fallon, Sally, and Enig, Mary. *Nourishing Traditions: The Cookbook that Challenges Politically Correct Nutrition and the Diet Dictocrats*. Washington, DC: NewTrends Publishing, Inc., 2001, page 5.

[171] "Multiple Risk Factor Intervention Trial; Risk Factor Changes and Mortality Results." *Journal of the American Medical Association*, September 24, 1982, 248:12:1465. Op cit. Fallon, Sally, and Enig, Mary. *Nourishing Traditions: The Cookbook that Challenges Politically Correct Nutrition and the Diet Dictocrats*. Washington, DC: NewTrends Publishing, Inc., 2001, pages 5-6.

[172] "The Lipid Research Clinics Coronary Primary Prevention Trial Results. I. Reduction in Incidence of Coronary Heart Disease," *Journal of the American Medical Association*, 1984, 251:359. Op cit. Fallon, Sally, and Enig, Mary. *Nourishing Traditions: The Cookbook that Challenges Politically Correct Nutrition and the Diet Dictocrats*. Washington, DC: NewTrends Publishing, Inc., 2001, page 6.

[173] Kronmal, R, *Journal of the American Medical Association*, April 12, 1985, 253:14:2091. Op cit. Fallon, Sally, and Enig, Mary. *Nourishing Traditions: The Cookbook that Challenges Politically Correct Nutrition and the Diet Dictocrats*. Washington, DC: NewTrends Publishing, Inc., 2001, page 6.

[174] Fallon, Sally, and Enig, Mary. *Nourishing Traditions: The Cookbook that Challenges Politically Correct Nutrition and the Diet Dictocrats*. Washington, DC: NewTrends Publishing, Inc., 2001, page 6.

[175] DeBakey, M, et al., Journal of the American Medical Association, 1964, 189:655-659. Op cit. Fallon, Sally, and Enig, Mary. *Nourishing Traditions: The Cookbook that Challenges Politically Correct Nutrition and the Diet Dictocrats*. Washington, DC: NewTrends Publishing, Inc., 2001, page 6.

Notes

176 Fallon, Sally, and Enig, Mary. *Nourishing Traditions: The Cookbook that Challenges Politically Correct Nutrition and the Diet Dictocrats*. Washington, DC: NewTrends Publishing, Inc., 2001, page 6.

177 Moore, Thomas J, Lifespan: *What Really Affects Human Longevity*, 1990, Simon and Schuster, New York, NY. Op cit. Fallon, Sally, and Enig, Mary. *Nourishing Traditions: The Cookbook that Challenges Politically Correct Nutrition and the Diet Dictocrats*. Washington, DC: NewTrends Publishing, Inc., 2001, page 7.

178 O'Neill, Molly, *New York Times*, Nov 17, 1991. Op cit. Fallon, Sally, and Enig, Mary. *Nourishing Traditions: The Cookbook that Challenges Politically Correct Nutrition and the Diet Dictocrats*. Washington, DC: NewTrends Publishing, Inc., 2001, page 7.

179 Fallon, Sally, and Enig, Mary. *Nourishing Traditions: The Cookbook that Challenges Politically Correct Nutrition and the Diet Dictocrats*. Washington, DC: NewTrends Publishing, Inc., 2001, page 7.

180 *Ibid*, pages 10-13.

181 Ancel Keys (January 26, 1904 - November 20, 2004). US physiologist whose research into the relationship between diet, metabolism and health earned him the sobriquet "Mr. Cholesterol." The researches of the US physiologist Ancel Keys—nicknamed "Mr. Cholesterol" after his findings gained public recognition—had a profound effect on society's attitude to food and exercise. He introduced many of the assumptions which we now take for granted about the relationship between diet, energy expenditure, metabolic rates and health. He led the way in the application of objectively quantifiable measurements to such physiological processes as the effects of ageing and responses to heat, cold or starvation; he applied mathematics to human biology, studying, for instance, the relationships between height and weight, diet and blood fats, blood fats and the incidence of heart attacks. For his obituary, see the American Physiological Society's page at http://www.the-aps.org/membership/obituaries/ancel_keys.htm. Retrieved on 1/26/08. For a good biography, see http://en.wikipedia.org/wiki/Ancel_Keys. Retrieved on 5/30/08.

182 See "Coronary Heart Disease among Minnesota Business and Professional Men Followed Fifteen Years," Ancel Keys, Ph.D.; Henry Longstreet Taylor, Ph.D.; Henry Blackburn, M.D.; Josef Brozek, Ph.D.; Joseph T. Anderson, PH.D.; Ernst Simonson, M.D; from the Laboratory of Physiological Hygiene, University of Minnesota, Minneapolis, Minnesota. *Circulation. 1963;28:381-395.* Available online at http://circ.ahajournals.org/cgi/content/abstract/28/3/381. Retrieved on 1/26/08.

183 "Prevention of Coronary Heart Disease: Official Recommendations from Scandinavia." Ancel Keys. *Circulation.* 1968;38;227-228. *Circulation* is published by the American Heart Association. 7272 Greenville Avenue, Dallas, TX 72514. Print ISSN: 0009-7322. Accessible online at http://circ.ahajournals.org/cgi/reprint/38/2/227?maxtoshow=&HITS=10&hits=10&RESULTFORMAT=&fulltext=ancel+keyes&searchid=1&FIRSTINDEX=10&resourcetype=HWCIT. Retrieved on 1/26/08.

184 *Ibid.*

185 Bier DM, Brosnan JT, Flatt JP, et al. Report of the IDECG Working Group on lower and upper limits of carbohydrate and fat intake. *Eur J Clin Nutr* 1999;53(suppl):S177-8.

186 Cahill GF. "Starvation in man," *N Engl J Med* 1970;282:668-75.

187 Palgi A, Read JL, Greenberg I, Hoefer MA, Bistrian BR, Blackburn GL. Multidisciplinary treatment of obesity with a protein-sparing modified fast: results in 668 outpatients. *Am J Public Health* 1985;75:1190-4.

188 Follis RH, Straight WM. The effect of a purified diet deficient in carbohydrate on the rat. Bull Johns Hopkins Hosp 1943;72:39–41. See also Renner R, Elcombe AM. Metabolic effects of feeding "carbohydrate-free" diets to chicks. *J Nutr* 1967;93:31–6. See also Renner R, Elcombe AM. Protein as a carbohydrate precursor in the chick. *J Nutr* 1967;93:25-30. See also Renner R. Effectiveness of various sources of nonessential nitrogen in promoting growth of chicks fed carbohydrate-containing and "carbohydrate-free"

diets. *J Nutr* 1968;98:297–302. See also Renner R. Factors affecting the utilization of "carbohydrate-free" diets by the chick. I. Level of protein. *J Nutr* 1964;84:322–6.

[189] Renner R, Elcombe AM. Factors affecting the utilization of "carbohydrate-free" diets by the chick. II. Level of glycerol. *J Nutr* 1964;84:327–30.

[190] Harper AE. Defining the essentiality of nutrients. In: Shils MD, Olson JA, Shihe M, Ross AC, eds. *Modern nutrition in health and disease*. 9th ed. Boston: William and Wilkins, 1999:3–10.

[191] *Ibid.*

[192] Shaffer PA. Antiketogenesis. II. The ketogenic antiketogenic balance in man. *J Biol Chem* 1921;47:463–73.

[193] Hoyt CS, Billson FA. Low-carbohydrate diet optic neuropathy. *Med J Aust* 1977;1:65–6.

[194] Quiroz-Kendall E, Wilson FA, King LE Jr. Acute variegate porphyria following a Scarsdale Gourmet Diet. *J Am Acad Dermatol* 1983;8:46–9.

[195] Palgi A, Read JL, Greenberg I, Hoefer MA, Bistrian BR, Blackburn GL. Multidisciplinary treatment of obesity with a protein-sparing modified fast: results in 668 outpatients. *Am J Public Health* 1985;75:1190-4.

[196] See "Is Dietary Carbohydrate Essential for Human Nutrition?" Eric C Westman. Department of Medicine Duke University Medical Center. *American Journal of Clinical Nutrition*, Vol. 75, No. 5, 951-953, May 2002.

[197] See the article "William Banting Father of the Low-Carbohydrate Diet," at the website of Barry Groves, PhD, online at http://www.second-opinions.co.uk/banting.html. Retrieved on 6/17/09. Used by permission.

[198] Adapted from the Wikipedia article entitled "Low-Carbohydrate Diet," available online at http://en.wikipedia.org/wiki/Low-carbohydrate_diet. Retrieved on 12/15/08.

[199] "The Stillman Diet—History Of Diets, Part 12—Protein Diet." *Men's Fitness*. June 2003. Available online at http://findarticles.com/p/articles/mi_m1608/is_6_19/ai_102140891. Retrieved on 5/25/08.

[200] Air Force Diet. Toronto, Canada, Air Force Diet Publishers, 1960.

[201] Gardner Jameson and Elliot Williams (1964) *The Drinking Man's Diet*. San Francisco: Cameron. (2004) Revised Ed. ISBN 978-0918684653. See also Alan Farnham (2004) "The Drinking Man's Diet," on Forbes.com, at http://www.forbes.com/2004/04/21/cz_af_0421feat.html. Retrieved on 6/28/09.

[202] Lutz, Wolfgang; Allan, C.B. *Life Without Bread*. McGraw-Hill; 2000. ISBN 978-0658001703. English language, 1st Ed.

[203] Adapted from the Wikipedia article entitled "Low-Carbohydrate Diet," available online at http://en.wikipedia.org/wiki/Low-carbohydrate_diet. Retrieved on 12/15/08.

[204] See "The History of the Atkins Diet, A Revolutionary Lifestyle." Available online at http://www.thehistoryof.net/history-of-the-atkins-diet.html. Retrieved on 5/25/08.

[205] Adapted from the Wikipedia article entitled "Low-Carbohydrate Diet," available online at http://en.wikipedia.org/wiki/Low-carbohydrate_diet. Retrieved on 12/15/08.

[206] DJ Jenkins et al (1981) "Glycemic index of foods: a physiological basis for carbohydrate exchange." *Am J Clin Nutr* 34; 362-366.

[207] PBS News Hour: Low Carb Craze.

Notes

208 Americans Look for Health on the Menu: Survey finds nutrition plays increasing role in dining-out choices. Available online at http://www.diningstyle.com/press.htm. Retrieved on 3/19/08.

209 American Heart Association Statement on High-Protein, Low-Carbohydrate Diet Study Presented at Scientific Sessions. See also Research Reaffirms Role of Complex Carbohydrates in Weight Loss. See also The American Kidney Fund: American Kidney Fund Warns About Impact of High-Protein Diets on Kidney Health: 25 April 2002.

210 Adapted from the Wikipedia article entitled "Low-Carbohydrate Diet," available online at http://en.wikipedia.org/wiki/Low-carbohydrate_diet. Retrieved on 12/15/08.

211 Ibid.

212 Ibid.

213 Linda Stern, MD; Nayyar Iqbal, MD; Prakash Seshadri, MD; Kathryn L. Chicano, CRNP; Denise A. Daily, RD; Joyce McGrory, CRNP; Monica Williams, BS; Edward J. Gracely, PhD; and Frederick F. Samaha, MD (2004). "The Effects of Low-Carbohydrate versus Conventional Weight Loss Diets in Severely Obese Adults: One-Year Follow-up of a Randomized Trial." Annals of Internal Medicine 140 (10): 778–785. See also William S. Yancy, Jr., MD, MHS; Maren K. Olsen, PhD; John R. Guyton, MD; Ronna P. Bakst, RD; and Eric C. Westman, MD, MHS (2004). "A Low-Carbohydrate, Ketogenic Diet versus a Low-Fat Diet To Treat Obesity and Hyperlipidemia." Annals of Internal Medicine 140 (10): 769–777.

214 Adapted from the Wikipedia article entitled "Low-Carbohydrate Diet," available online at http://en.wikipedia.org/wiki/Low-carbohydrate_diet. Retrieved on 12/15/08.

215 Ibid.

216 Ibid.

217 See "An insulin index of foods: the insulin demand generated by 1000-kJ portions of common foods," by SH Holt, JC Miller and P Petocz. American Journal of Clinical Nutrition 66, 1997.

218 Adapted from the Wikipedia article entitled "Low-Carbohydrate Diet," available online at http://en.wikipedia.org/wiki/Low-carbohydrate_diet. Retrieved on 12/15/08.

219 Ibid.

220 Ibid.

221 Ibid.

222 Ibid.

223 Ibid.

224 "Ketogenic low-carbohydrate diets have no metabolic advantage over nonketogenic low-carbohydrate diets," by Johnson et al., American Journal of Clinical Nutrition, Vol. 83, No. 5, 1055-1061, May, 2006. Available online at http://www.ajcn.org/cgi/content/abstract/83/5/1055. Retrieved on 3/19/08.

225 Adapted from the Wikipedia article entitled "Low-Carbohydrate Diet," available online at http://en.wikipedia.org/wiki/Low-carbohydrate_diet. Retrieved on 12/15/08.

226 Protections for human subjects of research are required under Department of Health and Human Services (HHS) regulations at 45 CFR 46. Subpart A of the HHS regulations constitutes the Federal Policy (Common Rule) for the Protection of Human Subjects, which has been adopted by an additional 16

Executive Branch Departments and Agencies. Each institution engaged in (non-exempt) HHS-supported human subjects research must provide a written Assurance of Compliance, satisfactory to the Office for Protection from Research Risks (OPRR), that it will comply with the HHS human subjects regulations. - 45 CFR 46.103(a)

Institutions conducting (non-exempt) HHS-supported human subjects research must provide Certification to the supporting agency that the research has been reviewed and approved by an Institutional Review Board (IRB) designated under an OPRR-approved Assurance. Under no circumstances may (non-exempt) human subjects research be supported prior to Certification. - 45 CFR 46.103(f). Except where the IRB specifically approves a waiver in accordance with HHS regulations, no investigator may involve a human being as a subject in (non-exempt) research unless the investigator has obtained the legally effective informed consent of the subject, or the subject's legally authorized representative. The meaning of "legally effective" and "legally authorized" is determined in part by applicable State law. See "Summary of Basic Protections for Human Subjects," December 23, 1997, Office for Protection from Research Risks. Available online at http://www.hhs.gov/ohrp/humansubjects/guidance/basics.htm. Retrieved on 2/15/08.

[227] Thomas L. Halton, Sc. D., Walter C. Willett, M.D., Dr. P.H., Simin Liu, M.D., Sc. D., JoAnn E. Manson, M.D., Dr. P.H., Christine M. Albert, M.D., M.P.H., Kathryn Rexrode, M.D., and Frank B. Hu, M.D., Ph. D. (2006). "Low-carbohydrate diet score and the risk of coronary heart disease in women". *New England Journal of Medicine* 355:1991-2002. PMID 17093250. Available online at http://www.ncbi.nlm.nih.gov/pubmed/17093250?dopt=Abstract. Retrieved on 3/18/08.

[228] Yancy, W.S.; Foy M, Chalecki AM, Vernon MC, Westman EC. (2005). "A low-carbohydrate, ketogenic diet to treat Type 2 diabetes," *Nutrition & Metabolism* 1 (2): 34; doi: 10.1186/1743-7075-2-34. PMID 16318637. Available online at http://www.pubmedcentral.nih.gov/articlerender.fcgi?artid=1325029. Retrieved on 3/14/08.

[229] Bravi, F.; Bosetti C, Scotti L, Talamini R, Montella M, Ramazzotti V, Negri E, Franceschi S, & La Vecchia C (2007). "Food groups and renal cell carcinoma: A case-control study from Italy," *International Journal of Cancer* 120 (3): 681-5. PMID 17058282. Available online at http://www.ncbi.nlm.nih.gov/pubmed/17058282?dopt=Abstract. Retrieved on 3/18/08.

[230] Evangeliou, A; Vlachonikolis I, Mihailidou H, Spilioti M, Skarpalezou A, Makaronas N, Prokopiou A, Christodoulou P, Liapi-Adamidou G, Helidonis E, Sbyrakis S, Smeitink J. (2003). "Application of a ketogenic diet in children with autistic behavior: pilot study," *Journal of Child Neurology* 18 (2): 113-8. PMID 12693778. Available online at http://www.ncbi.nlm.nih.gov/pubmed/12693778?dopt=Abstract. Retrieved on 3/18/08.

[231] See Benoit FL, Martin RL, Watten RH. "Changes in body composition during weight reduction in obesity. Balance studies comparing effects of fasting and a ketogenic diet," *Ann Intern Med* 1965, 63:604-12.

[232] See Young CM, Scanlan SS, Im HS, Lutwak L. "Effect of body composition and other parameters in obese young men of carbohydrate level of reduction diet," *Am J Clin Nutr.* 1971 Mar;24(3):290-6. PMID: 5548734. Available online at http://www.ncbi.nlm.nih.gov/pubmed/5548734?dopt=Abstract. Retrieved on 2/3/08.

[233] See "Effects of Varying Carbohydrate Content of Diet in Patients with Non-Insulin-Dependent Diabetes Mellitus," by Garg A, Bantle JP, Henry RR, Coulston AM, Griver KA, Raatz SK, Brinkley L, Chen YD, Grundy SM, Huet BA, et al. *JAMA.* 1994 May 11;271(18):1421-8. Available online at: http://www.ncbi.nlm.nih.gov/pubmed/7848401?ordinalpos=1&itool=EntrezSystem2.PEntrez.Pubmed.P ubmed_ResultsPanel.Pubmed_RVAbstractPlusDrugs1. Retrieved on 2/9/08.

[234] See "Deleterious Metabolic Effects of High-Carbohydrate, Sucrose-Containing Diets in Patients with Non-Insulin-Dependent Diabetes Mellitus," by Coulston AM, Hollenbeck CB, Swislocki AL, Chen YD, Reaven GM. *Am J Med.* 1987 Feb;82(2):213-20. Available online at http://www.ncbi.nlm.nih.gov/pubmed/3544839?ordinalpos=1&itool=EntrezSystem2.PEntrez.Pubmed.P ubmed_ResultsPanel.Pubmed_RVAbstractPlusDrugs1. Retrieved on 2/9/08.

Notes

[235] See Christopher D. Gardner; Alexandre Kiazand; Sofiya Alhassan; Soowon Kim; Randall S. Stafford; Raymond R. Balise; Helena C. Kraemer; Abby C. King. Comparison of the Atkins, Zone, Ornish, and LEARN Diets for Change in Weight and Related Risk Factors Among Overweight Premenopausal Women: The A TO Z Weight Loss Study: A Randomized Trial. *JAMA*. 2007;297(9):969-977. Available online at http://jama.ama-assn.org/cgi/content/full/297/9/969. Retrieved on 12/3/08.

[236] See William S. Yancy, Jr, Marjorie Foy, Allison M. Chalecki, Mary C. Vernon, and Eric C. Westman. A low-carbohydrate, ketogenic diet to treat Type 2 diabetes. *Nutr Metab* (Lond). 2005; 2: 34. Available online at http://www.pubmedcentral.nih.gov/articlerender.fcgi?tool=pubmed&pubmedid=16318637. Accessed on 2/3/08.

[237] Dena M. Bravata, MD, MS; Lisa Sanders, MD; Jane Huang, MD; Harlan M. Krumholz, MD, SM; Ingram Olkin, PhD; Christopher D. Gardner, PhD; Dawn M. Bravata, MD (2003). "Efficacy and Safety of Low-Carbohydrate Diets" 289. Available online at http://jama.ama-assn.org/cgi/content/abstract/289/14/1837. Retrieved on 3/22/08.

[238] Linda Stern, MD; Nayyar Iqbal, MD; Prakash Seshadri, MD; Kathryn L. Chicano, CRNP; Denise A. Daily, RD; Joyce McGrory, CRNP; Monica Williams, BS; Edward J. Gracely, PhD; and Frederick F. Samaha, MD (2004). "The Effects of Low-Carbohydrate versus Conventional Weight Loss Diets in Severely Obese Adults: One-Year Follow-up of a Randomized Trial". *Annals of Internal Medicine* 140 (10): 778–785. Available online at http://www.annals.org/cgi/content/abstract/140/10/778?etoc. Retrieved on 3/22/08

[239] From an outpatient clinic, the study recruited 28 overweight participants with Type 2 diabetes for a 16-week single-arm pilot diet intervention trial. They provided LCKD counseling, with an initial goal of <20 g carbohydrate/day, while reducing diabetes medication dosages at diet initiation. Participants returned every other week for measurements, counseling, and further medication adjustment. The primary outcome was hemoglobin A_{1c}. Diabetes medications were discontinued in 7 participants, reduced in 10 participants, and unchanged in 4 participants. The mean body weight decreased by 6.6% from 131.4 ± 18.3 kg to 122.7 ± 18.9 kg. Fasting serum triglyceride decreased 42% from 2.69 ± 2.87 mmol/L to 1.57 ± 1.38 mmol/L while other serum lipid measurements did not change significantly. See *"A low-carbohydrate, ketogenic diet to treat Type 2 diabetes"* by William S Yancy Jr., Marjorie Foy, Allison M Chalecki, Mary C Vernon and Eric C Westman. *Nutrition & Metabolism* 2005, 2:34; doi: 10.1186/1743-7075-2-34. The electronic version of this article is the complete one and can be found online at: http://www.nutritionandmetabolism.com/content/2/1/34. Retrieved on 3/18/08.

[240] See "Low-Carbohydrate Nutrition and Metabolism," by Eric C Westman, Richard D Feinman, John C Mavropoulos, Mary C Vernon, Jeff S Volek, James A Wortman, William S Yancy and Stephen D Phinney. *American Journal of Clinical Nutrition*, Vol. 86, No. 2, 276-284, August 2007. © 2007 American Society for Nutrition. Available online at http://www.ajcn.org/cgi/content/full/86/2/276. Retrieved on 1/24/08.

[241] See "Comparison of low fat and low carbohydrate diets on circulating Fatty Acid composition and markers of inflammation," by Forsythe CE, Phinney SD, Fernandez ML, Quann EE, Wood RJ, Bibus DM, Kraemer WJ, Feinman RD, Volek JS. Department of Kinesiology, University of Connecticut, 2095 Hillside Road, Unit 1110, Storrs, CT, 06269-1110, USA. *Lipids*. 2008 Jan; 43(1): 65-77. Epub 2007. Nov 29.

[242] See "Restricted-Carbohydrate Diets in Patients with Type 2 Diabetes: A Meta-Analysis," *Journal of the American Dietetic Association*, Volume 108, Issue 1, 2007, pages 91-100 J. KIRK. Available online at http://www.sciencedirect.com/science?_ob=ArticleURL&_udi=B758G-4RDH61V-P&_user=10&_coverDate=01%2F31%2F2008&_alid=680233855&_rdoc=1&_fmt=summary&_orig=browse&_cdi=12926&_sort=d&_docanchor=&view=c&_acct=C000050221&_version=1&_urlVersion=0&_userid=10&md5=4213ea9afbc2f2c16837d768598cdf07#. Retrieved on 1/24/08.

[243] *Ibid*.

[244] Pirozzo S, Summerbell C, Cameron C, Glasziou P (2002). "Advice on low-fat diets for obesity," *Cochrane database of systematic reviews (Online)* (2): CD003640. PMID 12076496. Available online at http://www.ncbi.nlm.nih.gov/pubmed/12076496?dopt=Abstract. Retrieved on 3/18/08.

[245] See "A low-carbohydrate as compared with a low-fat diet in severe obesity," by Samaha FF, Iqbal N, Seshadri P, et al., *N. Engl. J. Med.* 348 (21): 2074–81, 2003. doi: 10.1056/NEJMoa022637. PMID 12761364. Available online at http://www.ncbi.nlm.nih.gov/pubmed/12761364?dopt=Abstract. Retrieved on 3/18/08. See also "A randomized trial of a low-carbohydrate diet for obesity," by Foster GD, Wyatt HR, Hill JO, et al., *N. Engl. J. Med.* 348 (21): 2082–90, 2003. doi: 10.1056/NEJMoa022207. PMID 12761365. Available online at http://www.ncbi.nlm.nih.gov/pubmed/12761365?dopt=Abstract. Retrieved on 3/18/08. See also "Comparison of the Atkins, Ornish, Weight Watchers, and Zone diets for weight loss and heart disease risk reduction: a randomized trial," by Dansinger ML, Gleason JA, Griffith JL, et al., *JAMA* 293 (1): 43-53, 2005. doi: 10.1001/jama.293.1.43. PMID 12761365. Available online at http://www.ncbi.nlm.nih.gov/pubmed/12761365?dopt=Abstract. Retrieved on 3/18/08.

[246] See "Effects of low-carbohydrate vs. low-fat diets on weight loss and cardiovascular risk factors: a meta-analysis of randomized controlled trials," by Nordmann AJ, Nordmann A, Briel M, et al., *Arch. Intern. Med.* 166 (3): 285-93, 2006. doi: 10.1001/archinte.166.3.285. PMID 16476868. Available online at http://www.ncbi.nlm.nih.gov/pubmed/16476868?dopt=Abstract. Retrieved on 3/18/08.

[247] See Stanford Diet Study Tips Scale In Favor of Atkins Plan. Available online at http://nutrition.stanford.edu/pdfs/AZ_press.pdf. Retrieved on 3/18/08. See also "Study Shows Low-Carb Diet Improves Cholesterol," available online at http://www.dukemednews.duke.edu/news/article.php?id=9412. Retrieved on 3/18/08.

[248] Effects of variations in dietary fat and carbohydrate content on various aspects of glucose, insulin, and lipoprotein metabolism were evaluated in 11 patients with hypertension, who also had non-insulin-dependent diabetes mellitus (NIDDM). All of these patients were being treated with sulfonylureas, thiazides, and beta-adrenergic receptor antagonists. The comparison diets contained either 40 or 60% of total calories as carbohydrate, with reciprocal changes in fat content from 40 to 20%. The diets were consumed in a random order for 15 days in a crossover experimental design. The ratio of polyunsaturated to saturated fat and total cholesterol intake were held constant in the two diets.

See "Effect of low fat-high carbohydrate diets in hypertensive patients with non-insulin-dependent diabetes mellitus," by Fuh MM, Lee MM, Jeng CY, Ma F, Chen YD, and Reaven GM, *Am J Hypertens.* 1990 Jul;3(7):527-32. Available online at http://www.ncbi.nlm.nih.gov/pubmed/2194509. Retrieved on 5/5/09.

[249] See "A low-carbohydrate diet may prevent end-stage renal failure in type 2 diabetes. A case report," by Jørgen Vesti Nielsen, Per Westerlund, and Per Bygren, *Nutrition & Metabolism* 2006, 3:23; doi: 10.1186/1743-7075-3-23. Available online at http://www.nutritionandmetabolism.com/content/3/1/23#B17. Retrieved on 5/5/09.

[250] *Ibid.*

[251] *Ibid.*

[252] See "Low-carbohydrate diet in type 2 diabetes. Stable improvement of bodyweight and glycemic control during 22 months follow-up," by Jørgen Vesti Nielsen and Eva Joensson, *Nutrition & Metabolism,* 2006, 3:22; doi: 10.1186/1743-7075-3-22. Available online at http://www.nutritionandmetabolism.com/content/3/1/22. Retrieved on 5/5/09.

[253] *Ibid.*

[254] *Ibid.*

255 See Kauffman, Ph.D., Joel M. *Malignant Medical Myths: Why Medical Treatment Causes 200,000 Deaths in the USA Each Year, and How to Protect Yourself.* West Conshohocken, PA: Infinity, 2006. Joel M. Kauffman obtained a BS in Chemistry from the Philadelphia College of Pharmacy and Science, now called University of the Sciences in Philadelphia (USP), and a PhD in Organic Chemistry from the Massachusetts Institute of Technology. After 11 years of experience in the chemical industry, Dr. Kauffman joined USP in 1979, rising to Professor of Chemistry in 1990. His experience includes about 10 years of exploratory drug development at USP and 4 years at the Massachusetts College of Pharmacy and Health Sciences. He obtained grants and contracts from many sources including the National Institutes of Health, the Department of Energy, the Office of Naval Research and the Army Research Office and several manufacturing companies. Dr. Kauffman has written 80 papers on chemical and medical topics, and 11 patents, including 2 on antituberculosis drugs. He has also posted reviews on more than 100 books on Amazon.com.

256 Control of dental caries by a low carbohydrate diet," by Pankey LD. *J Fla State Dent Soc.* 1948 Oct;19(10):5-7. PMID: 18889992. Available online at http://www.ncbi.nlm.nih.gov/pubmed/18889992. Retrieved on 7/15/09.

257 P. Hujoel. "Dietary Carbohydrates and Dental-Systemic Diseases." *J Dent Res* 88(6):490-502, 2009. doi: 10.1177/0022034509337700. Available online at http://jdr.sagepub.com/cgi/content/abstract/88/6/490. Retrieved on 7/15/09. Used by permission.

258 *Ibid.*

259 See the Weston A Price Foundation website, available online at http://www.westonaprice.org/nutritiongreats/price.html. Retrieved on 7/15/09.

260 Adapted from the Wikipedia article entitled "Weston Price," available online at http://en.wikipedia.org/wiki/Weston_Price. Retrieved on 7/15/09. See also the Price-Pottenger Nutrition Foundation website at http://www.ppnf.org/catalog/ppnf/index.htm and the Weston A Price Foundation website at http://www.westonaprice.org/splash_2.htm.

THE WAY THINGS OUGHT TO BE (PART II)

261 See http://www.mercola.com/2005/may/31/diabetes_disease.htm. Retrieved on 3/18/08. See also http://www.mercola.com/2001/jul/14/insulin.htm. Retrieved on 3/18/08. See *The Rosedale Diet* (2004), by Dr. Ron Rosedale and Carol Colman, HarperCollins Publishers, NY. In addition to the selected quotes appearing in this book, Dr. Ron Rosedale writes lucidly on insulin in general and its direct and indirect influence on all the body's organs and hormones. Dr. Rosedale includes discussions on aging, centenarian studies, cardiovascular disease, osteoporosis, the negative effects of sugar, glycation, Advanced Glycated End Products (A.G.E.s), insulin resistance, and insulin sensitivity.

Dr. Ron Rosedale is an internationally renowned expert in nutritional and metabolic medicine and an anti-aging specialist. He is founder of the Rosedale Center in Denver, Colorado; co-founder of the Colorado Center for Metabolic Medicine in Boulder, Colorado; and founder of the Carolina Center of Metabolic Medicine in Asheville, North Carolina. As a keynote speaker, he has appeared before such prestigious groups as the Eighth Congressional International Medical Conference on Molecular Medicine, the First European Conference on Longevity Medicine and Quality of Life, and many more. He has been a guest on numerous national radio and television news shows. He lives in Denver, Colorado.

262 See http://www.mercola.com/2005/may/31/diabetes_disease.htm. Retrieved on 3/22/08. See also http://www.mercola.com/2001/jul/14/insulin.htm. Retrieved on 3/22/08. See also Rosedale, Ron, and Colman, Carol. *The Rosedale Diet.* HarperCollins Publishers Inc. New York, NY. 2004.

[263] See http://www.mercola.com/2005/may/31/diabetes_disease.htm. Retrieved on 3/18/08. See also http://www.mercola.com/2001/jul/14/insulin.htm. Retrieved on 3/18/08. See also *The Rosedale Diet* (2004), by Dr. Ron Rosedale and Carol Colman, HarperCollins Publishers, NY.

[264] For a particularly good discussion of the Dawn Phenomenon, as cited in my first book, see "Anti-Aging Teleclinic," with Dr. Ron Rosedale and Dr. Joseph Mercola, pages 32-34. Available online at the Mercola.com website at http://www.mercola.com/forms/downloads/antiagingteleclinic.htm. Retrieved on 1/31/08.

[265] Biography courtesy of Wikipedia. See http://en.wikipedia.org/wiki/Richard_K._Bernstein. Retrieved on 5/12/08.

[266] Every year since 1901 the Nobel Prize has been awarded for achievements in physics, chemistry, physiology or medicine, literature and for peace. The Nobel Prize is an international award administered by the Nobel Foundation in Stockholm, Sweden. Each year the respective Nobel Committees send individual invitations to thousands of members of academies, university professors, scientists from numerous countries, previous Nobel Laureates, members of parliamentary assemblies and others, asking them to submit candidates for the Nobel Prizes for the coming year. These nominators are chosen in such a way that as many countries and universities as possible are represented over time. Around 200-300 names are submitted since the same candidate can be nominated by several persons. See http://nobelprize.org/index.html. Retrieved on 3/18/08.

[267] Dr.Bernstein's four published books are: (1) *Dr. Bernstein's Diabetes Solution: The Complete Guide to Achieving Normal Blood Sugars (Hardcover)*. Little, Brown & Company. 2007. (2) *Diabetes Type II: Living a Long, Healthy Life Through Blood Sugar Normalization*. Prentice Hall Trade, 1st ed. edition. 1990. (3) *The Diabetes Diet: Dr. Bernstein's Low-Carbohydrate Solution*. Little, Brown & Company. 2005. (4) *Diabetes: The GlucograF Method for Normalizing Blood Sugar*. Crown. 1981. Dr. Bernstein also posts articles and free excerpts of his and other authors' works online at: http://www.thebernsteinconnection.com/about.php and http://www.diabetesincontrol.com/categoryresults.php?recordID=2. Retrieved on 6/17/09.

[268] For one example of the American Diabetes Association's dietary recommendations, their "Diabetes Food Pyramid" see http://www.diabetes.org/nutrition-and-recipes/nutrition/foodpyramid.jsp. Retrieved on 1/4/08. This pyramid groups foods based on their carbohydrate and protein content instead of their classification as a food. The largest group—grains, beans, and starchy vegetables—is on the bottom. They recommend that you should eat more servings of grains, beans, and starchy vegetables than of any of the other foods, 6-11 servings per day.

[269] Bernstein, Richard K. *The Diabetes Diet*. New York: Little, Brown and Company, 2005, pages 20-21.

[270] See http://www.diabetesincontrol.com/categoryresults.php?recordID=2. Retrieved on 6/17/09.
.

[271] Bernstein, Richard K. *The Diabetes Diet*. New York: Little, Brown and Company, 2005, author's note, page ix.

[272] See Mary G. Enig, Ph. D. *Know Your Fats: The Complete Primer for Understanding the Nutrition of Fats, Oils, and Cholesterol*. Silver Spring, MD: Bethesda Press, 2000. There is a remarkable summary of vitamins, minerals, enzymes, additives, and more information about carbohydrates, proteins, and fat in the introduction to the book *Nourishing Traditions: The Cookbook that Challenges Politically Correct Nutrition and the Diet Dictocrat* by Sally Fallon with Mary G, Enig, Ph.D. Washington, DC: NewTrends Publishing, October, 1999. Mary G. Enig, Ph.D., is an expert of international renown in the field of lipid biochemistry. She has headed a number of studies on the content and effects of *trans* fatty acids in America and Israel, and has successfully challenged government assertions that dietary animal fat causes cancer and heart disease. Recent scientific and media attention on the possible adverse health effects of *trans* fatty acids has brought increased attention to her work. She is a licensed nutritionist, certified by the Certification Board for Nutrition Specialists, a qualified expert witness, nutrition consultant to individuals, industry and state and federal governments, contributing editor to a number of scientific publications, Fellow of the American College of Nutrition and President of the Maryland Nutritionists Association. She is the author

of over 60 technical papers and presentations, as well as a popular lecturer. Dr. Enig is currently working on the exploratory development of an adjunct therapy for AIDS using complete medium chain saturated fatty acids from whole foods. She is Vice-President of the Weston A Price Foundation and Scientific Editor of *Wise Traditions* as well as the author of Know Your Fats: The Complete Primer for Understanding the Nutrition of Fats, Oils, and Cholesterol, Bethesda Press, May, 2000. She is the mother of three healthy children brought up on whole foods including butter, cream, eggs and meat. Her books include: Dr Mary Enig, *Know Your Fats: The Complete Primer for Understanding the Nutrition of Fats, Oils and Cholesterol,* (Bethesda Press, May, 2000); Sally Fallon, with Dr Mary Enig (contributing editor), *Nourishing Traditions: The Cookbook that Challenges Politically Correct Nutrition and the Diet Dictocrats,* (NewTrends Publishing, October, 1999); and Dr Mary Enig, *Trans fatty acids in the food supply: A comprehensive report covering 60 years of research,* (Enig Associates, 1993).

273 The best online reference to search for information about supplements can be found at http://www.mercola.com.

274 Cheese is a food made from milk, usually of cows, buffalos, goats, or sheep, by coagulation. The milk is acidified, typically with a bacterial culture, then the addition of the enzyme rennet or a substitute (e.g. acetic acid or vinegar) causes coagulation, to give "curds and whey". Some cheeses also have molds, either on the outer rind (similar to a fruit peel) or throughout. Hundreds of types of cheese are produced. Their different styles, textures and flavors depend on the origin of the milk (including the animal's diet), whether it has been pasteurized, butterfat content, the species of bacteria and mold, and the processing including the length of aging. Herbs, spices, or wood smoke may be used as flavoring agents. The yellow to red color of many cheeses is a result of adding annatto.   For more information, see http://en.wikipedia.org/wiki/Cheese. Retrieved on 5/31/08. For a comprehensive list of cheeses by place of origin, see http://en.wikipedia.org/wiki/List_of_cheeses. Retrieved on 5/31/08.

275 See Groves, Barry. *Trick and Treat: How 'Healthy Eating' is Making us Ill.* London, UK: Hammersmith Press Ltd., 2008, page 94. The study referred to is "Formation of modified fatty acids and oxyphytosterols during refining of low erucic acid rapeseed oil," by Lambelet P. et al., *J Agric Food Chem* 2003; 51: 4284-4290. *Op cit.* Groves. Available online at http://pubs.acs.org/doi/abs/10.1021/jf030091u. Retrieved on 5/7/09. Used by permission.

In his book, Mr. Groves presents an excellent discussion of fats and oils, and, relating to polyunsaturated oils, presents the evidence of a cancer link and risk (see pages 95-102).

276 "Addition of saturated fat and removal of starch from a high-monounsaturated fat and starch-restricted diet improved glycemic control and were associated with weight loss without detectable adverse effects on serum lipids." See "Results of use of metformin and replacement of starch with saturated fat in diets of patients with type 2 diabetes," by Hays JH, Gorman RT, Shakir KM. *Endocr Pract.* 2002 May-Jun;8(3):177-83. Available online at http://www.ncbi.nlm.nih.gov/pubmed/12113629. I first found this article posted on one of Dr. Barry Groves's websites at http://www.diabetes-diet.org.uk/index.html. Retrieved on 10/24/09.

For a great discussion of various mammalian diets, see "Should All Animals Eat a High-Fat, Low-Carb Diet?" posted on another one of Dr. Barry Groves's websites at http://www.second-opinions.co.uk/index.html. Retrieved on 10/24/09. From the article: "If we look at the various natural diets of all mammals, we find the same pattern: all of the diets are high in fat, and most of that fat is saturated. Apart from the saturated fats found in meat, all the short chain fatty acids produced by fermentative bacteria are 100% saturated. Also, all mammals' natural diets are very low in carbohydrate in the case of herbivores, and practically carbohydrate free in the case of carnivores. There is no reason to suppose that we 'civilised' humans should eat any differently."

277 Canola is one of two cultivars of rapeseed or *Brassica campestris* (*Brassica napus* L. and *B. campestris* L.). Their seeds are used to produce edible oil that is fit for human consumption because it has lower levels of erucic acid than traditional rapeseed oils and to produce livestock feed because it has reduced levels of the toxin glucosin. Canola was originally naturally bred from rapeseed in Canada by Keith Downey and Baldur R. Stefansson in the early 1970s, but it has a very different nutritional profile in addition to much

less erucic acid. The name "canola" was derived from "Canadian oil, low acid" in 1978. A product known as LEAR (for *low erucic acid rapeseed*) derived from cross-breeding of multiple lines of *Brassica juncea* is also referred to as canola oil and is considered safe for consumption. Adapted from the Wikipedia article entitled "Canola," available online at http://en.wikipedia.org/wiki/Canola. Retrieved on 3/4/09.

278 Enig, Mary, and Fallon, Sally. *Eat Fat, Lose Fat.* New York: Penguin Group, First Plume Printing, 2006, page 17.

279 *Ibid*, page 33.

280 *Ibid*, page 48.

281 See "Change in dietary saturated fat intake is correlated with change in mass of large low-density-lipoprotein particles in men," by Dreon DM, Fernstrom HA, Campos H, Blanche P, Williams PT, Krauss RM. *Am J Clin Nutr* 1998, 67(5):828-836. Available online at http://www.ajcn.org/cgi/reprint/67/5/828. Retrieved on 5/8/09. Op cit. Accurso et al., (2008).

282 See "Dietary fats, carbohydrate, and progression of coronary atherosclerosis in postmenopausal women," by Mozaffarian D, Rimm EB, Herrington DM. *Am J Clin Nutr* 2004, 80(5):1175-1184. Available online at http://www.ajcn.org/cgi/content/full/80/5/1175. Retrieved on 5/8/09. Op cit. Accurso et al., (2008).

283 See "Dietary carbohydrate restriction in type 2 diabetes mellitus and metabolic syndrome: time for a critical appraisal," by Anthony Accurso, Richard K Bernstein, Annika Dahlqvist, Boris Draznin, Richard D Feinman, Eugene J Fine, Amy Gleed, David B Jacobs, Gabriel Larson, Robert H Lustig, Anssi H Manninen, Samy I McFarlane, Katharine Morrison, Jørgen Vesti Nielsen, Uffe Ravnskov, Karl S Roth, Ricardo Silvestre, James R Sowers, Ralf Sundberg,, Jeff S Volek, Eric C Westman, Richard J Wood, Jay Wortman, and Mary C Vernon. *Nutrition & Metabolism* 2008, 5:9; doi: 10.1186/1743-7075-5-9. Available online at http://www.nutritionandmetabolism.com/content/5/1/9#B29. Retrieved on 5/8/09.

284 Ravnskov U. High cholesterol may protect against infections and atherosclerosis. *Q J Med* 2003;96:927-34. Available online at http://cel.isiknowledge.com/InboundService.do?product=CEL&action=retrieve&SrcApp=Highwire&UT =000187231900008&SID=1AHedPKn74BIbjiHOIc&Init=Yes&SrcAuth=Highwire&mode=FullRecord&cust omersID=Highwire. Retrieved on 4/28/09.

285 Ravnskov U. High cholesterol may protect against infections and atherosclerosis. *Q J Med* 2003;96:927-34. Available online at http://cel.isiknowledge.com/InboundService.do?product=CEL&action=retrieve&SrcApp=Highwire&UT =000187231900008&SID=1AHedPKn74BIbjiHOIc&Init=Yes&SrcAuth=Highwire&mode=FullRecord&cust omersID=Highwire. Retrieved on 4/28/09.

286 Ravnskov U. The questionable role of saturated and polyunsaturated fatty acids in cardiovascular disease. *J Clin Epidemiol* 1998;51:443-60. Available online at http://www.ncbi.nlm.nih.gov/pubmed/9635993?dopt=Abstract. Retrieved on 4/28/09.

287 Ravnskov U. High cholesterol may protect against infections and atherosclerosis. *Q J Med* 2003;96:927-34. Available online at http://cel.isiknowledge.com/InboundService.do?product=CEL&action=retrieve&SrcApp=Highwire&UT =000187231900008&SID=1AHedPKn74BIbjiHOIc&Init=Yes&SrcAuth=Highwire&mode=FullRecord&cust omersID=Highwire. Retrieved on 4/28/09.

288 Ravnskov U. The questionable role of saturated and polyunsaturated fatty acids in cardiovascular disease. *J Clin Epidemiol* 1998;51:443-60. Available online at http://www.ncbi.nlm.nih.gov/pubmed/9635993?dopt=Abstract. Retrieved on 4/28/09.

[289] Ravnskov U. High cholesterol may protect against infections and atherosclerosis. *Q J Med* 2003;96:927-34.   Available   online   at http://cel.isiknowledge.com/InboundService.do?product=CEL&action=retrieve&SrcApp=Highwire&UT =000187231900008&SID=1AHedPKn74BIbjiHOIc&Init=Yes&SrcAuth=Highwire&mode=FullRecord&cust omersID=Highwire. Retrieved on 4/28/09.

[290] Ravnskov U, Rosch PJ, Sutter MC, Houston MC. Should we lower cholesterol as much as possible? *BMJ* 2006;332:1330-2. Available online at http://www.bmj.com/cgi/content/full/332/7553/1330. Retrieved on 4/28/09.

[291] See "*Hypercholesterolaemia:* Should medical science ignore the past?" by Uffe Ravnskov, *BMJ* 2008;337:a1681.   Available   online   at http://www.bmj.com/cgi/content/full/337/sep16_3/a1681?ijkey=rIAxXmCReGu9zU7&keytype=ref. Retrieved on 4/28/09. Used by permission.

[292] See de Lorgeril M, Salen P. Cholesterol lowering, sudden cardiac death and mortality. *Scand Cardiovasc J* 2008;42:264–7. Available online at http://www.ncbi.nlm.nih.gov/pubmed/18615354. Retrieved on 6/31/09.

See also Ware WR. The mainstream hypothesis that LDL cholesterol drives atherosclerosis may have been falsified by non-invasive imaging of coronary artery plaque burden and progression. *Med Hypotheses* (2009), doi: 10.1016/j.mehy.2009.05.030.

This article provided 19 questions, and "These inconvenient questions, which are based [on] 19 studies, unless provided with satisfactory evidence-based answers, appear to falsify the hypothesis that LDL cholesterol is the driving force behind atherosclerosis. This large number of null results based on direct observation of both calcified and non-calcified plaque in the appropriate vascular bed, and involving large numbers of men and women over a wide range of age, ethnic background, plaque burden, and cholesterol levels cannot be easily dismissed. To paraphrase Karl Popper, hypotheses survive by not being falsified."

[293] And diabetes is not a coronary risk equivalent. See "Is diabetes a coronary risk equivalent? Systematic review and meta-analysis," by U. Bulugahapitiya, S. Siyambalapitiya, J. Sithole and I. Idris, *Diabetic Medicine*, Volume 26, Issue 2, pages 142-148. doi: 10.1111/j.1464-5491.2008.02640.x. Available online at http://www3.interscience.wiley.com/journal/121567674/abstract?CRETRY=1&SRETRY=0. Retrieved on 6/24/09. "This meta-analysis did not support the hypothesis that diabetes is a 'coronary heart disease equivalent.' Public health decisions to initiate cardio-protective drugs in patients with diabetes for primary CHD prevention should therefore be based on appropriate patients' CHD risk estimates rather than a 'blanket' approach of treatment."

[294] Uffe Ravnskov (born 1934) is a Danish independent researcher, a member of various international scientific organisations, and a former private medical practitioner in Sweden. In recent years he has gained international recognition for his research into numerous scientific studies, leading to the publication of a book which stated that the widely popularised Lipid Hypothesis is scientifically invalid.

He was born in Copenhagen, Denmark, and received his medical doctorate from the University of Copenhagen in 1961. Over the following seven years, he worked at various surgical, roentgenological, neurological, paediatric and medical departments in Denmark and Sweden. He then began scientific studies at the Departments of Nephrology and Clinical Chemistry at the Lund University Hospital in Lund, Sweden. He was awarded his doctorate of philosophy (specialising in internal medicine and nephrology) there in 1973, and was assistant professor at the university's Department of Nephrology from 1975 to 1979.

Dr Ravnskov entered private medical practice as a specialist in internal medicine and nephrology in 1979, and worked in Lund in this capacity and as a family doctor until retiring in 2000. Since 1979, he has worked as an independent scientific researcher and since 2000, continues to do so on a full-time basis.

While not the first scientific researcher to question the validity of the Lipid Hypothesis (which has become increasingly fashionable in corporate, media and certain medical circles in many countries due to the work of doctors such as Ancel Keys in the 1950s), when this came to be promoted strongly in Sweden Dr Ravnskov felt there was an incongruity between the Diet-Heart Idea and scientific literature he could recall.

He began to collect and examine the data from past scientific studies, and discovered sufficient evidence to enable him to assert that the scientific foundations of the Diet-Heart Idea were scientifically flawed, and thus the Lipid Hypothesis had no validity. The amount of conflicting statements he had assembled on the topic made him realise an entire book was necessary to publicly question all the "inaccuracies, misinterpretations, exaggerations and misleading quotations in this research area." His book *Kolesterolmyten* ("The Cholesterol Myths") was subsequently published in Sweden in 1991 and in Finland in 1992. It received adverse attention from the local media when they consulted the researchers and health authorities that it criticised; in the 2003 edition of the book, Ravnskov recalls how it was belittled in a television programme on Finland's Channel 2 television station and a copy of the book literally set on fire. Suppression of the work by media-generated ridicule and hysteria, rather than by scientifically valid refutation proved to be generally effective, and distribution of the book languished.

With the popularisation of the internet in the late 1990s, Dr Ravnskov saw the opportunity to inform the general public of his findings and, in 1997, published selected sections of *The Cholesterol Myths* on the world wide web. According to the search engine Direct Hit (since acquired by Ask.com in 1999), Ravnskov's website soon became ranked as one of the top ten most popular websites about cholesterol. As a result of this worldwide interest, his book was translated into English and published in the United States as *The Cholesterol Myths: Exposing the Fallacy that Saturated Fat and Cholesterol cause Heart Disease* in September, 2000, by a publishing house established by the head of the Weston A. Price Foundation, Sally Fallon. It was later published in Germany in 2002, under the title *Mythos Cholesterin. Die zehn größten Irrtümer* ("Cholesterol Myth: The Ten Biggest Errors").

Since 1990, Dr Ravnskov has published over 80 scientific papers critical of the Diet-Heart Idea, proposing new hypotheses and also showing that "the successful dissemination of the diet-heart idea is due to authors systematically ignoring or misquoting discordant (contradictory) studies." He was the first to suggest that the positive effect of the statins may be due to other effects than cholesterol-lowering (a view which Ravnskov notes has gained widespread acceptance). In a meta-analysis of cholesterol-lowering trials published in the *British Medical Journal* in 1992, he demonstrated that coronary mortality was not lowered by cholesterol lowering, but total mortality was increased.

In 2003 he published a review of the many studies that have shown low density lipoprotein (LDL) to be protective against infections, and put forward the hypothesis that high cholesterol, rather than promoting atherosclerosis, in fact may protect against it.

Dr Ravnskov continues to actively investigate scientific communications on cholesterol and heart disease for misinformation, and in the *British Medical Journal* in October, 2005, refuted statements contained in a July, 2005, paper on coronary heart disease in Poland, printed in the same journal.

In a 2005 interview with a representative from Health Myths Publishing, Dr Ravnskov was asked for his viewpoint on what causes heart disease, and remarked:

> "Most researchers today in this field agree that inflammation of the arterial wall is the start. The crucial question is, what starts the inflammation? As cholesterol has been demonized for so many years we have not been able to clear the blackboard and rethink... all studies of dead people have failed to show an association between their intake of saturated fat, or their serum cholesterol, and the degree of atherosclerosis. People who avoid all saturated fat and who have low cholesterol become just as atherosclerotic as people who gorge in animal food and whose cholesterol is high.

> Another misconception is that atherosclerosis is a disease. When arteries become inflamed the body immediately starts a repair process to strengthen the vascular wall. Smooth muscle cells

proliferate, fibrosis follows, and later, if necessary for further strength, cholesterol and calcium are used for reinforcement. This is in particular important in the coronary arteries because due to the steady movements of the heart and the negative pressure at their outside they have to be stronger than for instance arteries running to the intestines or inside bony channels. Inflammatory processes go on now and then already from childhood; it is a natural defence mechanism and atherosclerosis should therefore be considered as scars, remnants from a long life's combat with noxious chemicals or microorganisms…I think that the final attack is caused by microorganisms, but this is not the only answer. Any factor that weakens our immune defense may facilitate the growth of microorganisms, also at the inside of our vessels. These factors may be environmental (toxic compounds) or nutritional. There is much evidence that microorganisms may play a role. I published a review about this issue a few years ago. This paper has since long been one of the most-frequently read article in that journal."

Dr Ravnskov has received the Skrabanek Award in 1999 from Trinity College, Dublin, Ireland, for original contributions in the field of medical skepticism. He was also honoured with the Integrity In Science Award 2003 given by The Weston A. Price Foundation.

He is a member of the free panel of the Journal of the Swedish Medical Association (the medical journal *Läkartidningen*), the International Science Oversight Board, the International Society for the Study of Fatty Acids and Lipids, and is the spokesman for THINCS, The International Network of Cholesterol Skeptics. He resides in Lund, Sweden.

Biography courtesy of the Wikipedia article entitled "Uffe Ravnskov," available online at http://en.wikipedia.org/wiki/Uffe_Ravnskov. Retrieved on 4/29/09.

[295] McCully, Kilmer S. *The Heart Revolution: The Extraordinary Discovery That Finally Laid the Cholesterol Myth to Rest*. New York: Perennial, 1999, pages 10-11.

[296] See Uffe Ravnskov and Kilmer S. McCully, "Vulnerable Plaque Formation from Obstruction of *Vasa Vasorum* by Homocysteinylated and Oxidized Lipoprotein Aggregates Complexed with Microbial Remnants and LDL Autoantibodies," *Ann. Clin. Lab. Sci.*, Winter 2009; 39: 3 - 16. Available online at http://www.annclinlabsci.org/cgi/content/abstract/39/1/3. Retrieved on 4/29/09.

[297] Colpo, Anthony. *The Great Cholesterol Con: Why Everything You've Been Told About Cholesterol, Diet and Heart Disease is Wrong!* Distributed by Lulu, 2006, page 188.

[298] See Enig, Mary and Fallon, Sally. *Eat Fat Lose Fat*. New York: Plume, 2006, page 68. For the Ornish study, see Ornish D, Brown SE, Scherwitz LW, et al. "Can lifestyle changes reverse coronary heart disease? The Lifestyle Heart Trial." *Lancet*. 1990;336(8708):129-133.

[299] The wide variety of Sashimi is typically categorized as either Finfish, Shellfish, Roe, or Ascidians (sea squirts). Finfish include: Aji (Japanese jack mackerel), Aka-yagara (Cornetfish), Anago (Saltwater eel, Conger eel), Ankimo (Monkfish liver), Ayu (Sweetfish), Buri (Adult Yellowtail), Chūtoro (Medium-fat Bluefin tuna belly), Gindara (Sablefish), Hamachi (Young Yellowtail), Hamo (Daggertooth pike conger), Hatahata (Sandfish), Hikari-mono (Various kinds of "shiny" (silvery scales) fish, such as Mackerel), Hiramasa (Yellowtail amberjack (*Seriola lalandi*)), Hirame (Flounder), Hoshigarei (Spotted halibut), Ibodai (Japanese butterfish), Inada (Very young Yellowtail), Isaki (Striped pigfish), Ishigarei (Stone flounder), Iwashi (Sardine), Kajiki (Swordfish), Kanpachi (Greater amberjack, *Seriola dumerili*), Karei (Flatfish), Kasugo (young Sea bream), Katsuo (Skipjack tuna), Kawahagi (Filefish), Kibinago (Banded Blue sprat), Kihada (Yellowfin tuna), Kisu (Sillago), Kohada (Japanese gizzard Shad), Kurodai (Snapper), Maguro (top loin of Bluefin tuna), Makajiki (blue Marlin), Mamakari (Sprat), Masu (Trout), Meji (maguro, Young tuna), Mekajiki (Swordfish) Mutsu (Bluefish), Negi-toro (Bluefin tuna belly and chopped green onion), Nijimasu (Rainbow trout), Noresore (baby Anago), Ohyou (Halibut), Okoze (Stonefish), Ōtoro (Fattiest portion of Bluefin tuna belly), Saba (Chub mackerel or Blue mackerel), Sake (Salmon), Samma (Pacific saury or Mackerel pike), Sawara (Spanish mackerel), Sayori (Halfbeak (Springtime)), Seigo (young Sea bass), Shima-aji (White trevally), Shime-saba (Marinated Chub mackerel or Blue mackerel), Shira-uo (Salangid), Shiro maguro (Albacore or "white tuna"), Shiromi (Seasonal "white meat" fish), Suzuki (Sea bass), Tai (Red

sea bream, *Pagrus major*), Tara (Cod), Toro (fatty Bluefin tuna belly), Unagi (Freshwater eel, often broiled or grilled with a sweet sauce, so ask for it without the sauce if possible).

Shellfish include: Akagai (Ark shell), Ama-ebi (Raw Pink shrimp (*Pandalus borealis*)), Aoyagi (Round clam), Awabi (Abalone), Conch, Dungeness crab, Ebi (Boiled shrimp), Hamaguri (Clam, *Meretrix lusoria*), Himejako (Giant clam), Himo ("fringe" around an Akagai), Hokkigai (Surf clam), Hotategai (Scallop), Ika (Cuttlefish or Squid), Ise ebi (A Spiny lobster, *Panulirus japonicus*), Kaibashira (Valve muscles of Scallop or Shellfish), Kani (Crab, also refers to imitation crab), Kuruma-ebi (Prawn species *Penaeus japonicus*), Mategai (Razor clam), Matsubagani (Snow crab), Mirugai (Geoduck clam), Namako (Sea cucumber), Ni-ika (Squid simmered in a soy-flavored stock), Sazae (Horned turban shell), Shako (Mantis shrimp or "Squilla"), Shiba ebi (Grey prawn), Soft shell crab, Tairagai (Pen-shell clam), Tako (Octopus), Tarabagani (King crab), Torigai (Cockle), Tsubugai (Whelk (*Neptunea, Buccinum, Babylonia japonica*)).

Roe, a mass of fish eggs, include: Ikura (Salmon roe), Kazunoko (Herring roe), Masago (Smelt roe), Tarako (Alaska pollock roe), Tobiko (roe of Flying fish), Uni (Gonad of Sea urchin; different colors). Ascidians (sea squirts) include Hoya (Sea pineapple). For further information, see http://en.wikipedia.org/wiki/List_of_sushi_and_sashimi_ingredients_and_styles. Retrieved on 5/25/08.

[300] For a good comparison of fermented soy products such as tempeh, versus non-fermented soy products such as tofu, see the numerous articles on the "Soy index Page" hosted by Mercola.com at http://www.mercola.com/article/soy/index.htm. Retrieved on 7/25/08. Eating high levels of some soy products, such as tofu, could raise the risk of memory loss. A study that examined more than 700 elderly Indonesians found that high tofu consumption (at least once a day) was associated with worse memory, particularly among those over age 68. Soy contains phytoestrogens, which may heighten the risk of dementia. However, tempeh, a fermented soy product made from the whole soy bean, has been associated with better memory. This could be related to the fact that it contains high levels of the vitamin folate, which is known to reduce dementia risk. See "High Tofu Intake Is Associated with Worse Memory in Elderly Indonesian Men and Women," By Hogervorst E, Sadjimim T, Yesufu A, Kreager P, and Rahardjo TB. *Dement Geriatr Cogn Disord*. 2008 Jun 27;26(1):50-57. Op cit. Mercola.com. Available online at http://www.ncbi.nlm.nih.gov/sites/entrez?orig_db=PubMed&db=pubmed&cmd=Search&term=%22De mentia%20and%20geriatric%20cognitive%20disorders%22%5BJour%5D%20AND%202008%5Bpdat%5D% 20AND%20Hogervorst%5Bauthor%5D. Retrieved on 7/25/08.

[301] Notably absent from nearly every on- and off-line reference regarding sources of protein are insects. Entomophagy (the eating of insects) has yet to become a day-to-day activity for most people in the United States and Europe in spite of the superior nutritional content of edible insects compared to other animals. See "Insects as Human Food (Microlivestock)" by William F. Lyon, HYG-2160-96, Ohio State University Extension Fact Sheet, Entomology. Available online at http://ohioline.osu.edu/hyg-fact/2000/2160.html. Retrieved on 5/3/08. See also http://en.wikipedia.org/wiki/Entomophagy. Retrieved on 5/3/08.

[302] The effect of eating asparagus on one's urine has long been known. Certain constituents of asparagus are metabolized giving urine a distinctive smell due to various sulfur-containing degradation products, including various thiols, thioesters, and ammonia. Derivatives of asparagusic acid are also found in urine. The speed of onset of urine smell has been estimated to occur within 15-30 minutes of ingestion. All individuals produce the odorous compounds after eating asparagus, but only about 40% of the population have the autosomal genes required to smell them. See http://en.wikipedia.org/wiki/Asparagus. Retrieved on 4/27/08.

[303] Thomas Stearns Eliot, OM (Order of Merit) (26 September 1888–4 January 1965), was a poet, playwright and literary critic. He received the Nobel Prize in Literature in 1948. Among his most famous writings are the poems *The Love Song of J. Alfred Prufrock*, *The Waste Land*, *The Hollow Men*, *Ash Wednesday* and *Four Quartets*; the plays *Murder in the Cathedral* and *The Cocktail Party*; and the essay "Tradition and the Individual Talent."

Eliot was born in the United States, moved to the United Kingdom in 1914 (at age 25), and became a British subject in 1927 at the age of 39. Of his nationality and its role in his work, Eliot said: "My poetry wouldn't be what it is if I'd been born in England, and it wouldn't be what it is if I'd stayed in America. It's a combination of things. But in its sources, in its emotional springs, it comes from America."

Little Gidding is the fourth and final poem of T. S. Eliot's *Four Quartets*. It was first published in September, 1942, after being delayed for over a year because of the air-raids on Great Britain and Eliot's declining health. The title refers to a small Anglican community in Huntingdonshire, established by Nicholas Ferrar in the 17th century and scattered during the English Civil War.

The poem uses the image of fire and Pentecostal fire to emphasize the need for purification and purgation. Humanity's flawed understanding of life and turning away from God leads to a cycle of warfare, but this can be overcome when mankind is able to recognize the lessons of the past. Within the poem, the narrator meets a ghost that is a combination of various poets and literary figures that represents how the past, present, and future are really merged together and that understanding this truth is the way to salvation.

Biography and synopsis abridged from the Wikipedia articles entitled "T. S. Eliot," and "Little Gidding (poem)," available online at http://en.wikipedia.org/wiki/Ts_eliot and http://en.wikipedia.org/wiki/Little_Gidding_(poem), respectively. Retrieved on 5/12/09.

[304] See the article "Insulin and its Metabolic Effects," by Dr. Ron Rosedale, presented at Designs for Health Institute's BoulderFest, August 1999 Seminar, available online at http://articles.mercola.com/sites/articles/archive/2001/07/14/insulin-part-one.aspx. Retrieved on 6/19/08.

[305] The current methodology for those "naïve to treatment," and "treated patients," is part of an entire "Road Map to Achieve Glycemic Goals" based upon HbA$_{1c}$ levels of type 2 diabetics as positioned by the American Association of Clinical Endocrinologists. See the American Association of Clinical Endocrinologists' homepage at http://www.aace.com/index.php. Retrieved on 4/24/08. In particular, see the roadmap at http://www.aace.com/pub/roadmap/. Retrieved on 4/24/08.

[306] The *Physicians' Desk Reference* (*PDR*) is a commercially published compilation of manufacturers' prescribing information on prescription drugs, updated annually. While designed to provide physicians with the full legally mandated information relevant to writing prescriptions, it is widely available in libraries and bookstores, widely used by other medical specialists, and in significant part valuable to consumers. It is financially supported in part by pharmaceutical manufacturing corporations which create drugs listed within its pages. For the online version, free for US medical professionals only, see http://www.pdr.net/login/Login.aspx. Retrieved on 4/25/08. For the free consumer drug and medical information site, see http://www.pdrhealth.com/home/home.aspx. Retrieved on 4/25/08.

[307] See the video "How Does Leptin Impact Your Level of Health?" by Dr. Ron Rosedale and Dr. Joseph Mercola on Youtube at http://www.youtube.com/watch?v=ZN8ptwaRm5Q. Retrieved on 6/25/08. The mammalian target of rapamycin, commonly known as mTOR, is a serine/threonine protein kinase that regulates cell growth, cell proliferation, cell motility, cell survival, protein synthesis, and transcription. mTOR inhibitors are already used in the treatment of transplant rejection. They are also beginning to be used in the treatment of cancer. mTOR inhibitors may also be useful for treating several age-associated diseases. Kaeberlein and colleagues have proposed the hypothesis that decreased TOR activity accounts for lifespan extension by caloric restriction. For further reading and references, see http://en.wikipedia.org/wiki/Mammalian_target_of_rapamycin. Retrieved on 4/25/08.

[308] In his book *Authentic Happiness*, Martin Seligman, one of the founders of Positive psychology, describes happiness as consisting of "positive emotions" and "positive activities." See http://en.wikipedia.org/wiki/Happiness. Retrieved on 5/30/08. Positive psychology is a recent branch of psychology that "studies the strengths and virtues that enable individuals and communities to thrive." Positive psychologists seek "to find and nurture genius and talent," and "to make normal life more fulfilling," not to cure mental illness. Several humanistic psychologists—such as Abraham Maslow, Carl Rogers, and Erich Fromm—developed successful theories and practices that involved human happiness, despite a lack of solid empirical evidence at the time behind their work, and especially that of their successors, who chose to emphasize phenomenology and individual case histories. Recently the theories

of human flourishing developed by these humanistic psychologists have found empirical support from studies by humanistic and positive psychologists, especially in the area of self-determination theory. Current empirical researchers in this sub-field include Martin Seligman, Ed Diener, Mihaly Csikszentmihalyi, C. R. Snyder, Christopher Peterson, Barbara Fredrickson, Donald Clifton, Albert Bandura, Shelley Taylor, Charles S. Carver, Michael F. Scheier, Daniel Gilbert, and Jonathan Haidt. See http://en.wikipedia.org/wiki/Positive_psychology. Retrieved on 5/30/08.

[309] The quote is from the conclusion of "Frederick G. Banting, Nobel Lecture, September 15, 1925," The Nobel Prize in Physiology or Medicine 1923. Accessed from Nobelprize.org at http://nobelprize.org/nobel_prizes/medicine/laureates/1923/banting-lecture.html. Accessed on December 29, 2007. The Nobel Prize in Physiology or Medicine in 1923 for the discovery of insulin was actually divided between Frederick G. Banting and John J. R. Macleod. The choice of this combination of Laureates has been much debated ever since the prize was awarded. Thus, for instance, Banting shared his part of the prize amount with his younger coworker Charles Best. See http://nobelprize.org/nobel_prizes/medicine/articles/lindsten/index.html. Retrieved on 12/29/07.

DILEMMAS

[310] The statements "This book is written..." and "shall continue to add footnotes..." and "I wrote this book..." are all from the first paragraph of the Preface to Dawkins, Richard. *The Blind Watchmaker: Why the Evidence of Evolution Reveals a Universe Without Design*. New York: W.W. Norton & Company, page XV. Of course, he was referring to "our own existence" and not an optimal solution to diabetes, however, the constructs fit so well in this book's context that I just had to use them.

[311] See Poundstone, William. *Prisoner's Dilemma; John Von Neumann, Game Theory, and the Puzzle of the Bomb*. New York: Doubleday, 1992, pages 117-119. The entire prisoner's dilemma discussion is Copyright © 1992 William Poundstone.

[312] For a particularly good discussion of Plato's *The Republic* and the role of doctors, see Terence Irwin's *Plato's Ethics* (Oxford University Press, 1995, pages 351-352). "Does Plato expect anything more from people with wisdom than he would expect from them if they simply had correct belief? In some striking and important passages of the Laws, Plato makes it clear that he expects them to display one distinguishing feature of knowledge in contrast to belief. They must understand why the things they are told are right and good really are right and good; they must not simply take other people's word for it. To explain this demand, Plato introduces a comparison with doctors. On the one hand, the slave doctor, who also gives treatment to slaves, just gives instructions without giving any reason for them. The free doctor, on the other hand, who treats free people, explains why the treatment prescribed is the best one for the patients. Instead of simply giving orders, the free doctor discusses the patients' conditions with them and tells them enough to persuade them that the treatment being prescribed is the best one for them (719e7-720e5 in *The Republic*). This discussion involves communicating some theoretical understanding to the patient..."

[313] Stell, L Two cheers for physicians' conflicts of interest. *Mt Sinai J Med* 2004;71,236-242. Available online at http://www.ncbi.nlm.nih.gov/pubmed/15365589?dopt=Abstract. Retrieved on 3/14/09.

[314] McDowell, TJ Physician self referral arrangements: legitimate business or unethical "entrepreneurialism." *Am J Law Med* 1989;15,61-109. Available online at http://www.ncbi.nlm.nih.gov/pubmed/2764015?dopt=Abstract. Retrieved on 3/14/09.

[315] Moore, N Entrepreneurial doctors and lawyers: regulating business activity in the medical and legal professions. Spece, R Shimm, D Buchanan, A eds. *Conflicts of interest in clinical practice and research* 1996,171-196, New York, NY: Oxford University Press.

[316] Kouri, B, Parsons, R, Alpert, H Physician self-referral for diagnostic imaging: review of the empiric literature. *AJR Am J Roentgenol* 2002;179,843-850. Available online at

Notes

http://www.ajronline.org/cgi/content/full/179/4/843?ijkey=9700ac1ab1459c8a27e2b9a0084d5137b80d8ec2&keytype 2=tf_ipsecsha. Retrieved on 3/14/09. See also Mitchell, J, Sass, T Physician ownership of ancillary services: indirect demand inducement or quality assurance? *J Health Econ* 1995;14,263-289. Available online at http://www.ncbi.nlm.nih.gov/pubmed/10145136?dopt=Abstract. Retrieved on 3/14/09. See also Nallamothu, B, Rogers, M, Chernew, M, et al Opening of specialty cardiac hospitals and use of coronary revascularization in Medicare beneficiaries. *JAMA* 2007;297,962-968. Available online at http://jama.ama-assn.org/cgi/content/abstract/297/9/962?ijkey=bfc824f70f476933c2c4d63f1fa858999211ce44&keytype2=tf_ipsecsha. Retrieved on 3/14/09.

[317] See Tonelli, M.D., M.A., FCCP, Mark R. "Conflict of Interest in Clinical Practice," *Chest* August, 2007, vol. 132, no. 2, 664-670. doi: 10.1378/chest.07-0315. Available online at http://www.chestjournal.org/content/132/2/664.full#ref-21. Retrieved on 3/14/09.

[318] Angell, M *The truth about drug companies*. 2004 Random House. New York, NY. See also Kassirer, J *On the take: how medicine's complicity with big business can endanger your health*. 2004 Oxford University Press. New York, NY. See also Blumenthal, D Doctors and drug companies. *N Engl J Med* 2004;351,1885-1890. Available online at http://content.nejm.org/cgi/content/full/351/18/1885?ijkey=0423b68ab05b7d39ec9e9bbd72d1f905e82f10 da&keytype2=tf_ipsecsha. Retrieved on 3/14/09. "Interactions between drug companies and doctors are pervasive. Relationships begin in medical school, continue during residency training, and persist throughout physicians' careers. The pervasiveness of these interactions results in part from a huge investment by the pharmaceutical industry in marketing. In 2002, the industry expended 33 percent of its revenues on "selling and administration." In 2001, one company, Novartis, reported spending 36 percent of its revenues on marketing alone. The marketing expenditures of the drug industry have been estimated variously at \$12 billion to \$15 billion yearly, or \$8,000 to \$15,000 per physician. In 2001, the industry's sales force of drug detailers, whose job is to meet individually with physicians and promote company products, numbered nearly 90,000 in the United States–1 salesperson for every 4.7 office-based physicians."

[319] Kassirer, J. *On the Take: How Medicine's Complicity with Big Business Can Endanger Your Health*. New York: Oxford University Press, 2004.

[320] Moynihan, R Who pays for the pizza? Redefining the relationships between doctors and drug companies: 1. Entanglement. *BMJ* 2003;326,1189-1192. Available online at http://www.bmj.com/cgi/content/full/326/7400/1189?ijkey=1d0ba84bbe6c5e26d9cc59d1ab5e10bef47b6 921&keytype2=tf_ipsecsha. Retrieved on 3/14/09.

[321] See Tonelli, M.D., M.A., FCCP, Mark R. "Conflict of Interest in Clinical Practice," *Chest* August, 2007, vol. 132, no. 2, 664-670. doi: 10.1378/chest.07-0315. Available online at http://www.chestjournal.org/content/132/2/664.full#ref-21. Retrieved on 3/14/09.

[322] See "A National Survey of Physician-Industry Relationship," Campbell EG, Gruen RL, Mountford J, Miller LG, Cleary PD, Blumenthal D. *N Engl J Med.* 2007 Apr 26;356(17):1742-50. Available online at http://content.nejm.org/cgi/content/full/356/17/1742. Retrieved on 3/14/09.

[323] See "Why do Doctors Use Treatments That Don't Work?" online at http://articles.mercola.com/sites/articles/archive/2004/03/13/doctor-treatments.aspx. Retrieved on 4/18/08. There are many more articles available on Dr. Mercola's website on point. See, for example, "Medical Research or Drug Company Secrets?" online at http://articles.mercola.com/sites/articles/archive/2002/11/20/drug-companies-part-nine.aspx; "The Doors Of Perception: Why Americans Will Believe Almost Anything," at http://articles.mercola.com/sites/articles/archive/2001/08/15/perception.aspx; "Drugs and Doctors May be the Leading Cause of Death in U.S." at http://articles.mercola.com/sites/articles/archive/2003/01/15/doctors-drugs-part-two.aspx; "Doctors Are The Third Leading Cause of Death in the US, Causing 250,000 Deaths Every Year," at http://articles.mercola.com/sites/articles/archive/2000/07/30/doctors-death-part-one.aspx; "Why Doctors Are 9,000 Times More Likely to Accidentally Kill You Than Gun Owners," at http://articles.mercola.com/sites/articles/archive/2000/05/14/doctor-accidents.aspx; and "Shame: A

Major Reason Why Most Medical Doctors Don't Change Their Views," at http://articles.mercola.com/sites/articles/archive/2002/03/30/doctors-shame.aspx. All online articles retrieved on 4/18/09.

[324] See Groves, Barry. *Trick and Treat: How 'Healthy Eating' is Making us Ill.* London, UK: Hammersmith Press Limited, 2008, pages 30-31. Used by permission

[325] For a compeling discussion from the point of view of a practicing medical doctor and ethicist, see Lantos, John D. *Do We Still Need Doctors: A Physician's Personal Account of Practicing Medicine Today.* New York: Routledge, 1997.

[326] See La Puma J, Szapary P, Maki KC. Physicians recommendations for and personal use of low-fat and low-carbohydrate diets. *Int J Obes Relat Metab Disord.* 2005;29:251–253. doi: 10.1038/sj.ijo.0802840. Available online at http://www.ncbi.nlm.nih.gov/pubmed/15534615. Retrieved on 7/29/09.

I am grateful to the authors Surender K Arora and Samy I McFarlane, as the quote comes from their article entitled: "The Case for Low Carbohydrate Diets in Diabetes Management," *Nutr Metab* (Lond). 2005; 2: 16. Published online 2005 July 14. doi: 10.1186/1743-7075-2-16. PMCID: PMC1188071. Available online at http://www.pubmedcentral.nih.gov/articlerender.fcgi?tool=pmcentrez&artid=1188071. Retrieved on 7/29/09.

[327] The subject of the film *A Beautiful Mind* was John Forbes Nash, Jr. Dr. Nash did not have diabetes, but he was the most notable of the schizophrenic patients treated in the Insulin Coma Unit at Trenton Psychiatric Hospital (TPH) in West Trenton, New Jersey, in 1961. An American mathematician and economist whose works in game theory, differential geometry, and partial differential equations provided insight into the forces that govern chance and events inside complex systems in daily life, his theories are still used today in market economics, computing, accounting and military theory. Serving as a Senior Research Mathematician at Princeton University during the later part of his life, he shared the 1994 Nobel Memorial Prize in Economic Sciences with game theorists Reinhard Selten and John Harsanyi.

In 1961, John was committed by Alicia and his sisters to Trenton State Hospital in New Jersey. There, he was subjected to insulin-coma therapy, which involved injecting the patient with large amounts of insulin to put them into a coma, often causing seizures. His colleagues in mathematics were outraged and wrote a letter to the hospital, urging the doctors to protect his mind for the good of humanity. He was discharged after six months of the insulin treatment and looked absolutely terrible to his family members.

Dr. Manfred Sakel, a Viennese psychiatrist, developed the technique of Insulin Coma Therapy (ICT) in 1928 and introduced it to the United States in 1936. Nondiabetic patients with schizophrenia and major depression were treated with ICT 5 days a week for 6 weeks.

The insulin unit at TPH treated 24 males and 24 females daily in separate wards. The initial dose of regular insulin was 10–20 units administered intramuscularly at 7:00 a.m. in the unit; the dose was increased by about 10 units per day to about 90–100 units until hypoglycemic coma developed. A team of trained nurses and physicians supervised the care of the patients, who rested on litters. In some patients, more than 100 units of insulin were needed to produce coma.

After 30–60 minutes of hypoglycemic coma, nurses reversed the condition by intragastric glucose solution or Karo syrup. Patients were carefully observed until cognitive, returned to their room, and then provided meals and snacks.

In her book *A Beautiful Mind*, Sylvia Nasar reports that Dr. Nash first showed the overt signs of schizophrenia in 1959 when he began to see encrypted messages in newspaper stories. He was teaching at the Massachusetts Institute of Technology and after a poorly presented lecture in March, he was involuntarily committed to the McLean Hospital, a private hospital for wealthy patients affiliated with the Harvard Medical School in Boston.

Notes

He received injections of chlorpromazine but the principal treatments offered were psychotherapy, group therapy, and counseling. After a stay of 50 days, he was released. In May, his wife gave birth to a son. He was not able to return to work, and for the next two years, in the grip of a persistent psychosis, he roamed Europe.

He underwent 6 weeks of insulin coma treatment. When he was released from the hospital, he was much improved. His thoughts were under control and he was able to once again work on a scientific paper. From July of 1961 to August 1962, he worked at Princeton.

His illness recurred and sadly, further treatment was refused. He spent the next decades as a shadowy figure on the Princeton University campus.

Why was Dr. Nash treated with ICT? In 1961, the options available for patients with schizophrenia were antipsychotic drugs, Electroconvulsive Therapy (ECT), insulin coma, and lobotomy. The optimal treatment was believed to be chlorpromazine, although many psychiatrists still looked to ECT for its benefits. When chlorpromazine failed, ECT was the realistic option. While most psychiatric hospitals had abandoned ICT, it had persisted at Trenton State Hospital, and it was a logical offering when these other treatments were refused. (Lobotomy was no longer a realistic option, having been replaced by antipsychotic drugs.)

For biographical information see the Wikipedia article entitled "John Forbes Nash, Jr." online at http://en.wikipedia.org/wiki/John_Forbes_Nash; see also http://nobelprize.org/nobel_prizes/economics/laureates/1994/nash-autobio.html. Both retrieved on 3/14/09. See also http://www.pbs.org/wgbh/amex/nash/filmmore/ps_ict.html. Retrieved on 3/1/09.

For information about IST, see Sakel M: *The Pharmacological Shock Treatment of Schizophrenia*. New York, Nervous and Mental Diseases Publishing Co., 1938. See also Sakel M: The Insulin Treatment of Schizophrenia. In *An Introduction to Physical Methods of Treatment in Psychiatry*. 1st edition. Sargent W, Slater E, Eds. Edinburgh, U.K., E. & S. Livingstone, 1944. See also Fink, M., Shaw, R., Gross, G., and F. S. Coleman. "Comparative study of chlorpromazine and insulin coma in the therapy of psychosis." *Journal of the American Medical Association*. 1958; 166:1846-50. See also Rinkel, M., and H. E. Himwich. *Insulin Treatment in Psychiatry*. New York: Philosophical Library, 1959.

See also Arthur Krosnick, MD, FACP, CDE, "Five Decades of Diabetes Patient Care: The Time of My Life," *Clinical Diabetes* 20:173-178, 2002.

And see Nasar S. *A Beautiful Mind*. New York: Simon & Schuster, 1961, pages 288-294.

[328] See "Guidelines and the Pharmaceutical Industry Relationships Between Authors of Clinical Practice," by Niteesh K. Choudhry, Henry Thomas Stelfox, and Allan S. Detsky. *JAMA*. 2002;287(5):612-617; doi: 10.1001/jama.287.5.612. Available online at http://jama.ama-assn.org/cgi/reprint/287/5/612.pdf. Retrieved on 6/13/09.

[329] "One hundred twenty CPGs were identified by our search strategy, of which 35 were excluded because a major North American or European society did not endorse the CPG and 38 were excluded because they were editorials about CPGs or comparisons of different CPGs. Therefore, 47 CPGs were initially included. Subsequently, 1 CPG was excluded because the authors could not be identified and 2 CPGs were excluded after the authors had been surveyed since these were evaluations of CPGs rather than actual CPGs. Therefore, 44 CPGs with 192 authors were included in the study.

Current addresses of 13 authors could not be located and 3 authors had died, resulting in a total of 176 potentially contactable authors. Of these, 107 authors (61%) responded representing 37 of the 44 CPGs included in our study. Therefore, 7 guidelines were not represented in our final sample. Despite this, all of the disease states that were initially included in our study protocol were still represented by at least 2 CPGs, with the exception of depression, for which there was only 1 CPG included in the sample and for which we received a response. Seven respondents refused to participate, all of whom were involved with different guidelines. Three of these 7 authors were from Europe, 2 were from the United States, and 2 were from Canada. This left 100 completed surveys, which form the basis of our results. Overall, the response rate was 57% of potentially contactable authors and 52% of all authors initially included in our sample. The distribution of sex and disease to which the guidelines pertained was similar for respondents and nonrespondents; however, the distribution of current country of residence was not. Sixty-three percent of authors currently residing in the United States did not respond whereas 29% of authors living in Canada did not respond (P=.001). Twenty-eight (26%) of 107 authors responded with a letter attached to their survey. These letters could be interpreted as being supportive (21%), neutral (57%), or critical (21%) of our study. Of the 100 authors who completed the first survey, 1 had died and 1 had moved and was unreachable, leaving 98 potentially contactable authors for the second survey. Of these, 82 (83%) responded. One of these authors refused to participate and 1 could not recall the nature of the disclosure process and, therefore, left the survey blank. Consequently, the response rate for the second survey was 82%." See *Ibid.*

330 See "Clinical Practice Guidelines. Management of Type 2 Diabetes Mellitus (4th Edition)," May, 2009. Malaysian Endocrine & Metabolic Society, Ministry of Health Malaysia, Academy of Medicine Malaysia, and Persatuan Diabetes Malaysia. Available online at http://www.diabetes.org.my/article.php?aid=590. Retrieved on 7/27/09.

331 Available online at http://www.diabetes.org/aboutus.jsp?WTLPromo=HEADER_aboutus&vms=302103524165. Retrieved on 7/28/09.

332 See the ADA 2008 Consolidated Financials online at http://www.diabetes.org/uedocuments/2008_ADA_ConsolidatedFinancialsFS_Final.pdf. Retrieved on 7/38/09.

333 See the American Diabetes Association "About Us" page online at http://www.diabetes.org/aboutus.jsp?WTLPromo=HEADER_aboutus&vms=302103523106. Retrieved on 7/28/09.

334 American Diabetes Association 2008-2011 Strategic Plan. Available online at http://www.diabetes.org/uedocuments/2008-2011ADAStrategicPlan.pdf. Retrieved on 7/28/09.

335 What limits the liver's capacity to convert amino acids to glucose? "Conversion of amino acids to glucose involves several metabolic processes; deamination or transamination, conversion of the released NH4+ to urea and finally synthesis of glucose from amino acid residues. The key to understanding the physiological limitation of glucose formation from amino acids lies in the large amount of energy required to fuel these processes. Energy in the sense used here means the hydrolysis of adenosinetriphosphate (ATP) to either AMP + PPi or ADP + Pi. Four ATP molecules are used to convert two NH4+ to urea and six more are required to convert the carbon skeletons of these amino acids to glucose. One ATP is also required to add a glucosyl group to a glycogen molecule so, you see, a lot of energy is used in this process. All cells and tissues are built up such that ATP levels are relatively stable. This is a basic prerequisite for life. Under gluconeogenesis the liver must rely upon aerobic metabolism to replace the ATP that is consumed. By definition this is an oxygen-dependent process. The "catch" is that the liver obtains most of its oxygen from the portal vein where the partial pressure of oxygen is rather low. This limits uptake of oxygen, limits ATP production and, therefore, the synthesis of glucose from amino acids. We have data about the total amount of oxygen supplied to the human liver. Calculations based on this (and assuming that all of this oxygen goes to support conversion of amino acids to glucose) suggest that the maximum capacity of hepatic glucose synthesis from amino acids lies around 400 grams/day. This is the equivalent of approximately 1600 kcal..." See "Rabbit Starvation: High Protein and High Fat Diets," by Professor Emeritus Robert S. Horn. Available online at http://www.medbio.info/Horn/PDF%20files/rabbit%20starvation.pdf. Retrieved on 12/16.09.

336 See "Standards of Medical Care in Diabetes—2006," *Diabetes Care*, January, 2006, vol. 29, no. suppl 1 s4-s42. Available online at http://care.diabetesjournals.org/content/29/suppl_1/s4.full. Retrieved on 7/27/09.

337 *Ibid.*

338 *Ibid.*

339 *Ibid.*

340 See "Standards of Medical Care in Diabetes—2007,"doi: 10.2337/dc07-S004. *Diabetes Care,* January, 2007, vol. 30, no. suppl 1 S4-S41. Available online at http://care.diabetesjournals.org/content/30/suppl_1/S4.full. Retrieved on 7/28/09.

341 See "Standards of Medical Care in Diabetes—2008," doi: 10.2337/dc08-S012. *Diabetes Care,* January, 2008, vol. 31, no. Supplement 1 S12-S54. Available online at http://care.diabetesjournals.org/content/31/Supplement_1/S12.full. Retrieved on 7/28/09.

342 *Ibid.*

343 *Ibid.*

344 *Ibid.*

345 *Ibid.*

346 Poundstone, William. *Prisoner's Dilem*ma: *John Von Neumann, Game Theory, and the Puzzle of the Bomb.* New York: Doubleday, 1992, page 278.

347 See "GAD Treatment and Insulin Secretion in Recent-Onset Type 1 Diabetes," by Johnny Ludvigsson, M.D., Ph.D., Maria Faresjö, Ph.D., Maria Hjorth, M.Sc., Stina Axelsson, M.Sc., Mikael Chéramy, M.Sc., Mikael Pihl, M.Sc., Outi Vaarala, M.D., Ph.D., Gun Forsander, M.D., Ph.D., Sten Ivarsson, M.D., Ph.D., Calle Johansson, M.D., Agne Lindh, M.D., Nils-Östen Nilsson, M.D., Jan Åman, M.D., Ph.D., Eva Örtqvist, M.D., Ph.D., Peter Zerhouni, M.Sc., and Rosaura Casas, Ph.D. *The New England Journal of Medicine,* Volume 359:1909-1920, October 30, 2008, Number 18. Available online at http://content.nejm.org/cgi/content/full/359/18/1909. Retrieved on 5/30/09. See also http://www.dvdc.org.au/. Retrieved on 5/30/09. See also http://www.jdrf.org.au/news/view/research-breakthrough-type-1-diabetes-vaccine-a-step-closer. Retrieved on 5/30/09.

EPILOGUE

348 Huxley, Professor T.H., "On the Reception of the Origin of Species," 1887. In Darwin, Francis. *The life and letters of Charles Darwin, including an autobiographical chapter.* London: John Murray. Volume 2, ed. 1887. Available online at http://darwin-online.org.uk/converted/published/1887_Letters_F1452/1887_Letters_F1452.2.html. Retrieved on 7/26/09.

"If T.H. Huxley (May 4, 1825 to June 29, 1895) is known at all, it is as "Darwin's bulldog." This self-imposed nickname recognizes the collegiate defense and enthusiastic offense—he undertook in support of the theory of evolution. In November of 1859, after reading the newly-published *Origin of Species,* he warned Charles Darwin that there would be mischief from anti-evolutionists, and that he himself, T.H. Huxley, was sharpening up his claws preparing to annihilate these creationist critics. He devoted himself for most of his career defending Darwinism and related notorious subversive subjects." See The Huxley File online at http://aleph0.clarku.edu/huxley/. Retrieved on 7/25/09.

[349] See Covey, Stephen R. *The 7 Habits of Highly Effective People with Diabetes.* Tarrytown, NY: Bayer Healthcare, LLC Diabetes Care, 2007, Habit No 2.

[350] For more information about the UN's Millennium Development Goals, see http://www.unmillenniumproject.org/goals/index.htm. Retrieved on 3/8/08.

[351] To see the online Resolution adopted by the General Assembly, [*without reference to a Main Committee (A/55/L.2)*], 55/2, United Nations Millennium Declaration, see http://www.un.org/millennium/declaration/ares552e.htm. Retrieved on 3/22/08.

[352] A common, often altruistic, theme amongst many is to be able to solve world hunger via some method that may produce more food. However, often missed is the relationship between poverty and hunger. Hunger is an effect of poverty and poverty is largely a political issue (While manifesting itself as an economic issue, conditions causing poverty are political and end up being economic.). People are hungry not due to lack of availability of food, but because people do not have the ability to purchase food and because distribution of food is not equitable. In addition, there is also a lot of politics influencing how food is produced, who it is produced by (and who benefits), and for what purposes the food is produced (such as exporting rather than for the hungry, feedstuff, etc.). See, for example, http://www.globalissues.org/TradeRelated/Poverty/Hunger/Solutions.asp. Of particular interest to a diabetic, is how to get the right food, i.e., less emphasis on carbohydrates, and more on essential proteins and fats, to the right people.

[353] A diverse committee of experts from around the world, convened at the request of the National Science Foundation (NSF), and announced 14 grand challenges for engineering in the 21st century that, if met, would improve how we live.

"Tremendous advances in quality of life have come from improved technology in areas such as farming and manufacturing," said committee member and GOOGLE co-founder Larry Page. "If we focus our effort on the important grand challenges of our age, we can hugely improve the future."

The panel, some of the most accomplished engineers and scientists of their generation, was established in 2006 and met several times to discuss and develop the list of challenges. Through an interactive Web site, the effort received worldwide input from prominent engineers and scientists, as well as from the general public, over a one-year period. The panel's conclusions were reviewed by more than 50 subject-matter experts.

The final choices fall into four themes that are essential for humanity to flourish: sustainability, health, reducing vulnerability and increasing joy of living. The committee did not attempt to include every important challenge, nor did it endorse particular approaches to meeting those selected. Rather than focusing on predictions or gee-whiz gadgets, the goal was to identify what needs to be done to help people and the planet thrive.

"We chose engineering challenges that we feel can, through creativity and commitment, be realistically met, most of them early in this century," said committee chair and former U.S. Secretary of Defense William J. Perry. "Some can be, and should be, achieved as soon as possible."

The National Science Foundation (NSF) is an independent federal agency that supports fundamental research and education across all fields of science and engineering, with an annual budget of $5.92 billion. NSF funds reach all 50 states through grants to over 1,700 universities and institutions. Each year, NSF receives about 42,000 competitive requests for funding, and makes over 10,000 new funding awards. The NSF also awards over $400 million in professional and service contracts yearly. The NSF website is http://www.nsf.gov/index.jsp. Retrieved on 3/4/08.

The National Academy of Engineering website is located at: http://www.nae.edu/nae/naehome.nsf. Retrieved on 3/4/08. The Grand Challenges site features a five-minute video overview of the project along with committee member interview excerpts.

Notes

[354] Although this meme is highly visible in nearly every industrialized nation, this challenge may be the least important of the 14 grand challenges.

"Claimed human-caused warming of the Earth to dangerous and unprecedented levels by human-related emissions of carbon dioxide is contradicted by a non-correlation of carbon dioxide levels with warming.

The Anthropogenic Global Warming Hypothesis states that sunlight radiation warms the Earth by being absorbed at its surface. Then some of the absorbed heat is reradiated into the atmosphere. Some gases in the atmosphere, called "greenhouse gases," absorb much of this heat, and then reradiate it, some toward the surface of the Earth, making the Earth warmer than it would be without a heat-absorbing atmosphere. The primary "greenhouse gases" by far is said to be carbon dioxide, with some hints about methane, ozone, and traces of halocarbons.

Many serious scientists cite evidence that it's the variations in solar output, solar distance and number of sunspots that are primarily responsible for temperature changes on Earth. This makes up the Solar Output Variation Hypothesis.

The predominant greenhouse gas is water vapor, not carbon dioxide. More water vapor also limits the day/night temperature range. This should not be construed as condoning wasteful use of hydrocarbon fuels. For the obvious economic reasons, not an unthreatening global warming, hydrocarbon fuels should be conserved or substituted when possible."

See "Climate Change Reexamined," by Joel M. Kauffman, Emeritus, Department of Chemistry & Biochemistry, University of the Sciences in Philadelphia, PA. Available online at http://www.scribd.com/doc/14299932/Climate-change-reexamined-joel-m. Retrieved on 5/15/09.

[355] Perhaps no one has influenced our knowledge of life on Earth as much as the English naturalist Charles Robert Darwin (1809-1882). His theory of evolution by natural selection, now the unifying theory of the life sciences, explained where all of the astonishingly diverse kinds of living things came from and how they became exquisitely adapted to their particular environments. His theory reconciled a host of diverse kinds of evidence such as the succession of fossil forms in the geological record, the geographical distribution of species, recapitulative appearances in embryology, homologous structures, vestigial organs and nesting taxonomic relationships. No other explanation before or since has made sense of these facts. In further works Darwin demonstrated that the difference between humans and other animals is one of degree not kind. In geology, zoology, taxonomy, botany, paleontology, philosophy, anthropology, psychology, literature and theology Darwin's writings produced profound reactions, many of which are still ongoing. Yet even without his evolutionary works, Darwin's accomplishments would be difficult to match. His brilliantly original work in geology, botany, biogeography, invertebrate zoology, psychology and scientific travel writing would still make him one of the most original and influential workers in the history of science. Darwin's writings are consequently of interest to an extremely wide variety of readers.

For more on Darwin, see *The Complete Work of Charles Darwin Online* (or *Darwin Online*) at http://darwin-online.org.uk/. The site contains over 79,000 pages of searchable text and 190,000 electronic images.

[356] To read the article "Nothing in Biology Makes Sense Except in the Light of Evolution," see http://www.pbs.org/wgbh/evolution/library/10/2/text_pop/l_102_01.html. Retrieved on 5/17/09.

[357] Theodosius Grygorovych Dobzhansky, also known as T. G. Dobzhansky, and sometimes Anglicized to Theodore Dobzhansky (Ukrainian—January 24, 1900 - December 18, 1975) was a noted geneticist and evolutionary biologist, and a central figure in the field of evolutionary biology for his work in shaping the unifying modern evolutionary synthesis. Dobzhansky was born in Ukraine (then part of Imperial Russia) and emigrated to the United States in 1927.

Dobzhansky was born on January 24, 1900 in Nemyriv, Ukraine (then in the Russian Empire). An only child, his father Grigory Dobzhansky was a mathematics teacher, and his mother was Sophia Voinarsky. In 1910 the family moved to Kiev, Ukraine. At high school, Dobzhansky collected butterflies and decided to become a biologist. In 1915, he met Victor Luchnik who convinced him to specialize in beetles instead.

Dobzhansky attended the University of Kiev between 1917 and 1921, where he then studied until 1924. He then moved to Leningrad, Russia, to study under Yuri Filipchenko, where a *Drosophila melanogaster* lab had been established.

In 1937 he published one of the major works of the modern evolutionary synthesis, the synthesis of evolutionary biology with genetics, entitled *Genetics and the Origin of Species*, which amongst other things defined evolution as "a change in the frequency of an allele within a gene pool." Dobzhansky's work was instrumental in spreading the idea that it is through mutations in genes that natural selection takes place. Also in 1937, he became a naturalized citizen of the United States. During this time he had a very public falling out with one of his *Drosophila* collaborators, Alfred Sturtevant, based primarily in professional competition.

Dobzhansky returned to Columbia University from 1940 to 1962. He was one of the signatories of the 1950 UNESCO statement *The Race Question*. He then moved to the Rockefeller Institute (shortly to become Rockefeller University) until his retirement in 1971.

On June 1, 1968 it was discovered that Dobzhansky was suffering from lymphocytic leukemia, a chronic form of leukemia, and given a few months to a few years to live. Natasha died of coronary thrombosis on February 22, 1969. In 1971 he retired but continued working as an emeritus professor, moving to the University of California, Davis where his student Francisco Jose Ayala was made assistant professor.

Meanwhile, he continued working and published a famous essay "Nothing in Biology Makes Sense Except in the Light of Evolution." A loyal defender of Darwinian evolution, Dobzhansky, according to Francisco J. Ayala "was a religious man." Dobzhansky himself spoke of God as creating through evolution, and considered himself a communicant of the Eastern Orthodox Church.

His leukemia became more serious in the summer of 1975; on November 11 he made a trip to San Jacinto, California where he died of heart failure on December 18. He was cremated and his ashes were scattered in the Californian wilderness.

Abridged biography courtesy of the Wikipedia article entitled "Theodosius Dobzhansky." Available online at http://en.wikipedia.org/wiki/Theodosius_Dobzhansky. Retrieved on 5/17/09.

[358] *American Biology Teacher*, volume 35, pages 125-129.

[359] Abridged description courtesy of the Wikipedia article entitled "Nothing in Biology Makes Sense Except in the Light of Evolution." Available online at http://en.wikipedia.org/wiki/Nothing_in_Biology_Makes_Sense_Except_in_the_Light_of_Evolution. Retrieved on 5/17/09.

[360] "Why Are People?" is the title of the first chapter of Richard Dawkin's book *The Selfish Gene* (New York: Oxford University Press, 30th Anniversary edition, 2006).

[361] Dawkins, Richard. *The Ancestor's Tale: A Pilgrimage to the Dawn of Evolution*. New York: Houghton Mifflin Company, 2005, page 7.

[362] *Ibid*, page 530.

[363] *Ibid*.

[364] Masur K, Thévenod F, Zänker KS (eds): Diabetes and Cancer. Epidemiological Evidence and Molecular Links. *Frontiers in Diabetes*. Basel; Karger, 2008, Vol 19, page 50.

[365] *Ibid*, page 51.

[366] *Ibid*, page 44.

Notes

367 Calle EE, Kaaks R (2004) Overweight, obesity and cancer: epidemiological evidence and proposed mechanisms. *Nature Reviews: Cancer* 4(8): 579-91. Op cit. Smyth D, and Smyth T., "The Relationship Between Diabetes and Cancer," *Journal of Diabetes Nursing*, July-August, 2005. Available online at http://findarticles.com/p/articles/mi_m0MDR/is_7_9/ai_n15727529/?tag=content;col1. Retrieved on 5/20/09.

368 Shi R, Yu H, McLarty, J, Glass J (2004) IGF-I and breast cancer: a meta-analysis. *International Journal of Cancer* 111(3): 418-23. Op cit. Smyth D, and Smyth T. (2005).

369 Stattin P, Rinaldi S, Biessy C, Stenman UH, Hallmans G, Kaaks R (2004) High levels of circulating insulin-like growth factor-1 increase prostate cancer risk: a prospective study in a population-based nonscreened cohort. *Journal of Clinical Oncology* 22(15): 3104-12. Op cit. Smyth D, and Smyth T. (2005).

370 Richardson LC, Pollack LA (2005) Therapy Insight: influence of type 2 diabetes on the development, treatment and outcomes of cancer. *Nature Clinical Practice Oncology* 2(1): 48-53. Op cit. Smyth D, and Smyth T. (2005).

371 Anderson KE, Anderson E, Mink PJ, Hong CP, Kushi LH, Sellers TA et al (2001) Diabetes and endometrial cancer in the Iowa women's health study. *Cancer Epidemiology, Biomarkers & Prevention* 10(6): 611-6. Op cit. Smyth D, and Smyth T. (2005).

372 Michels KB, Solomon CG, Hu FB, Rosner BA, Hankinson SE, Colditz GA et al (2003) Type 2 diabetes and subsequent incidence of breast cancer in the Nurses' Health Study. *Diabetes Care* 26(6): 1752-8. Op cit. Smyth D, and Smyth T. (2005).

373 Khaw KT, Wareham N, Bingham S, Luben R, Welch A, Day N (2004) Preliminary communication: glycated hemoglobin, diabetes, and incident colorectal cancer in men and women: a prospective analysis from the European prospective investigation into cancer-Norfolk study. *Cancer Epidemiology, Biomarkers & Prevention* 13(6): 915-9. See also Jee SH, Ohrr H, Sull JW, Yun JE, Ji M, Samet JM (2005) Fasting serum glucose level and cancer risk in Korean men and women. *Journal of the American Medical Association* 293(2): 194-202. Op cit. Smyth D, and Smyth T. (2005).

374 Jee SH, Ohrr H, Sull JW, Yun JE, Ji M, Samet JM (2005) Fasting serum glucose level and cancer risk in Korean men and women. *Journal of the American Medical Association* 293(2): 194-202. Op cit. Smyth D, and Smyth T. (2005).

375 Khaw KT, Wareham N, Bingham S, Luben R, Welch A, Day N (2004) Preliminary communication: glycated hemoglobin, diabetes, and incident colorectal cancer in men and women: a prospective analysis from the European prospective investigation into cancer-Norfolk study. *Cancer Epidemiology, Biomarkers & Prevention* 13(6): 915-9. Op cit. Smyth D, and Smyth T. (2005).

376 National Cancer Institute: Diabetes increases men's risk of liver, pancreatic cancer, study finds. *NCI Cancer Bulletin.* NCI, Bethesda, MD. Available online at http://www.cancer.gov/NCICancerBulletin/NCI_Cancer_Bulletin_102604/page4. Retrieved on 5/20/09. Op cit. Smyth D, and Smyth T. (2005).

377 Yang YX, Hennessy S, Lewis JD (2004) Insulin therapy and colorectal cancer risk among type 2 diabetes mellitus patients. *Gastroenterology* 127(4): 1044-50. Op cit. Smyth D, and Smyth T. (2005).

378 Having diabetes when given a cancer diagnosis increases the risk of death by 41%, researchers here said. That finding comes from the first systematic assessment of long-term, all-cause mortality in newly diagnosed cancer patients with or without diabetes, according to Frederick Brancati, M.D., and colleagues at Johns Hopkins University.

All told, they found 48 articles that evaluated the effect of pre-existing diabetes on cancer outcome, including 23 that could be combined in a meta-analysis.

Possible explanations include interactions between the two disease types, treatment effects, poorer response to therapy, and sub-optimal cancer screening that leads diabetic patients to be diagnosed later, the researchers said.

It's even possible that the observed increase in risk of death is just a result of the effect of diabetes on cardiovascular health and has nothing to do with cancer at all, Dr. Brancati and colleagues said.

See the online article "Diabetes Increases Cancer Death Risk," By Michael Smith, North American Correspondent, *MedPage Today*, Published: December 16, 2008. Reviewed by Dori F. Zaleznik, MD; Associate Clinical Professor of Medicine, Harvard Medical School, Boston. Available online at http://www.medpagetoday.com/Endocrinology/Diabetes/12177. Retrieved on 5/24/09.

The above source comments on the original article by Barone BB, et al., "Long-term all-cause mortality in cancer patients with preexisting diabetes mellitus: a systematic review and meta-analysis," *JAMA* 2008; 300(23): 2754-2764. Available online at http://jama.ama-assn.org/cgi/content/short/300/23/2754. Retrieved on 5/24/09.

[379] The authors performed a prospective cohort study using data from the Second National Health and Nutrition Examination Survey and the Second National Health and Nutrition Examination Survey Mortality Study to determine this relation.

This analysis focused upon a nationally representative sample of 3,054 adults aged 30-74 years who underwent an oral glucose tolerance test at baseline (1976-1980). Deaths were identified by searching national mortality files through 1992. Adults were classified as having either previously diagnosed diabetes (n = 247), undiagnosed diabetes (n = 180), impaired glucose tolerance (n = 477), or normal glucose tolerance (n = 2250). There were 195 cancer deaths during 40,024 person-years of follow-up. Compared with those having normal glucose tolerance, adults with impaired glucose tolerance had the greatest adjusted relative hazard of cancer mortality (relative hazard = 1.87, 95% confidence interval (CI): 1.06, 3.31), followed by those with undiagnosed diabetes (relative hazard = 1.31, 95% CI: 0.48, 3.56) and diabetes (relative hazard = 1.13, 95% CI: 0.49, 2.62).

See "Abnormal glucose tolerance and the risk of cancer death in the United States," by Saydah SH, Loria CM, Eberhardt MS, Brancati FL. *Am J Epidemiol.* 2003 Jun 15;157(12):1092-100. Available online at http://www.ncbi.nlm.nih.gov/pubmed/12796045?ordinalpos=87&itool=EntrezSystem2.PEntrez.Pubmed. Pubmed_ResultsPanel.Pubmed_DefaultReportPanel.Pubmed_RVDocSum. Retrieved on 5/20/09.

[380] Coughlin SS, Calle EE, Teras LR, Petrelli J, Thun M, "Diabetes Mellitus as a Predictor of Cancer Mortality in a Large Cohort of US Adults," *Am J Epidemiol,* 2004;159:1160-1167. Available online at http://aje.oxfordjournals.org/cgi/content/full/159/12/1160. Retrieved on 5/20/09.

[381] See "Prospective Study of Hyperglycemia and Cancer Risk," by Pär Stattin, MD, PHD, Ove Björ, BSC, Pietro Ferrari, BSC, Annekatrin Lukanova, MD, PHD, Per Lenner, MD, PHD, Bernt Lindahl, MD, PHD, Göran Hallmans, MD, PHD and Rudolf Kaaks, PHD. *Diabetes Care,* March, 2007, vol. 30, no. 3, 561-567. doi: 10.2337/dc06-0922. Available online at http://care.diabetesjournals.org/content/30/3/561.full. Retrieved on 5/20/09.

[382] See http://www.cancer.gov/cancertopics/what-is-cancer. Retrieved on 5/23/09.

[383] Abridged from the Wikipedia article entitled "Cancer," available online at http://en.wikipedia.org/wiki/Cancer. Retrieved on 6/08/09.

[384] Darwin, Charles. *On the Origin of Species by Means of Natural Selection,* or *The Preservation of Favoured Races in the Struggle for Life.* London: John Murray, Albemarle Street, 1859. In *Darwin: The Indelible Stamp. Four Essential Volumes in One.* Edited, with commentary, by James D. Watson. Philadelphia: Running Press, 2005, page 600. Please note that this is not a first edition quote, as preferred by more scholarly writers, but the gist of the message is just as clear in any edition.

385 I had originally written "…at a level much higher than the individual," however, after further reading, most notably, Richard Dawkins's *Unweaving the Rainbow*, I came to realize that evolution, whether through domestication, sexual selection, or natural selection, unfolds gradually from the level of the individual. Being American, most of my knowledge was shaped by the American-based writer Stephen Jay Gould. "Ironically, Gould is one of the few Darwinians who still think of natural selection as working at levels higher than the individual organism." See Dawkins, Richard. *Unweaving the Rainbow*. Boston & New York: A Mariner Book, Houghton Mifflin Company, 1998, p. 199.

For two great, recent overviews of the *fact* of evolution, see Dawkins, Richard. *The Greatest Show on Earth: The Evidence for Evolution*. New York: Free Press, 2009; and Coyne, Jerry A. *Why Evolution is True*. New York: Viking, the Penguin Group, 2009. According to Coyne, "Life on Earth evolved gradually beginning with one primitive species—perhaps a self-replicating molecule—that lived more than 3.5 billions years ago; it then branched out over time, throwing off many new and diverse species; and the mechanism for most (but not all) of evolutionary change is natural selection." (Page 3)

386 For a good discussion of arms races, manipulation, and descriptions of the five different types of fitness, see the chapters entitled "Arms Races and Manipulation," and "An Agony in Five Fits," in Dawkins, Richard. *The Extended Phenotype: The Long Reach of the Gene*. New York: Oxford University Press, 2008.

Note that all these concepts, namely, parasitism, symbiosis, conflict, cooperation, and co-evolution—which were developed with reference to whole organisms—are relevant to genes within an organism. See *Ibid*, page 178.

387 For a fascinating article detailing how cancer is not an "it" but a "they," see "Evolution of Cooperation Among Tumor Cells," by Robert Axelrod, David E. Axelrod, and Kenneth J. Pienta. Published online before print August 28, 2006, doi: 10.1073/pnas.0606053103. *Proceedings of the National Academy of Sciences of the United States of America (PNAS)*, September 5, 2006 vol. 103 no. 36 13474-13479. Available online at http://www.pnas.org/content/103/36/13474.full#sec-3. Retrieved on 5/21/09.

"…We marshal evidence that tumor cells overcome certain host defenses by means of diffusible products. Our original contribution is to raise the possibility that two nearby cells can protect each other from a set of host defenses that neither could survive alone. Cooperation can evolve as by-product mutualism among genetically diverse tumor cells. Our hypothesis supplements, but does not supplant, the traditional view of carcinogenesis in which one clonal population of cells develops all of the necessary genetic traits independently to form a tumor. Cooperation through the sharing of diffusible products raises new questions about tumorigenesis and has implications for understanding observed phenomena, designing new experiments, and developing new therapeutic approaches."

388 See The Wistar Institute (2006, November 17). Does Natural Selection Drive The Evolution Of Cancer? *ScienceDaily*. Available online at http://www.sciencedaily.com/releases/2006/11/061117114616.htm. Retrieved on 5/24/09.

389 For percentage breakdown by geography, see the Disease Control Priorities Project online at http://www.ncbi.nlm.nih.gov/books/bv.fcgi?rid=dcp2.table.4313. Retrieved on 5/31/09.

For actual numbers of diabetics worldwide, see the World Health Organization's diabetes pages online at http://www.who.int/diabetes/facts/world_figures/en/index.html. Retrieved on 5/31/09.

"The reasons for the uneven worldwide distribution of Type 1 diabetes mellitus have yet to be fully explained. Epidemiological studies have shown a higher prevalence of Type 1 diabetes in northern Europe, particularly in Scandinavian countries, and Sardinia. Recent animal research has uncovered the importance of the generation of elevated levels of glucose, glycerol and other sugar derivatives as a physiological means for cold adaptation. High concentrations of these substances depress the freezing point of body fluids and prevent the formation of ice crystals in cells through supercooling, thus acting as a cryoprotectant or antifreeze for vital organs as well as in their muscle tissue. In this paper, we hypothesize that factors predisposing to elevated levels of glucose, glycerol and other sugar derivatives may have been selected for, in part, as adaptive measures in exceedingly cold climates."

See "The sweet thing about Type 1 diabetes: a cryoprotective evolutionary adaptation," by Moalem S, Storey KB, Percy ME, Peros MC, Perl DP. *Med Hypotheses*, 2005;65(1):8-16. Available online at http://www.ncbi.nlm.nih.gov/sites/entrez?Db=pubmed&Cmd=ShowDetailView&TermToSearch=15893 109. Retrieved on 5/31/09.

[390] Over the last decade, an abundance of evidence has emerged demonstrating a close link between metabolism and immunity. It is now clear that obesity is associated with a state of chronic low-level inflammation. In the below cited article, the authors discuss the molecular and cellular underpinnings of obesity-induced inflammation and the signaling pathways at the intersection of metabolism and inflammation that contribute to diabetes. They also consider mechanisms through which the inflammatory response may be initiated and discuss the reasons for the inflammatory response in obesity. The authors put forth for consideration some hypotheses regarding important unanswered questions in the field and suggest a model for the integration of inflammatory and metabolic pathways in metabolic disease."

See "Inflammation, stress, and diabetes," by Kathryn E. Wellen and Gökhan S. Hotamisligil. *J. Clin. Invest.* 115(5): 1111-1119 (2005). doi: 10.1172/JCI25102. Available online at http://www.jci.org/articles/view/25102/version/1. Retrieved on 6/10/09.

[391] "...genes are named after the conditions and abnormalities that led to their discovery. This, inevitably, means that their name commemorates what happens when they *don't* work. The gene that triggers the development of eyes in fruit flies — discovered in 1915 — is called 'eyeless'." See Ings, Simon. *A Natural History of Seeing: The Art and Science of Vision*. New York: W.W. Norton & Company, 2008, p. 83.

Researchers have found nearly 20 different genes that can affect one's risk for developing diabetes. See GeneticHealth online at http://www.genetichealth.com/dbts_genetics_of_type_1_diabetes.shtml. Retrieved on 5/31/09.

There are hundreds, more, thousands of articles in the medical literature pertaining to the genetic associations with diabetes. Here I'll provide just two such recent articles that you may find interesting:

Regarding type 2 diabetes, see for example "Genetic Basis of Beta-Cell Dysfunction in Man," by Groop L and Lyssenko V. *Diabetes Obes Metab* 2009 Nov;11 Suppl 4():149-58. "Although the genetic causes of monogenic disorders have been successfully identified in the past, the success in dissecting the genetics of complex polygenic diseases has until now been limited. With the introduction of whole genome wide association studies (WGAS) in 2007, the picture has been dramatically changed. Today we know of about 20 genetic variants increasing the risk of type 2 diabetes (T2D). Most of them seem to influence the capacity of beta-cells to increase insulin secretion to meet the demands imposed by an increase in body weight and insulin resistance. This probably represents only the tip of the iceberg, and over the next few years refined tools will provide a more complete picture of the genetic complexity of T2D. This will not only include the current dissection of common variants increasing the susceptibility of the disease but also rare variants with stronger effects, copy number variations and epigenetic effects like DNA methylation and histone acetylation. For the first time, we can anticipate with some confidence that the genetics of a complex disease like T2D really can be dissected." Available online at http://www.ncbi.nlm.nih.gov/pubmed/19817797?itool=EntrezSystem2.PEntrez.Pubmed.Pubmed_Result sPanel.Pubmed_RVDocSum&ordinalpos=3. PMID: 19817797; doi: 10.1111/j.1463-1326.2009.01117.x. Retrieved on 12/8/09.

Regarding type 1 diabetes, see for example "Genetic Basis of Type 1 Diabetes: Similarities and Differences between East and West," by Ikegami H, Noso S, Babaya N, Hiromine Y, and Kawabata Y. *Rev Diabet Stud* 2008 Summer;5(2):64-72. "Type 1 diabetes is a multifactorial disease caused by a complex interaction of genetic and environmental factors. The genetic factors involved consist of multiple susceptibility genes, at least five of which, *HLA*, *INS*, *CTLA4*, *PTPN22* and *IL2RA/CD25*, have been shown to be associated with type 1 diabetes in Caucasian (Western) populations, as has recently been confirmed by genome-wide association studies. It has been proposed, however, that the contribution of these genes to type 1 diabetes susceptibility may be different in Asian (Eastern) populations." Available online at

http://www.ncbi.nlm.nih.gov/pmc/articles/PMC2556443/?tool=docline.   PMID: 18795209;   doi:
10.1900/RDS.2008.5.64. Retrieved on 12/8/09.

[392] The famous quotation describing life in the state of war of every man against every man: "...the life of
man, solitary, poor, nasty, brutish, and short," is from Chapter XIII "Of the Natural Condition of Mankind,
as concerning their Felicity, and Misery," from *Leviathan, The Matter, Forme and Power of a Common Wealth
Ecclesiasticall and Civil*, commonly called *Leviathan*, a book written by Thomas Hobbes which was
published in 1651. It is titled after the biblical Leviathan. The book concerns the structure of society and
legitimate government, and is regarded as one of the earliest and most influential examples of social
contract theory. Adapted from the Wikipedia article entitled "Leviathan (book)," available online at
http://en.wikipedia.org/wiki/Leviathan_(book). Retrieved on 5/30/09.

[393] See "Diabetes induced by Coxsackie virus: Initiation by bystander damage and not molecular mimicry,"
by Horwitz, et al. *Nature Medicine* 4, 781 - 785 (1998), doi: 10.1038/nm0798-781. Available online at
http://www.nature.com/nm/journal/v4/n7/abs/nm0798-781.html. Retrieved on 6/13/09. For the first
prospective study, see "A prospective study of the role of coxsackie B and other enterovirus infections in
the pathogenesis of IDDM. Childhood Diabetes in Finland (DiMe) Study Group," by Hyöty, et al. *Diabetes*
June, 1995, vol. 44, no. 6, 652-657.   doi: 10.2337/diabetes.44.6.652.   Available online at
http://diabetes.diabetesjournals.org/content/44/6/652.abstract. Retrieved on 6/13/09.

[394] See "Innate immunity and intestinal microbiota in the development of Type 1 diabetes," by Li Wen, et
al. *Nature*. 2008, October 23; 455(7216): 1109–1113. Published online, September 21.   doi:
10.1038/nature07336.   PMCID: PMC2574766; NIHMSID: NIHMS67288.   Available online at
http://www.pubmedcentral.nih.gov/articlerender.fcgi?artid=2574766. Retrieved on 6/13/09.

"Humans consist of about a trillion cells, but there are some 10 trillion bacterial cells on or in us at any
given time. Bacteria digest our food, make our vitamins, educate our immune system to keep harmful
antigens   out.   But   there   are   also   notorius   and   harmful   bacteria."   See
http://www.ted.com/talks/bonnie_bassler_on_how_bacteria_communicate.html. Retrieved on 6/10/09.

Bonnie Bassler discovered that bacteria "talk" to each other, using a chemical language that lets them
coordinate defense and mount attacks. The find has stunning implications for medicine and industry. See
http://www.molbio.princeton.edu/index.php?option=content&task=view&id=27. Retrieved on 6/10/09.

For more on quorum sensing see the Wikipedia article entitled "Quorum Sensing," online at
http://en.wikipedia.org/wiki/Quorum_sensing. Retrieved on 6/10/09.

[395] In summary, high serum selenium concentrations were associated with higher prevalence of diabetes in
a representative survey of US adults conducted in 2003-2004. These findings are consistent with an earlier
National Health and Nutrition Examination Survey (NHANES) survey conducted in 1988-1994. See
"Serum Selenium Concentrations and Diabetes in US Adults: National Health and Nutrition Examination
Survey (NHANES) 2003-2004," by Martin Laclaustra, Ana Navas-Acien, Saverio Stranges, Jose M Ordovas,
and Eliseo Guallar. *Environmental Health Perspectives*, doi: 10.1289/ehp.0900704. Aavailable online at
http://ehp.niehs.nih.gov/docs/2009/0900704/abstract.html. Retrieved on 6/23/09.

[396] American Diabetes Association; American Psychiatric Association; American Association of Clinical
Endocrinologists; North American Association for the Study of Obesity (February 2004). "Consensus
development conference on antipsychotic drugs and obesity and diabetes." *Diabetes Care* 27 (2): 596–601.
doi: 10.2337/diacare.27.2.596.   PMID   14747245.   Available   online   at
http://care.diabetesjournals.org/cgi/content/full/27/2/596. Retrieved on 6/13/09.

[397] See "Incident Diabetes and Pesticide Exposure among Licensed Pesticide Applicators: Agricultural
Health Study, 1993–2003," by M. P. Montgomery, F. Kamel, T. M. Saldana, M. C. R. Alavanja, and D. P.
Sandler. *American Journal of Epidemiology*, March 14, 2008. doi: 10.1093/aje/kwn028. Available online at
http://www.toxfree.net/chlordane/Education/Healthrisk/Applicators.pdf. Retrieved on 6/25/09.

"The authors' aim was to investigate the relation between lifetime exposure to specific agricultural pesticides and diabetes incidence among pesticide applicators. The study included 33,457 licensed applicators, predominantly non-Hispanic White males, enrolled in the Agricultural Health Study. Incident diabetes was self-reported in a 5-year follow-up interview (1999–2003), giving 1,176 diabetics and 30,611 nondiabetics for analysis. Lifetime exposure to pesticides and covariate information were reported by participants at enrollment (1993–1997). Using logistic regression, the authors considered two primary measures of pesticide exposure: ever use and cumulative lifetime days of use. They found seven specific pesticides (aldrin, chlordane, heptachlor, dichlorvos, trichlorfon, alachlor, and cyanazine) for which the odds of diabetes incidence increased with both ever use and cumulative days of use. Applicators who had used the organochlorine insecticides aldrin, chlordane, and heptachlor more than 100 lifetime days had 51%, 63%, and 94% increased odds of diabetes, respectively. The observed association of organochlorine and organophosphate insecticides with diabetes is consistent with results from previous human and animal studies. Long-term exposure from handling certain pesticides, in particular, organochlorine and organophosphate insecticides, may be associated with increased risk of diabetes.

This study is to our knowledge the largest study to evaluate the potential effects of pesticides on diabetes incidence in adults. The prospective design of the study ensures that exposures were reported prior to the diagnosis of diabetes and reduces the potential for recall bias. Of the 50 pesticides evaluated, seven displayed evidence suggesting an association with diabetes incidence in both ever-use and cumulative days-of-use models: aldrin, chlordane, heptachlor, dichlorvos, trichlorfon, alachlor, and cyanazine. It is noteworthy that all of these pesticides are chlorinated compounds, while only half of the pesticides investigated were chlorinated. Few studies, if any, have considered the potential diabetogenic effects of alachlor and cyanazine, which both showed a dose-response association with diabetes in the present study. However, the biologic plausibility of a diabetogenic effect of exposure to persistent organic pollutants (e.g., dioxins, polychlorinated biphenyls, and organochlorine insecticides) and organophosphate insecticides is supported by numerous studies."

See also "Treatment of Homes for Termites Decades Ago May Cause Diabetes Today," by Dr. Richard Cassidy, *DiabetesHealth*, Mar 13, 2009. Available online at http://www.diabeteshealth.com/read/2009/03/12/6117/treatment-of-homes-for-termites-decades-ago-may-cause-diabetes-today/. Retrieved on 6/25/09.

"Recently, the Centers for Disease Control mapped the incidence of diabetes by state. There is a striking correlation between the incidence of diabetes and the use of chlordane for termite control in these states. Southern states with the highest temperatures and humidity have not only the highest rates of termite infestations and chlordane use, but also the highest rate of diabetes. States from the midsection of the United States, with moderate temperatures and humidity and lower chlordane applications, have lower rates of diabetes. In northern states such as Minnesota, where chlordane was rarely used, the incidence of diabetes is less than 50 percent that of southern states."

Because of concern about damage to the environment and harm to human health, the United States Environmental Protection Agency (EPA) banned all uses of chlordane in 1983 except termite control. The EPA banned all uses of chlordane in 1988.

[398] See, for example, "Blood levels of alloxan in children with insulin-dependent diabetes mellitus," by A. Mrozikiewicz, D. Kielstrokczewska-Mrozikiewicz, Z. Lstrokowicki, E. Chmara, K. Korzeniowska and P. M. Mrozikiewicz. *Acta Diabetologica*, Volume 31, Number 4, December, 1994, pages 236-237. doi: 10.1007/BF00571958. Available online at http://www.springerlink.com/content/r001211h96j18266/. Retrieved on 6/08/09.

The mechanisms underlying alloxan and streptozotocin diabetes are a major research topic of the Institute of Clinical Biochemistry of Hannover Medical School. For the full list of publications addressing this topic, which can all be downloaded via PubMed, see http://www.mh-hannover.de/8750.html. Retrieved on 6/08/09.

[399] See "Diabetes mellitus and orthostatic hypotension resulting from ingestion of Vacor rat poison: endocrine and autonomic function studies," by K S Peters, T G Tong, K Kutz, and N L Benowitz. *West J*

Med. 1981 January; 134(1): 65–68. Available online at http://www.pubmedcentral.nih.gov/articlerender.fcgi?artid=1272465. Retrieved on 6/08/09.

[400] According to Nicholas P. Money, in *Mr. Bloomfield's Orchard*, "In England in 1960, 100,000 turkeys died following loss of appetite, lethargy, and liver failure. It was discovered that they had been fed aflatoxin-contaminated peanut meal, and the name turkey X-disease was coined for their plague...It is unlikely that turkeys, or any other animals, are the targets for aflatoxins in an evolutionary sense. It has been suggested that animals compete with fungi for the same food—harvested grain, for example—and that aflatoxins would reduce the number of these rivals. But I'm not convinced; other microorganisms are probably the "intended" victims. While fungi produce mycotoxins in minute quantities in the soil and in plant tissues, local concentrations may be high enough in the immediate vicinity of the growing hyphae to clear the territory for the mold." See Money, Nicholas P. *Mr. Bloomfield's Orchard: The Mysterious World of Mushrooms, Molds, and Mycologists.* New York: Oxford University Press, 2002, Page 162.

Regarding another mycotoxin, amatoxin, Dr. Money writes: "Insects and fungi have interacted with one another for 400 million years or more, an expanse of time that has offered ample opportunity for the evolution of defense and counter-defense mechanisms in both groups of organisms. If insect larvae are the real targets of amatoxins, then human casualties were "unintended" by evolution. In every sense, then, mushrooms couldn't care less about *Homo sapiens*." See page 156.

Interestingly, in this book he wrote about Curtis Gates Lloyd, one of Cincinnati's most eligible bachelors, and a millionaire obsessed with fungi. Mr. Lloyd became a self-taught expert in fungal identification and had undertaken the publication of his own mycological work. "Mr. Lloyd had suffered from diabetes for many years, and with little in the contemporary pharmacopia to prolong his life, he died of complications from the disease in 1926." See page 102.

See also Money, Nicholas P. *Carpet Monsters and Killer Spores: A Natural history of Toxic Mold.* New York: Oxford University Press, 2004.

"Fungi never intended to inflame or poison humans. After all, black molds spent hundreds of millions of years rotting dead plants before the evolution of wheezing authors and bleeding babies. Their spores were designed for drifting in air, not for swimming in lung mucous, so problems with molds are rooted in our insistence on breathing rather than any microbial malevolence." See page 58.

"Fungi produce hundreds of different kinds of toxins, a few of proven harm to humans, most of dubious significance. Everyone is familiar with poisonous mushrooms. A single fruiting body of a death cap or a destroying angel contains a few thousandths of a gram of amatoxins, which is adequate to kill an adult. Amatoxins are peptides that block protein synthesis in cells. The reason that the mushroom accumulates these poisonous molecules is unclear, but the most satisfying answer is that they defend the fruiting body against insect grubs." See page 59.

[401] See The *Garden of Eden Longevity Diet Antifungal/Antimycotoxin,Anti-Cancer, Anti-Atherosclerosis*; see also *The Fungal/Mycotoxin Etiology of Breast Cancer Foods That Cause & Foods that Prevent*; see also *The Fungal/Mycotoxin Etiology of Prostate Cancer Foods That Cause & Foods That Prevent*; and *The Fungal/Mycotoxin Etiology of Atherosclerosis Foods That Cause & Foods that Prevent* all written by A.V. Costantini, M.D., H. Wieland, M.D., and Lars Qvick, M.D. For excerpts, see http://www.fungalbionicbookseries.com/index.htm. Retrieved on 6/08/09.

In describing the strength of mycotoxins, the above authors wrote the following:

"As many as 1,000 compounds, classifiable as mycotoxins, were studied by the pharmacology industry as potential antibiotics in the 1930s and 1940s only to be discarded as being too toxic for higher life forms to be of value in treating bacterial diseases in humans. Little, if any of the discarded data was published. Yet what these toxicity studies actually documented was the existence of a large number of fungal-derived toxins which caused serious target organ injury in various animal models. Obviously, in retrospect, what was being seen was the pathology produced by the mycotoxins. In order to understand this toxicity, one only has to look at what some of these mycotoxins, used as medications, causes in humans: The mycotoxin cyclosporin used for transplantation causes cancer and atherosclerosis, complete with hyperlipidemia, in ALL humans who have received it. Many others develop gout and other diseases."

Prof. Dr. A.V. Costantini, MD was the keynote speaker at the 1993 conference of the American Academy of Environmental Medicine held in Reno, Nevada, where he stated the following:

"Auto-immune diseases are characterized by the finding of so-called auto-antibodies. It is a most popular concept but biologically fatally defective in that no species of life can make an antibody against itself; particularly causing fatal disease such as scleroderma. Scleroderma is considered to prove the validity of the auto-immune concept with the presence of auto-antibodies. However these are now documented to be antibodies against ubiquitin which is present in many species including fungi. Scleroderma responds well to the antifungal agent griseofulvin. Against whose ubiquitin is the host raising antibodies to, its own, or fungal-derived, in a disease state which responds to an antifungal drug? The auto-immune diseases appearing to have a fungal and mycotoxin origin are: scleroderma, diabetes mellitus, HLA-related disease, rheumatoid arthritis, Sjogren's syndrome, psoriasis & systemic lupus erythematosus. All of the drugs effective in the treatment of these diseases possess antifungal or anti-mycotoxin activity. This includes all NSAIDs [Non-Steroidal Anti-Inflammatory Drugs]."

From the Chesser-Naugle International Lectureship Grant: The Fungal/Mycotoxin Connections: Autoimmune Diseases, Malignancies, Atherosclerosis, Hyperllpldemias, and Gout, October 11, 1993. Twenty-eighth annual meeting entitled "New horizons in Chemical Sensitivities: State of the Art Diagnosis and Treatment. Available online at http://www.arthritistrust.org/Articles/Fungal-Mycotoxin%20Connection/index.htm. Retrieved on 6/08/09.

[402] See Kaufmann, Doug and Holland, David. *The Fungus Link to Diabetes: A Cutting-Edge Approach to Stopping One of America's Fastest Growing Epidemics in Its Tracks.* Rockwall, Texas: MediaTrition, Inc., 2003.

[403] See Maas, Laurens. *The Hidden Cure: The Five Laws of Perfect Health.* Wheatmark: Tuscan, Arizona, 2009.

[404] The most outraged and formidable opponent of Charles Darwin was Richard Owen, Hunterian Professor at the Royal College of Surgeons, who examined the fossil bones Darwin had had brought back from South America. Owen acted largely behind the scenes, and was the one who provided material for Bishop Wilberforce's scathing review in the *Quarterly Review*, where Wilberforce referred to Darwin's ideas as "his utterly rotten fabric of guess and speculation." See "Commentary: On the Origin of Species," in *Darwin: The Indelible Stamp. Four Essential Volumes in One.* Edited, with commentary, by James D. Watson. Philadelphia: Running Press, 2005, page 342.

The four volumes include: *The Voyage of the Beagle* (no publication information given); *On the Origin of Species by Means of Natural Selection* (London: John Murray, Albemarle Street, 1859); *The Descent of Man, and Selection in Relation to Sex* (Second Edition, London: John Murray, Albemarle Street, 1882); and *The Expression of the Emotions in Man and Animals* (London: John Murray, Albemarle Street, 1872).

The Voyage of the Beagle is a title commonly given to the book written by Charles Darwin published in 1839 as his *Journal and Remarks*, which brought him considerable fame and respect. The title refers to the second survey expedition of the ship HMS *Beagle*, which set sail from Plymouth Sound on December 27, 1831, under the command of captain Robert FitzRoy.

[405] Appendix C contains scores of low-carbohydrate, ketogenic diet articles, including several on point to ketogenic diet and cancer. See for example:

- Implementing a ketogenic diet based on medium-chain triglyceride oil in pediatric patients with cancer. Nebeling LC, Lerner E., *J Am Diet Assoc.* 1995 Jun;95(6):693-7. Available online at http://www.ncbi.nlm.nih.gov/pubmed/7759747. Retrieved on 5/27/09.

- Effects of a ketogenic diet on tumor metabolism and nutritional status in pediatric oncology patients: two case reports. Nebeling LC, Miraldi F, Shurin SB, Lerner E., *J Am Coll Nutr.* 1995 Apr;14(2):202-8. Available online at http://www.ncbi.nlm.nih.gov/pubmed/7790697. Retrieved on 5/27/09.

314

Notes

- The calorically restricted ketogenic diet, an effective alternative therapy for malignant brain cancer. Weihua Zhou, Purna Mukherjee, Michael A Kiebish, William T Markis, John G Mantis, and Thomas N Seyfried, *Nutr Metab* (Lond). 2007; 4: 5. Published online 2007 February 21. doi: 10.1186/1743-7075-4-5. Available online at http://www.ncbi.nlm.nih.gov/pubmed/17313687. Retrieved on 5/29/09.

- The Effects of Varying Dietary Carbohydrate and Fat Content on Survival in a Murine LNCaP Prostate Cancer Xenograft Model. Mavropoulos JC, Buschemeyer WC 3rd, Tewari AK, Rokhfeld D, Pollak M, Zhao Y, Febbo PG, Cohen P, Hwang D, Devi G, Demark-Wahnefried W, Westman EC, Peterson BL, Pizzo SV, Freedland SJ, *Cancer Prev Res* (Phila Pa). 2009 May 26. Available online at http://www.ncbi.nlm.nih.gov/pubmed/19470786. Retrieved on 5/29/09.

- Targeting energy metabolism in brain cancer with calorically restricted ketogenic diets. Seyfried TN, Kiebish M, Mukherjee P, Marsh J, *Epilepsia*. 2008 Nov;49 Suppl 8:114-6. Available online at http://www.ncbi.nlm.nih.gov/pubmed/19049606. Retrieved on 5/29/09.

The ketogenic diet has also been used successfully in the treatment of epilepsy.

The biggest modern study with an intent-to-treat prospective design was published in 1998. As with most studies of the ketogenic diet, there was no control group, which would be patients who were denied the treatment. A team from the Johns Hopkins Hospital studied 150 children for at least 12 months. By three months, 25 patients had dropped out, 26% had a good reduction in seizures (50–90% reduction), 31% had an excellent reduction (90–99% reduction) and 3% became seizure free. By twelve months, 67 patients had dropped out, 23% had a good reduction, 20% had an excellent reduction and 7% were seizure free. See Freeman JM, Vining EP, Pillas DJ, Pyzik PL, Casey JC, Kelly LM. The efficacy of the ketogenic diet–1998: a prospective evaluation of intervention in 150 children. *Pediatrics*. 1998 Dec;102(6):1358–63. PMID 9832569. Available online at http://www.ncbi.nlm.nih.gov/pubmed/9832569. Retrieved on 5/28/09.

In the same year, a multi-center study of 51 children showed similar efficacy, and proved that the results could be repeated by other institutions. See Vining EP, Freeman JM, Ballaban-Gil K, Camfield CS, Camfield PR, Holmes GL, *et al*. A multicenter study of the efficacy of the ketogenic diet. *Arch Neurol*. 1998 Nov;55(11):1433–7. PMID 9823827. Available online at http://www.ncbi.nlm.nih.gov/pubmed/9823827. Retrieved on 5/28/09. See also Hartman AL, Vining EP. Clinical aspects of the ketogenic diet. *Epilepsia*. 2007 Jan;48(1):31–42. PMID 17241206. doi: 10.1111/j.1528-1167.2007.00914.x. Available online at http://www.ncbi.nlm.nih.gov/pubmed/17241206. Retrieved on 5/28/09.

The first randomised controlled trial was published in 2008, which had an intent-to-treat prospective design, but no blinding. It studied 145 children, half of whom were randomly selected to start the ketogenic diet immediately, and half to start after a three-month delay. The children who were delayed treatment acted as a control, which is particularly important for medical conditions where patients may get better or worse regardless of treatment. Of the children in the diet group, 38% had at least a 50% reduction in seizure frequency, 7% had at least a 90% reduction; one child became seizure-free. Only 6% of the control group saw a greater than 50% reduction in seizure frequency and no children had a 90% reduction. The mean seizure frequency of the diet group fell by a third; the control group's mean seizure frequency actually got worse. See Neal EG, Chaffe H, Schwartz RH, Lawson MS, Edwards N, Fitzsimmons G, *et al*. The ketogenic diet for the treatment of childhood epilepsy: a randomised controlled trial. *Lancet Neurol*. 2008 Jun;7(6):500–6. PMID 18456557. doi: 10.1016/S1474-4422(08)70092-9. Available online at http://www.ncbi.nlm.nih.gov/pubmed/18456557. Retrieved on 5/28/09.

Abridged from the Wikipedia article entitled "Ketogenic Diet," available online at http://en.wikipedia.org/wiki/Ketogenic_diet. Retrieved on 5/28/09.

POSTSCRIPT

[406] In its original context, this quote refers to the 17th century comparative anatomist Tyson, who "Nevertheless after carefully reviewing the evidence which demonstrated conspiculously that the porpoise *must* be a mammal, Tyson nowhere has the courage to declare that it is *not* a fish, for once attaching more importance to habitat than to structure. He says he should *like* to think it was a mammal, but further than that he did not go." See Cole, F.J. *A History of Comparative Anatomy: From Aristotle to the Eighteenth Century.* London: Macmillan & Co. Ltd., 1944, p. 202.

[407] There are three main approaches to studying anatomy: systemic, regional, and clinical. Systemic anatomy is the study of the body as a series of organ systems. Although systemic anatomy textbooks typically cover all the human organ systems, they may group them differently, into from six to many more organ systems. This grouping difference is based on writers' specialty, preference and style, and editors' formatting concerns. Complicating the issue, some organ systems share significant functional overlap. For instance, the nervous and endocrine system both operate via a shared organ, the hypothalamus; thus the two systems are sometimes combined and studied as the neuroendocrine system. And the vestibular system, in fact all sense organs, are often covered in sections on the nervous system. The musculoskeletal system combines two as one; textbooks frequently include the immune with the lymphatic system.

The publication of Andreas Vesalius's *De Humani Corporis Fabrica* in 1543 ushered a new era in the history of medicine and marked the beginning of modern anatomy. This first anatomy book of 659 pages detailed *six* human systems: (1) skeletal, (2) muscles and ligaments, (3) circulatory, (4) cerebral and peripheral nerves, (5) abdominal and thoracic organs, and (6) brain and organs of special senses. See Persaud, T.V.N. *A History of Anatomy: The Post-Vesalian Era.* Springfield, IL: Charles C. Thomas Publisher, Ltd., 1997.

In the classic work *Anatomy of the Human Body* (Philadelphia: Lea & Febiger, 1918), Henry Gray (1827-1861, smallpox) posthumously grouped the various systems of the human body into the following *six* headings: "(1) Osteology — the bony system or skeleton, (2) Syndesmology — the articulations or joints, (3) Myology — the muscles. With the description of the muscles it is convenient to include that of the fasciæ which are so intimately connected with them, (4) Angiology — the vascular system, comprising the heart, blood vessels, lymphatic vessels, and lymph glands, (5) Neurology — the nervous system. The organs of sense may be included in this system, and (6) Splanchnology — the visceral system. Topographically the viscera form two groups, viz., the thoracic viscera and the abdomino-pelvic viscera. The heart, a thoracic viscus, is best considered with the vascular system. The rest of the viscera may be grouped according to their functions: (a) the respiratory apparatus; (b) the digestive apparatus; and (c) the urogenital apparatus. Strictly speaking, the third subgroup should include only such components of the urogenital apparatus as are included within the abdomino-pelvic cavity, but it is convenient to study under this heading certain parts which lie in relation to the surface of the body, e.g., the testes and the external organs of generation." The work, thoroughly revised and re-edited by Warren H. Lewis (New York: Bartleby.com, 2000) is available online at http://www.bartleby.com/107/.

"The shortcomings of existing anatomical textbooks probably impressed themselves upon Henry Gray when he was still a student at St. George's Hospital Medical School, near London's Hyde Park Corner, in the mid 1840's. He began thinking about creating a new anatomy textbook a decade later, while war was being fought in the Crimea. New legislation was being planned which would establish the General Medical Council (1858) to regulate professional education and standards.

Gray shared the idea for the new book with a gifted artistic colleague on the teaching staff at St. George's, Dr. Henry Vandyke Carter, in November, 1855. Neither was interested in producing a pretty book, or an expensive one. Their purpose was to supply an affordable, accurate teaching aid for students like their own, who might soon be required to operate on soldiers injured at Sebastopol or on some other battlefield. The book they planned together was a practical one, designed to encourage youngsters to study anatomy, help them pass exams, and assist them as budding surgeons.

The book Gray and Carter created, *Anatomy: Descriptive and Surgical,* published by JW Parker & Son, appeared in August, 1858, to immediate acclaim." (Condensed from Stranding, 2005, p. xvii).

Notes

The thirty-ninth edition of *Gray's Anatomy: The Anatomical Basis of Clinical Practice* (Edited by Susan Stranding, et al., New York: Elsevier Churchill Livingstone, 2005), an enormous reference book consisting of 1,627 pages, "...is radically different from earlier editions because the body is described in regions rather than in systems. In the real world, the editorial team for the 39th edition decided that a book which would be of the greatest benefit to practicing clinicians should mirror their daily practice and describe anatomy in the way in which they use it, i.e., regionally." However, it too describes *six* systems: the (1) nervous, (2) blood, lymphoid tissues and haemopoiesis (red and white blood cells), (3) musculoskeletal, (4) smooth muscle and the cardiovascular and lymphatic, (5) skin and its appendages, and (6) endocrine. Basic structure and function of cells, integrating cells into tissues, embryogenesis, prenatal and neonatal growth are also covered. Following the systemic overview, this compendium then describes seven sections: (1) neuroanatomy, (2) head and neck, (3) back and macroscopic anatomy of the spinal cord, (4) pectoral girdle and upper limb, (5) thorax, (6) abdomen and pelvis, and (7) pelvic girdle and lower limb.

A recent textbook, *Principles of Anatomy and Physiology*, by Professors Gerard J. Tortora and Bryan Derrickson (New Jersey: John Wiley & Sons, Inc., 12th edition, 2009) describes *eleven* systems of the human body: the (1) integumentary, (2) skeletal, (3) muscular, (4) nervous, (5) endocrine, (6) cardiovascular, (7) digestive, (8) urinary, (9) lymphatic and immunity, (10) respiratory, and (11) reproductive system. In what seems like the authors proudly going the extra mile, this textbook advocates a high-carbohydrate, low-fat diet in support of optimum health: "...many experts recommend the following distribution of calories: 50-60% from carbohydrates, with less than 15% from simple sugars; less than 30% from fats (triglycerides are the main type of dietary fat), with no more than 10% as saturated fats; and about 12-15% from proteins." (See page 1006).

[408] See Lorin, Henry. *Alzheimer's Solved (Condensed Edition).* South Carolina: BookSurge, LLC, 2005, p. 5.

[409] *Ibid*, p. 94.

[410] *Ibid*, p. 225.

[411] See McCleary, Larry. *The Brain Trust Program.* New York: Penguin Group (USA) Inc., 2007, pages 97-93.

[412] See "Ketogenic Diets and Physical Performance," by Stephen D Phinney. *Nutrition & Metabolism* 2004, 1:2. doi: 10.1186/1743-7075-1-2. Available online at http://www.nutritionandmetabolism.com/content/1/1/2. Retrieved on 12/10/09.

[413] *Ibid*.

[414] Dr. Appleton lists "146 Reasons Why Sugar Is Ruining Your Health," on her website at http://www.nancyappleton.com/NA144reasons.html. Retrieved on 12/10/09.

[415] See Ings, Simon. *A Natural History of Seeing: The Art & Science of Vision.* New York: W.W. Norton & Company, 2008, p. 65.

[416] See Diamond, Jared. *The Third Chimpanzee: The Evolution and Future of the Human Animal.* New York: Harper Perennial, 1992, p. 139

[417] "Whether diet may influence autoimmunity has been the subject of many unsolved debates. Interestingly, growing evidence indicates a large overlap between the mechanisms controlling tolerance to dietary antigens and autoimmunity. See "Autoimmunity and Diet," by Cerf-Bensussan N. *Nestle Nutr Workshop Ser Pediatr Program.* 2009;64:91-9; discussion 99-104, 251-7. Available online at http://www.ncbi.nlm.nih.gov/pubmed/19710517?itool=EntrezSystem2.PEntrez.Pubmed.Pubmed_Result sPanel.Pubmed_RVDocSum&ordinalpos=43. Retrieved on 12/11/09.

The use of omega-3 polyunsaturated fat—fish oil—has been known in small doses to aid the immune system. See "Dietary Fatty Acids and the Immune System," by Calder PC. *Lipids* 1999; 34:S137-S140. Available online at http://www.springerlink.com/content/0195rt84xr947wvt/fulltext.pdf. Retrieved on 12/13/09.

[418] As of 2009, proponents of evolution are 18-0 in US court cases. Although State v. Scopes (1925), the first and most famous court case, resulted in a loss for Scopes, who was then fined $100, the verdict was eventually set aside due to a technicality on appeal to the Supreme Court of Tennessee. The most recent case, Tammy Kitzmiller, et al. v. Dover Area School District, et al. (2005) was the first direct challenge brought in the United States federal courts against a public school district that required the presentation of intelligent design as an alternative to evolution as an "explanation of the origin of life." The plaintiffs successfully argued that intelligent design is a form of creationism, and that the school board policy thus violated the Establishment Clause of the First Amendment to the United States Constitution. The Decision of the Court in the matter of Kitzmiller, et al. v. Dover Area School District, et al., is available online at http://www.talkorigins.org/faqs/dover/kitzmiller_v_dover_decision.html. Retrieved on 12/10/09. For good background information and further references, see http://en.wikipedia.org/wiki/Kitzmiller_v._Dover_Area_School_District. Retrieved on 12/10/09.

[419] In 2006, Wilson Elser attorneys won a significant victory in US District Court, Southern District of New York, by securing the dismissal of a case charging the Atkins book and food products were defective and dangerous under product liability laws. The case involved a Florida man, and the lawsuit was commensed on the plaintiff's behalf by the Physicians Committee for Responsible Medicine, which publically advocates a vegan (no meat, no dairy, no fish) lifestyle and has long been an opponent of the Atkins diet, attacking it as unhealthy. Southern District Judge Denny Chin said the suit must be dismissed because the Atkins book and food products are not defective or dangerous under product liability law. See the archives of the Wilson Elser Moskowitz Edelman & Dicker LLP law firm online at http://www.wilsonelser.com/files/repository/Nextrounddietlit_FallWinter20042005.pdf and http://www.wilsonelser.com/files/repository/LeghornAtkins_Dec2006.pdf. Both retrieved on 12/14/09.

[420] John Washington Butler (1875 – 1952) was an American farmer and a member of the Tennessee House of Representatives. He is most noted for introducing the Butler Act, which prohibited teaching of evolution in public, i.e., state, schools, and which was challenged in the Scopes Trial. The Butler Act was a 1925 Tennessee law forbidding public school teachers from denying the Biblical account of man's origin. It was enacted as Tennessee Code Annotated Title 49 (Education) Section 1922. The law also prevented the teaching of the evolution of man from lower orders of animals in place of the Biblical account. However, the law did not prohibit the teaching of evolutionary theory for other species of plants or animals. The Butler Act was Introduced in the Tennessee House of Representatives as House Bill No. 185 by John Washington Butler on January 21, 1925; it passed the House on January 28, 1925 (Yeas: 71; Nays: 5); it passed the Senate on March 13, 1925 (Yeas: 24; Nays: 6); signed into law by Governor Peay on March 21, 1925; repealed on September 1, 1967 by Chapter No. 237, House Bill No. 48. See the Wikipedia article titled "Butler Act," available online at http://en.wikipedia.org/wiki/Butler_Act. Retrieved on 12/15/09.

[421] See "The Effects of a Low-Carbohydrate, Ketogenic Diet on the Polycystic Ovary Syndrome: A Pilot Study," by John C Mavropoulos, William S Yancy, Juanita Hepburn, and Eric C Westman. *Nutrition & Metabolism* 2005, 2:35. doi: 10.1186/1743-7075-2-35. Available online at http://www.nutritionandmetabolism.com/content/2/1/35. Retrieved on 12/10/09.

[422] See "The Effect of a Low-Carbohydrate Diet on Bone Turnover," by J. D. Carter, F. B. Vasey, and J. Valeriano. *Osteoporos Int* (2006) 17: 1398–1403. doi: 10.1007/s00198-006-0134-x. Available online at http://www.springerlink.com/content/ej54l85238623l57/. Retrieved on 12/10/09.

[423] See "Food Groups and Bone Health," by Susan A. New. In: *Nutrition and Bone Health*. Edited by M.F. Holick and B. Dawson-Hughes. New Jersey: Humana Press Inc., 2004.

[424] For a summary of the issues involved, see "Toward A Policy Agenda On Medical Research Funding: Results Of A Symposium," by Robert I. Field, Barbara J. Plager, Rebecca A. Baranowski, Mary Anne Healy and Margaret L. Longacre. *Health Affairs*, 22, no. 3 (2003): 224-230. doi: 10.1377/hlthaff.22.3.224. Available online at http://content.healthaffairs.org/cgi/content/full/22/3/224. Retrieved on 12/13/09.

[425] See "Sodium, Potassium, Phosphorous, and Magnesium," by Robert P. Heany. In: *Nutrition and Bone Health*. Edited by M.F. Holick and B. Dawson-Hughes. New Jersey: Humana Press Inc., 2004, p. 327.

[426] See "Calcium and Vitamin D for Bone Health in Adults," by Bess Dawson-Hughes. In: *Nutrition and Bone Health.* Edited by M.F. Holick and B. Dawson-Hughes. New Jersey: Humana Press Inc., 2004, p. 197.

[427] See "Vitamin A and Bone Health," by Peter Burckhardt. In: *Nutrition and Bone Health.* Edited by M.F. Holick and B. Dawson-Hughes. New Jersey: Humana Press Inc., 2004.

[428] See "Fluoride and Bone Health," by Johann D. Ringe. In: *Nutrition and Bone Health.* Edited by M.F. Holick and B. Dawson-Hughes. New Jersey: Humana Press Inc., 2004, p.345.

[429] See "Food Groups and Bone Health," by Susan A. New. In: *Nutrition and Bone Health.* Edited by M.F. Holick and B. Dawson-Hughes. New Jersey: Humana Press Inc., 2004, p. 237.

[430] *Ibid*, p. 245.

[431] *Ibid*, pages 236-237.

[432] *Ibid*, p. 237. See also the following: Macdonald HM, New SA, Grubb DA, Goloden MHN, Reid DM. "Impact of Food Groups on Perimenopausal Bone Loss." In: Burckhardt P, Dawson-Hughes B, Heaney RP, eds. Nutritional Aspects of Osteoporosis 2000 (4th International Symposium on Nutritional Aspects of Osteoporosis, Switzerland, 1997). Challenges of Modern Medicine. Ares-Serono, Academic, New York, 2001, pp. 399-408; Tucker KL, Chen H, Hannan MT, et al. "Bone Mineral Density and Dietary Patterns in Older Adults: the Framingham Osteoporosis Study." *Am J Clin Nutr* 2002; 76:245-252; New SA, Bolton-Smith C, Grubb DA, Reid DM. "Nutritional Influences on Bone Mineral Density: a Cross-Sectional Study in Premenopausal Women." *Am J Clin Nutr* 1997; 65:1831-1839; New SA, Robins Sp, Campbell MK, et al. "Dietary Influence on Bone Mass and Bone Metabolism: Further Evidence of a Positive Link Between Fruit and Vegetable Consumption and Bone Health?" *Am J Clin Nutr* 2000; 71:142-151; & Tucker KL, Hannan MT, Chen H, Cupples A, Wilson PWF, Kiel DP. "Potassium and Fruit & Vegetables are Associated with Greater Bone Mineral Density in Elderly Men and Women." *Am J Clin Nutr* 1999; 69:727-736. *Op cit.* "Food Groups and Bone Health," by Susan A. New. In: *Nutrition and Bone Health.* Edited by M.F. Holick and B. Dawson-Hughes. New Jersey: Humana Press Inc., 2004, p. 237.

[433] The authors followed coronary heart disease morbidity and mortality in a cohort of rural men (N = 1,752) participating in a prospective observational study. Dietary choices were assessed at baseline with a 15-item food questionnaire. 138 men were hospitalized or deceased owing to coronary heart disease during the 12 year follow-up. See "Food Choices and Coronary Heart Disease: A Population Based Cohort Study of Rural Swedish Men with 12 Years of Follow-up," by Sara Holmberg, Anders Thelin, and Eva-Lena Stiernström. *Int. J. Environ. Res. Public Health* 2009, 6, 2626-2638; doi: 10.3390/ijerph6102626. Available online at http://www.mdpi.com/1660-4601/6/10/2626/pdf. Retrieved on 12/13/09.

[434] See Taubes, Gary. *Good Calories, Bad Calories.* First Anchor Books Edition. New York: Anchor Books, 2008, p. 322.

[435] *Ibid*, p. 325. As it relates specifically to vitamin C, Gary Taubes states: "The vitamin C molecule is similar in configuration to glucose and other sugars in the body. It is shuttled from the bloodstream into the cells by the same insulin-dependent transport system used by glucose. Glucose and vitamin C compete in this *cellular-uptake* process, like strangers trying to flag down the same taxicab simultaneously. Because glucose is greatly favored in the contest, the uptake of vitamin C by cells is "globally inhibited" when blood sugar levels are elevated. In effect, glucose regulates how much vitamin C is taken up by the cells...In other words, there is significant reason to believe that the key factor determining the level of vitamin C in our cells and tissues is not how much or little we happen to be consuming in our diet, but whether the starches and refined carbohydrates in our diet serve to flush vitamin C out of our system, while simultaneously inhibiting the use of what vitamin C we do have."

www.ingramcontent.com/pod-product-compliance
Lightning Source LLC
Chambersburg PA
CBHW060613290526
45793CB00001B/19